Increasing Awareness of Child and Adolescent Mental Health

Increasing Awareness of Child and Adolescent Mental Health

Edited by
M. Elena Garralda, MD, FRCPsych
and Jean-Philippe Raynaud, MD, PhD

JASON ARONSON
Lanham • Boulder • New York • Toronto • Plymouth, UK

Published by Jason Aronson
An imprint of Rowman & Littlefield Publishers, Inc.
A wholly owned subsidiary of The Rowman & Littlefield Publishing Group, Inc.
4501 Forbes Boulevard, Suite 200, Lanham, Maryland 20706
http://www.rowmanlittlefield.com

Estover Road, Plymouth PL6 7PY, United Kingdom

British Library Cataloguing in Publication Information Available

Library of Congress Cataloging-in-Publication Data

Increasing awareness of child and adolescent mental health / edited by M. Elena
Garralda and Jean-Philippe Raynaud.
    p. cm. — (IACAPAP book series)
  Includes bibliographical references and index.
  ISBN 978-0-7657-0661-4 (cloth : alk. paper) — ISBN 978-0-7657-0662-1 (pbk. :
alk. paper) — ISBN 978-0-7657-0663-8 (electronic)
  1. Child mental health services. 2. Teenagers—Mental health services. 3. Child
psychiatry. 4. Adolescent psychiatry. I. Garralda, M. Elena. II. Raynaud, Jean-
Philippe, 1960–
  RJ499.I427 2010
  618.92'89—dc22   2009054105

∞™ The paper used in this publication meets the minimum requirements of
American National Standard for Information Sciences—Permanence of Paper for
Printed Library Materials, ANSI/NISO Z39.48-1992.
Printed in the United States of America

Contents

Part II: Individual Disorders/Problems

Part III: Treatment and Services

IACAPAP Book Series

The Child in His Family Series (1970–1994)

Vol	Year	Title	Publisher	Editors
1	1970	The Child in His Family	Wiley	
	1970	L'enfant dans la famille	Masson	E. J. Anthony and
2	1973	The Impact of Disease and Death	Wiley	C. Koupernik
	1974	L'enfant devant la maladie et la mort		
3	1974	Children at Psychiatric Risk	Wiley	E. J. Anthony,
	1980	L'enfant à haut risque psychiatrique	PUF	C. Chiland, and
4	1978	Vulnerable Children	Wiley	C. Koupernik
	1980	L'enfant vulnérable	PUF	
5	1978	Children and Their Parents in a Changing World	Wiley	
	1984	Parents et enfants dans un monde en changement	PUF	
6	1982	Preventive Child Psychiatry in an Age of Transitions	Wiley	E. J. Anthony
	1985	Prevention en psychiatrie de l'enfant dans un temps de transition	PUF	and C. Chiland
7	1982	Children in Turmoil: Tomorrow's Parents Enfants dans la tourmente: Parents de	Wiley	
	1985	demain	PUF	
8	1986	Perilous Development: Child Raising and Identity Formation under Stress	Wiley	
	1992	Le developpement en peril	PUF	

(continued)

9	1992	New Approaches to Infant, Child, Adolescent and Family Mental Health	Yale University Press	
	1990	Nouvelle approches de la sante mentale de la naissance a l'adolescence pour l'enfant et sa famille	PUF	
10	1990	Why Children Reject School: View from Seven Countries	Yale University Press	C. Chiland and J. G. Young
	1990	Le refus de l'ecole: Un apercu transculturel	PUF	
11	1994	Children and Violence	Jason Aronson	
	1998	Les enfants et la violence	PUF	

The Leadership Series (1998–2004)

Vol	Year	Title	Publisher	Editors
12	1998	Designing Mental Health Services and Systems for Children and Adolescents: A Shrewd Investment	Brunner/ Mezel	J. G. Young and P. Ferrari
13	2002	Brain, Culture and Development	MacMillan	J. G. Young, P. Ferrari, S. Malhotra, S. Tyano and E. Caffo
14	2002	The Infant and the Family in the 21st Century	Brunner-Routledge	J. Gomes-Pedro, K. Nugent, J. G. Young and T. B. Brazelton
15	2004	Facilitating Pathways: Care, Treatment and Prevention in Child and Adolescent Mental Health	Springer	H. Remschmidt, M. Belfer, and I. Goodyer

The Working with Children and Adolescents Series (2006–)

Vol	Year	Title	Publisher	Editors
16	2006	Working with Children and Adolescents: An Evidenced-Based Approach to Risk and Resilience	Jason Aronson	M. E. Garralda and M. Flament
17	2008	Culture and Conflict in Child and Adolescent Mental Health	Jason Aronson	M. E. Garralda and J.-P. Raynaud
18	2010	Increasing Awareness of Child and Adolescent Mental Health	Jason Aronson	

Acknowledgments

We would like to thank the authors for contributing to this volume of the IACAPAP book series and providing some interesting and thought provoking chapters. At Jason Aronson, Julie Kirsch and Melissa Wilks ensured a smooth pathway to publication. Finally, our grateful thanks are due to Nicole Hickey, who provided excellent administration to the editors.

Preface

The world of today is really complex and diverse. In some countries the population is rich and healthy, free and independent, and living under democratic rules, while in other countries the population is poor and starving and is living under dictatorships. The breakdown of the colonial system since the 1960s has really changed the world giving us a great number of new nations and new national identities. Social and family circumstances often differ between countries.

Today, communication is developing at a speed that was unbelievable only 30 years ago. To go between continents today is a question of hours instead of days, weeks, or months. The communication of ideas and thoughts is possible in seconds. Facts and fictions are continuously broadcast, day and night, by TV and satellites. People who suffer have lots of opportunities to learn from conditions in other parts of the world, inspiring them to look for shelter, protection, and a new life somewhere else—a true challenge for mental health professionals working with parents and children!

The theme of the 19th World Congress of the International Association for Child and Adolescent Psychiatry and Allied Professions—IACAPAP—is "Improving Child Mental Health: Increasing Awareness and New Pathways for Care." The aim of this congress book, to be presented in Beijing in the Spring of 2010, is to focus interest on enhancing knowledge and attention to the mental health problems of children and young people. It is necessary that both public health and mental health professionals actively plan how to meet the needs of children across different countries and continents, and that they develop the necessary services and methods to support those coming with a burden of psychiatric need.

August 2009, Stockholm

Per-Anders Rydelius, M.D., Ph.D.
President of IACAPAP, Professor of Child and Adolescent Psychiatry at Karolinska Institute, Stockholm, Sweden.

Introduction

M. Elena Garralda and Jean-Philippe Raynaud

The publication of this book marks the celebration of the 2010 World IACAPAP (International Association for Child and Adolescent Psychiatry and Allied Professions) Congress in Beijing, China, and as such continues a time honored tradition which has resulted in the IACAPAP Congress book series.

As in previous editions, the book aims to provide an update of recent empirically derived knowledge on themes that affect child and adolescent mental health and have an appeal for clinicians across cultures and countries. It also seeks to provide accounts of influences and initiatives that—whilst having general relevance—may be of specific interest to certain continents. Contributions represent the views of experts from around the world, supported by empirical and clinical experience.

In line with the aspiration of the Beijing Congress of increasing awareness of child and adolescent mental health, the first section of the book addresses epidemiological aspects of service use by children and young people with mental health problems and the effects on mental health of broad macroscopic social change such as industrialization and refugee status. It also addresses policies, behaviors, and attitudes affecting the microscopic world of the child's family, ranging from the one-child policy in China to the different parent combinations now prevalent in Western countries. The second section of the book focuses on individual disorders, with contributions on the boundaries of attention-deficit disorder across different cultures, changes in the nature of presenting symptoms in Japan, and the frequency of autism generally. The final section focuses on treatment and services: it outlines pediatric liaison services; the use of acupuncture in children with autism, an intriguing area of special relevance within the country hosting this Congress; and the development of services in Central and Eastern Europe.

INFLUENCES ON CHILD AND ADOLESCENT MENTAL HEALTH

It has long been documented that child and adolescent psychiatric disorders are common and present in one to ten/twenty children in the general population; nevertheless, the majority of children with disorders do not access specialist mental health care. Kapil Sayal and Tamsin Ford dissect the existing epidemiological data from the perspective of pathways to service use in children with psychiatric disorders, using information from the USA and Europe. Clearly, children with psychiatric disorders are in contact with a variety of non-specialist services including schools and social services, but also primary and secondary pediatric care, while the determinants of referral involve both psychopathological and psychosocial characteristics. Important tasks for future work remain, increasing the recognition and care provided in different settings and clarifying family attitudes on child mental health problems across different countries.

Western nuclear families are becoming increasingly complex; the marked increase in divorce rates over the past few decades has resulted in a range of different combinations in the care structures for children and young people. Rossana Bisceglia and colleagues outline these and review critically the evidence pertaining to effects on child mental health. This shows unequivocally that living with two natural parents is linked to optimal child adjustment. However, the effects of other combinations vary and depend on factors such as the number of transitions experienced by the child; the context of the biological and personality characteristics of parents that predate change; the child's experience of living in a particular family structure; the quality of the child's relationships with custodial and non-custodial parents; and the economics of the family.

China hosts almost one-quarter of the world's population, with a huge and ever-growing population. From the 1970s the country has been seeking to control growth and this led to the current one-child policy whereby couples are expected to only have one child. Yi Zheng outlines the rationale for this policy as well as its demographic, economic, and social consequences. There has been a recognition that the policy may have unintended consequences on child and family psychosocial adaptation; the chapter outlines research showing that children from one-parent families are in fact well in terms of mental health, and it reviews parenting interventions that are being put into place to counteract any adverse effects on parenting and child adjustment.

The rapidity of industrialization and globalization in the last half century is unprecedented in developing countries. In his chapter, Cornelio Banaag documents how this rapid evolution has brought positive but also negative changes for children and their families in countries like the Philippines and Indonesia.

The ease of travel and communication across countries together with the disparities in humanitarian and economic status underlies the increase in asylum seeking refugees. Refugee status involves a variety of psychosocial stressors, both before and after emigration, and affects children especially so in the case of unaccompanied young asylum seekers. Schuyler Henderson and colleagues argue that whereas the clinical goals of psychosocial interventions are to help children, families, and communities restore the world of childhood, they also have to navigate the politically, socially, and psychologically dangerous waters that go with being a "refugee" and help rearticulate what has been torn apart. Over and above empirical research and the building of clinical experience, they make the case for a narrative approach to include stories of development, resilience, vulnerability, trauma, parenting, schooling, and the future. They note that attending to these ethical dimensions would help enhance clinicians' capacity to build mental health and psychosocial interventions that are responsive to restoring the very human bonds that are under attack in political violence, as well as restoring the narrative milieus that allow people to live in a "relationship to the past in their history, and to the future in their hopes."

INDIVIDUAL DISORDERS

In their chapter, Guilherme Polanczyk and colleagues discuss the boundaries of the attention-deficit/hyperactivity disorder (ADHD) diagnosis, with a special focus on four aspects: culture and ADHD; ADHD as a dimensional or categorical entity; the overlap between ADHD and conduct disorder; and the overlap between ADHD and bipolar disorder.

Changes in society's attitudes and customs can influence the presentation of mental health problems in children and adolescents. Sadaaki Shirataki and Kazu Kobayashi describe striking changes over the past few decades in the problems reaching child and adolescent psychiatrists in Japan. Some, for example the increase in developmental disorders, are mirrored across countries; others, such as the marked shift from internalizing to externalizing problems, may be particular to Japan. Based on their experience of consultation to schools and their reflections on important changes in attitudes in Japanese society—whereby a strong previous emphasis on tight families and responsible social attitudes has been superseded by a focus on self-interest and fulfilment—the authors consider the contribution of societal attitudes to the observed changes in child psychopathology.

The answer to the question: "Is there an autistic epidemic?" is tackled by Mandy Steiman and colleagues. Theirs is a comprehensive, critical review of the literature on epidemiological surveys of pervasive developmental and autistic spectrum disorders, one that takes due note of crucial method-ological issues. They conclude that there is not enough evidence to support the idea of an epidemic. This may be due to the fact that many confounding factors and varying methodologies (i.e., changing diagnostic criteria, diag-nostic substitution, and different kinds of ascertainment methods) obscure the interpretation of possible contributing factors. The review does high-light changes in diagnostic practices, partly driven by educational adminis-trative imperatives, given that a diagnosis of autism opens the way to edu-cational help. This does not detract from the need for continuing efforts to be made to monitor the prevalence and incidence of autism and related disorders. To assess whether or not the incidence has increased, factors that account for variability in rates must be tightly controlled. As stated by the authors, the needs of children with autism and their families require ongo-ing attention and action within the spheres of public health and educa-tional institutions.

There is an increasing interest in psychotraumatology in children and adolescents. Reviewing the literature and their own experience, Charlotte Allenou and colleagues describe how mothers coping with severe trauma in their children can themselves present post-traumatic symptoms. This may have important consequences and add new perspectives to our understand-ing of interactions in these vulnerable families.

TREATMENT AND SERVICES

Using an historical perspective, Maryland Pao defines pediatric psychoso-matic medicine and describes its practice in the USA and Asia. She discusses how pediatric consultation-liaison should contribute to promoting public awareness of children's mental and physical health, to reducing stigma and the provision of mental health education and training to providers, as well as to research on children's disorders and treatments in the context of de-velopment and culture.

The recent striking increase in recognition of autistic spectrum disorders, already discussed in the chapter by Steiman and colleagues, has gone along-side a mushrooming of therapeutic techniques and Virginia Wong and Vanessa Chu outline the use of traditional Chinese medicine in relation to these disorders. They provide a detailed description of traditional Chinese medical concepts, such as the technique of acupuncture, and document the promising results arising out of their empirical trials on the use of acupunc-ture in children with autism. They highlight the fact that the current practice of acupuncture in China is still evolving and that there remains a lack of consensus on the best acupuncture techniques for treating autism. They also make a plea for more research to help establish functional acupuncture areas and validate their inclusion in an integrated treatment program that includes a Western medicine model.

In their chapter Dainius Puras and Robertas Povilaitis provide an overview of the situation regarding child and adolescent mental health in Central and Eastern Europe with special focus on contextual factors and prevention. They show that much has been achieved, particularly in developing services and prevention programs, and highlight the challenges and obstacles for the future in this dynamic and changing region.

Finally, Jean-Yves Hayez addresses promotion of child and adolescent mental health from a conceptual and historical perspective. He first defines his concept of child mental health and describes its constituent elements. He goes on to outline the reference models that form the basis of programs aimed at promoting child mental health and the chapter ends by summarizing the history of child and adolescent psychiatry and child mental health.

I

INFLUENCES ON CHILD AND ADOLESCENT MENTAL HEALTH

1

From Epidemiology of Child and Adolescent Mental Health Problems to Service Utilization

Kapil Sayal and Tamsin Ford

INTRODUCTION

Epidemiological approaches are useful for examining rates of child and adolescent mental health disorders and service use, quantifying the discrepancy between these, investigating reasons for this discrepancy, and suggesting methods to address this unmet need. Studies involving general population samples have found that few children with psychiatric disorders are recognized as having a disorder or receive services. For example, widely quoted figures from the United States suggest that although up to 20% of children can be regarded as meeting criteria for disorder, only 1% of children receive mental health services in specialist mental health settings and a further 6% receive these services in primary care and schools (Costello et al. 1993). In Great Britain, 43% of children with an impairing psychiatric disorder identified in an epidemiological survey had *NOT* been in contact with *any* professional in relation to their mental health in the subsequent three years following the initial assessment, while only 25% had been in contact with *mental health* services (Ford et al. 2007).

Conservative estimates suggest that the worldwide prevalence of child and adolescent mental health disorders is around 10% and that a further 10% of children have sub-threshold or impairing mental health problems (Costello et al. 1993). Most health services research has focused on children with disorders (defined according to diagnostic criteria). However, sub-threshold behavioral and emotional problems or associated impairment that may not meet criteria for a disorder are also risk factors for outcomes and are associated with service use (Sayal 2004). It is important to consider the wider range of child mental health problems, as most childhood psychopathology is normally distributed, with evidence to suggest that impairment and prognosis are related to psychopathology across the range, and not just at the extreme where children fit criteria for disorders (Goodman & Goodman 2009).

Differences in agreement about the definition of need result in controversy about the level of service provision that would be adequate to meet these needs; it should also be remembered that contact with services does not mean that needs are necessarily met. Epidemiological studies can help identify the level of difficulties in the community and factors associated with them as well as the barriers and facilitators to help-seeking and access to services. Although a considerable amount is known about the clinical and socio-demographic predictors of service use, the barriers to care that involve families' perceptions are also important areas of research in child psychiatric epidemiology (Costello et al. 1993). Children depend on adults to seek help on their behalf. Parents and other important adults, such as teachers and general practitioners, play a crucial role in determining whether help is sought and services are accessed. So a better understanding of parents' and first-line professionals' views about children's mental health is vital to aid access to services according to need. There are considerable public education and service planning implications.

OUTLINE

This chapter aims to provide a selective rather than exhaustive review of the literature and is organized into several sections. The initial sections focus on how the use of epidemiological approaches in child and adolescent mental health services research can aid service development; a brief background on international differences in service organization with a particular emphasis on the United States where most research has taken place; and concepts related to help-seeking and barriers to care for child mental health. More recent literature in this field has investigated children with a broad range of psychopathology defined either in terms of meeting criteria for disorder or scoring above cut-off scores on rating scales. In terms of awareness of child and adolescent mental health problems, we look at parental perceptions of problems and their role in determining service use. Finally, we describe the literature examining factors associated with referral to and use of specialist mental health services as well as the use of other services (such as primary care, school, and social services). Although most of the literature has investigated children with a broad range of psychopathology, where appropriate, findings relating to specific disorders are also drawn out.

EPIDEMIOLOGY IN CHILD AND ADOLESCENT
MENTAL HEALTH SERVICES RESEARCH

This section highlights a few of the main methodological issues in epidemiological aspects of health services research. Until the 1980s there was limited epidemiological research about factors affecting children's use of services for mental health problems (Rutter, Tizard, & Whitmore 1970). Subsequently, in many countries, the ascertainment of service-use information has been a minor aspect of population surveys. Often such information had been of limited reliability or validity and been accompanied by a restricted range of predictor measures. For example, even by the mid-1990s relatively little was known about the relationship between impairment and service use (Costello et al. 1993).

Estimates of prevalence rates of disorders may vary widely across studies because of differences in both the population that has been sampled (such as age, gender, ethnicity, social class distribution, deprivation levels, and type of geographical setting) and other methodological factors (such as the sampling method, case definition, diagnostic criteria, use of impairment criteria, and choice of informants and how their data are combined). Such variations in estimates of the prevalence of disorders might adversely influence findings relating to service use and subsequent recommendations for optimal levels of service provision. Even if prevalence rates were known precisely there is controversy about the level of service provision that would be adequate to meet needs (Jenkins 2001). Some children have more than one disorder and service use is affected by factors other than objectively defined need (such as meeting criteria for a disorder) as well as by differences in service availability. Not all children with disorders require services (for example, some disorders may be self-limiting), and for others the offer of services will not be accepted. In contrast, some children with symptoms or an impairment not meeting criteria for a disorder may benefit from services, while interventions for some disorders, such as autism, may alleviate but not remove "need" as defined by the presence of symptoms and impairments. However, the prevalence of impairing psychiatric disorder in the community can be used as a proxy indicator of the level of "need" for services (Jenkins 2001), and epidemiological approaches can be used to identify levels of "perceived" need and factors that influence demand for services. Studies investigating whether a particular factor is associated with service use whilst adjusting for the contribution of other factors can help to clarify which factors are independently involved in the help-seeking process (Sayal 2006).

Traditionally, child and adolescent mental health services have developed in an unplanned and ad-hoc manner (Harrington et al. 1999), often reflecting political priorities or individual preferences rather than need. Epidemiological findings can inform service development in terms of the allocation of limited resources and delivery of services. Improvements in the mental health of the population can be influenced by input from many public sector services, such as schools, housing, and social services, rather than being the particular remit of specialist mental health services (Jenkins 2001).

In addition to identifying how many children might need services, monitoring this over time, and reporting the prevalence and predictors of service use, epidemiological approaches can shed light on the etiology of psychopathology and exciting projects are beginning to use epidemiological tools in clinical practice (Ford 2008). Many valid and reliable measures of psychopathology are now available and their clinical utility is being explored (Costello et al. 2005; Foreman et al. 2009). The use of existing screening questionnaires in schools or primary health care settings presents challenges because of the tendency to identify many children as at risk who would not have the disorder after a fuller assessment (poor positive predictive power) and to miss too many children who would have a disorder (poor sensitivity) (Costello et al. 2005; Sayal, Letch & El Abd 2008). However, some measures might work better in high risk groups, particularly if followed up by a more detailed structured assessment for those who screened positive (Glazebrook et al. 2003; Goodman et al. 2004).

Standardized measures completed by young people and families as part of the referral process, or prior to first attendance, could speed access to the correct intervention and help signpost the rational allocation of cases to the professional(s) best trained to help. The Brief Child and Family Phone Interview, developed from the assessments used in the Ontario Child Health Survey, has scales for young people, parents, and teachers, and is designed to be administered by clinicians and takes about 30 minutes (Boyle et al. 2009). It has follow-up scales designed for outcome monitoring, and the use of such standardized questionnaires to evaluate clinical outcomes is being explored by several clinical and academic groups (Garralda 2009; Johnstone and Gower 2005; Ford et al. 2006). A study of a computerized screening in Australian adolescents revealed that computerized measures worked just as well as completing paper questionnaires (Patton et al. 1999). Yokley and Reuter (1989) reported that most clinicians were happy to incorporate computerized assessments in their clinical practice, reducing the time and resource constraints of data entry from paper questionnaires in clinical practice.

INTERNATIONAL DIFFERENCES

The way in which services are organized and the interface between primary and specialist care varies across countries. This means that research findings from one country may not fully generalize to countries with other types of health care systems. In some countries primary care physicians or general practitioners have a gate-keeping role. In many countries primary care services can be bypassed with direct access to specialists. Although most of the reported literature comes from the United States it is still possible to extract relevant principles for other health care systems. Primary health care providers for children and adolescents with mental health problems include primary care pediatricians and family (general) practitioners. In terms of specialist care, school mental health services are also a prominent provider in the United States.

The funding of health care will influence access with family economic circumstances having a smaller influence on access to services where services are centrally funded and free at the point of delivery. In the United States, health services are mainly funded by insurance. Although there are a variety of schemes the most common type involves private health insurance (often provided by employers) which allows access to managed care through structures such as a health maintenance organization. For children there are also state-funded insurance schemes. In recent years managed care organizations have encouraged a gate-keeping model in primary care whereby specialist referral incurs no additional cost to the patient (Bindman and Majeed 2003). This model enables some comparability of research findings with countries with freely accessible and centrally funded services.

PARENTAL AWARENESS AND PERCEPTIONS

For children with mental health problems, parental attitudes are crucial in acting as barriers or facilitators to accessing services (Farmer et al. 1999; Flisher et al. 1997; Owens et al. 2002; Pavuluri et al. 1996). Although many similar issues also apply to adolescents, some help-seeking may occur independently of parents. These issues are apparent in a number of countries despite organizational differences in health care systems. However, differences in parental interpretation of children's behavior and levels of concern may reflect cultural, gender, and age factors. Cultural factors may also influence the ways in which parents seek help and how professionals respond to the help-seeking (Weisz and Weiss 1991). For example, studies of ethnicity and socio-demographic status show conflicting results in relation to service use, as discussed in detail later in the chapter. Such contradictory findings may relate to the differential use of public sector providers as well as the complex interaction of culture, history, geography, and race that make up ethnicity and socio-demographic status. The influence of ethnic minority status on health and access to health care is unlikely to be the same for different ethnic groups in different locations at different times.

Although early research (e.g., Griest, Wells, & Forehand 1979) suggested that parental mental health may be more important than child factors in determining perceptions, subsequent work (Griest et al. 1980) clarified that this association was confounded by the child's referral status. Owens and colleagues (2002) defined "barriers to care" as parental perceptions about factors that reduce the likelihood of accessing services. A slight modification of their conceptual framework on barriers is useful in summarizing the literature. These perceptions can be considered in five domains, outlined below.

Domains of Parental Perceptions

Recognition of Symptoms or Impairment (Disorder)

This can be difficult to disentangle from the presence of a disorder since the latter is often established from parental accounts. Parents are the main informants in endorsing whether symptoms are present and in determining the type and severity of a possible disorder. This issue can be more clearly examined in adolescents; for example, parental recognition of their child's depressive symptoms is limited (Logan and King 2002).

Perceptions of Symptoms as a Problem

Parents might not think that their child has a problem or, if they do, that it is serious enough to warrant intervention (Staghezza-Jaramillo et al. 1995). This could reflect parental concern, estimation of whether their child has more problems than other children, caregiver strain, or whether the problem has any impact or burden for the parent or others. These perceptions are usually based on the child's functioning across situations.

Perceptions of Need for Services

Parents might think that the difficulties are manageable without services. For example, Pavuluri and colleagues (1996) described parents who thought that problems would improve spontaneously, or that they should be strong enough to handle the problems themselves. Considerable discrepancies have been found between symptom scores and perceived need for treatment (Zahner et al. 1992), suggesting that other factors play an important role in shaping parental perceptions.

Perceptions of Services

These include factors such as lack of trust; reluctance to discuss these problems with a professional; views of others; thinking treatment may be inappropriate, unhelpful, or harmful (Staghezza-Jaramillo et al. 1995); views about the availability of particular professionals; and, for adolescents, refusal to attend or wanting to solve the problem on their own (Flisher et al. 1997). For some child and adolescent mental health disorders, such as ADHD, there may be concerns about, or even fear of, drug treatments. Stigma about both mental health problems and services is likely to be a major reason for parents not reporting concerns. This can result in parental shame and guilt (Costello et al. 1993), anxiety, and denial of mental health problems. Attitudes of referrers, teachers, and the media can perpetuate the stigmatization of mental health issues. In particular, parents may be concerned that they will be regarded a failure or blamed for the child's difficulties.

The above perceptions may reflect limited or inaccurate knowledge about services. Lack of information and perceived stigma about both mental health problems and services are common barriers to the use of services.

FACTORS INFLUENCING PARENTAL PERCEPTIONS

The investigation of factors influencing whether parents perceive the presence of problems or the need for services may help explain the gap between service need and service use. However, Teagle (2002) identified only 11 studies published before 1999; some of which employed overlapping samples. Two community-based studies are described which examined both rates and predictors of different types of perceptions. First, in the Netherlands, Verhulst and Van der Ende (1997) simultaneously examined predictors of referrals and three types of perceptions: of service need, of problems, and of greater problems than other children. One-fifth of parents perceived that their child had an emotional or behavioral problem and 6% that this was worse than other children's problems. Predictors of these two types of perception were similar. Perceptions of greater levels of problems were associated with increased likelihood of referral. Specific factors associated with perception of service need, but not with perception of problems, included academic problems, family functioning, and older age. Of the eight sets of symptoms measured by the Child Behavior Checklist (CBCL) only attention problems and anxious/depressed symptoms were associated with all four outcomes. The main limitation was that the study excluded children who were not of Dutch nationality, which may have reduced the likelihood of finding socioeconomic predictors.

Second, re-analyzing data from an expanded sample of the Great Smoky Mountain Study in the United States, Teagle (2002) separated out parental problem recognition as having two components: "problem perception," which includes both perception of problems or need for help or services, and "impact" (burden for others). Overall, problem perception applied to

13% and impact to 11% of parents. For children with any one of six selected disorders (ADHD, oppositional defiant disorder, conduct disorder, depressive disorders, anxiety disorders, and substance abuse/dependence) these proportions increased to 39% and 32% respectively. Not surprisingly, problem perception and impact were the strongest predictors of each other suggesting that one could approximate for the other. As problem perception was associated with younger age and impact with older age, they may reflect similar concepts operating at different ages.

Although there is some consensus about predictors of parental perception of problems, some inconsistencies have also been reported. Findings vary as a function of methodology (choice of sample, age, types of services included, nature of predictors examined) and statistical approach. As well as the severity of the child's symptoms and level of impairment, the type of disorder is also important in predicting parental perception of problems. For example, compared to disruptive disorders, parents are less likely to regard internalizing disorders as burdensome (Angold et al. 1998) or perceive a need for mental health services (Wu et al. 1999). Teagle (2002) suggested that ADHD was the disorder most strongly associated with family impact. Parental mental health problems are also robust positive predictors of parental perception of the child's problems (Angold et al. 1998; Dulcan et al. 1990; Verhulst and van der Ende 1997; Teagle 2002). It is possible that maternal depression influences child service use by reducing mothers' confidence in their parenting ability and/or by increasing the perceived severity of their child's difficulties (Boyle and Pickles 1997). In a post-hoc analysis Zahner and Daskalakis (1997) found that the main socio-demographic predictor of perceived need for services was a lower level of maternal education. However, this finding should be interpreted with caution since a large number of analyses were carried out and other studies have not found this association (Owens et al. 2002; Verhulst and van der Ende 1997).

SUMMARY

In summary, following parental awareness of child symptoms, it appears that parental perception of problems is the key initial step in the help-seeking process. The frequent overlap between the predictors of perception of problems and of service need might occur because they can be regarded as successive steps in the help-seeking process. This might also explain why perception of service need has been found to be a strong predictor of mental health service use (Zahner and Daskalakis 1997). Although many similar issues also apply to adolescents some help-seeking may occur independently of parents.

FACTORS ASSOCIATED WITH SERVICE CONTACT

The bulk of the literature reviewed combines *"any service use"* and "contact with *specialist mental health services"* because many of the large epidemiological studies examined the correlates of the use of all combined services and included services such as pediatrics or social services together with mental health services, or failed to define what services they were studying (such as Anderson et al. 1987; Almquist et al. 1999; Feehan et al. 1990). Correlates of service use might vary according to the setting and ease of access. Where possible this chapter has separated out individual services as the few studies examining the correlates of contact with different types of services have reported that predictors vary according to the type of service.

When the range of services for mental health problems is considered, 5-21% of all children in the United States are reported to have used services in the previous year (Angold et al. 2002; Burns et al. 1995; Cunningham and Freiman 1996; Farmer et al. 1999; Leaf et al. 1996; Staghezza-Jaramillo et al. 1995). Reported lifetime rates are higher in the United States (28-54%; Farmer et al. 2003; Zahner et al. 1992) than elsewhere (10-20%; Almquist et al. 1999; Feehan et al. 1990).

In terms of predictors of service contact in general, the bulk of the literature is consistent in suggesting that the presence and severity of psychopathology is related to all service contact for mental health problems (Briggs-Gowan et al. 2000; Farmer et al. 1997; Ford et al. 2008; Koot and Verhulst 1992; Staghezza-Jaramillo et al. 1995; Zwaanswijk et al. 2003). Contact with key referrers, such as primary health care and teachers, is also strongly associated with service contact across most services (Ford et al. 2008), as is the perception of the young person and/or key adults such as parents and teachers in many but not all studies (Ford et al. 2008; Garralda and Bailey 1988; Griest et al. 1980; Sourander 2001; Staghezza-Jaramillo et al. 1995; Teagle 2002; Wu et al. 1999; Zahner and Daskalakis 1997).

Mental Health Services

Reported findings relating to referral to and the use of specialist mental health services overlap. Conceptually, they can be regarded respectively as inception into (incidence) and any service use over a period (prevalence). If considered over an extended period, such as two years or more, the two concepts are likely to converge. There are discrepancies between the United States and other countries in relation to rates of specialist mental health service use. Between 3-8% of children in the United States are reported to have used specialist services in the previous year (Angold et al. 2002; Cunningham and Freiman 1996; Farmer et al. 1999; Leaf et al. 1996; Staghezza-Jaramillo et al. 1995) compared to 7% in Canada (Offord et al. 1987), and 1-4% in Europe

(Rutter et al. 1970; Verhulst and van der Ende 1997). Over longer time periods the rates are 5-24% in the United States (Farmer et al. 2003; Zahner et al. 1992) and 5-8% in Europe (Koot and Verhulst 1992; Laitinen-Krispijn et al. 1999; Sayal 2004; Verhulst and van der Ende 1997).

Information about rates of service use also give an indication of how many children *with disorders* are in a position to potentially access evidence-based treatments. In the United States, 36-40% of children with disorders are in contact with *any* services (Angold et al. 2002; Burns et al. 1995); rates are 20-29% in other countries (Anderson et al. 1987; Rutter et al. 1970). For children with disorders, rates of specialist service use vary between 11-26% in the United States (Burns et al. 1995; Kataoka, et al. 2002; Leaf et al. 1996; Staghezza-Jaramillo et al. 1995; Zahner et al. 1992), and 10-17% elsewhere (Koot and Verhulst 1992; Offord et al. 1987; Rutter et al. 1970; Verhulst and van der Ende 1997). The follow-up of the 1999 British Child and Adolescent Mental Health Survey showed that 5% of the whole sample (or 25% of those with impairing psychiatric disorders) were in contact with mental health services over the three years following initial assessment (Ford et al. 2007).

The literature on the socio-demographic correlates of service use is complex and contradictory, possibly due to interactions and overlap between these characteristics. For instance, if a woman has her first child in her mid-to-late teens she is likely to drop out of education, thus limiting her income as well as her educational qualifications. Although the majority of studies report no gender effect in relation to service contact, those authors reporting a significant gender difference mostly find a preponderance of boys in contact with mental health services (Angold et al. 2002; Briggs-Gowan et al. 2000; Katoaka, Zthang and Wells 2002; Rutter et al. 1970; Wu et al. 1999; Zahner and Daskalakis 1997; Zwaanswijk et al. 2003). There may be complex interactions between gender and other characteristics including age, psychopathology, neighborhood, and service setting (Gasquet et al. 1999; Laitenjen-Krispijn et al. 1999). Studies examining ethnicity are evenly divided between the over- and under-representation of children from ethnic minorities in services; findings are likely to reflect the complex interaction of culture, history, geography, and race that make up ethnicity, as any influence of ethnic minority status on health and access to health care is unlikely to be the same for different ethnic groups in different locations at different times (Angold et al. 2002; Briggs-Gowan et al. 2000; Burns et al. 1995; Katoaka et al. 2002; Wu et al. 1999; Zahner and Daskalakis 1997; Zwaanswijk et al. 2003). When using epidemiological data to inform service provision for minority groups commissioners need to select recent studies of populations that resemble the children they plan to serve.

Most investigators have reported no statistical association between service use and socioeconomic status while significant findings have been evenly split between reports of more contact from advantaged or disadvantaged groups, which may be partly explained by families of different socioeconomic status tending to use different settings, such as middle class families opting for education-based services (Burns et al. 1995; Gasquet et al. 1999; Gunther et al. 2003; Jensen, Blodau & Davis 1990; Kumpulainen and Rasanen 2002; Laitenen-Krispijn et al. 1999; Stagehzza-Jaramillo et al. 1995; Zahner and Daskalakis 1997). Poor physical health, poor academic performance, non-traditional family structure, parental psychopathology, and the experience of life events have been associated with service contact in most studies, although these factors are also strongly associated with the presence of psychiatric disorder (Briggs-Gowan et al. 2000; Ford et al. 2008; Gasquet et al. 1999; Gunther et al. 2003; Sourander et al. 2001; Staghezza-Jaramillo et al. 1995; Teagle 2002; Verhulst and van der Ende 1997; Zahener and Daskalakis 1997; Zwaanswijk et al. 2003). The region in which the child lives may also influence service contact with several authors reporting that service provision in various areas is not actually related to the level of need in that area (Boyle and Offord 1988; Ford et al. 2008; Sturm, Ringel & Andreyva 2003; Thomas and Holzer 1999). Farmer and team (1997) reported that children entering the service system via specialist mental health services had higher levels of family impact than those entering via education or general medicine.

As many disorders tend to be persistent over time referral to specialist services can also be considered in terms of early or late referral. Longitudinal studies have potential advantages in investigating predictors of referral. Data such as the timing of referral can be collected prospectively, which minimizes the risk of recall bias, and predictor factors are present before service use occurs, which aids interpretation of findings. However, most longitudinal studies have relied on parent or teacher recall of service use (Koot and Verhulst 1992; Kumpulainen and Rasanen 2002; Lavigne et al. 1998; Sourander et al. 2001), and others (Gunther et al. 2003) have not adjusted for the severity of disorder. Two studies have used case register data to investigate baseline predictors of referrals over a four-year period (Laitenen-Krispijn et al. 1999; Sayal 2004). In the United Kingdom (UK) Sayal (2004) confirmed the role of parental burden in predicting referrals made during the first year. However, baseline symptom severity was the best predictor of referrals made in the subsequent three years.

In general the type of symptom also plays an important role in predicting service use. Compared to internalizing symptoms, externalizing symptoms are more strongly associated with service use (Anderson et al. 1987; Wu et al. 1999). For specific disorders such as ADHD, depression, and conduct disorder, factors such as severity, impairment, comorbidity, parental perception of problems, male gender, and Caucasian ethnicity are the main predictors of service use (Bussing, Zima, & Belin 1998; Sayal et al. 2003; Vostanis et al. 2003; Wu et al. 1999). When considering referrals from primary care to specialist services, in the United States Costello and Janiszewski

(1990) found that depression and conduct disorder (but not ADHD, anxiety, or oppositional disorders) were associated with referral. In the UK, when comparing children who were and were not referred from primary care to specialist services Garralda and Bailey (1988) found that the non-referred children had made significantly more primary care visits than the referred children, highlighting the important role of primary care as a mental health service provider for these children.

Primary Care

Most children and adolescents with mental health problems are seen within primary health care rather than specialist settings (Offord et al. 1987) and so are managed, to varying extents, within primary care. In the United Kingdom Garralda and Bailey (1986a, b) found that around a quarter of children attending primary care had mental health disorders. Most children attended for physical reasons; mental health symptoms were the main or secondary presenting complaint in only 2% of consultations. There are similar findings in other countries (Giel et al. 1981; Gureje et al. 1994). Amongst a general population sample in the United States, 10% of all children used general medical services for emotional or behavior problems over a three-year period (Farmer et al. 2003). The use of general health services for mental health problems is associated with older child age, severity of symptoms, related impairment, parental perception that the child needs help, and impact on the family (Angold et al. 2002; Teagle 2002; Zahner et al. 1992).

Few studies have examined prevalence rates of psychiatric disorder in both community and primary care samples and differences in measures used across studies limit the comparison of findings. Possible associations might reflect the population sampled; for example, Garralda and Bailey (1986a) only found higher prevalence rates in primary care in a socially advantaged area. Population studies that have compared rates of psychiatric disorder between recent attenders and non-attenders have not found an association between disorder and attendance (Offord et al. 1987). In contrast, there is more evidence to suggest that psychiatric disorder is associated with frequency of attendance (Bowman and Garalda 1993). Parental perceptions also make a considerable contribution to frequent attendance (Woodward et al. 1988). Early American studies suggested that children with psychiatric disorder were heavier users of ambulatory medical care, defined by Woodward and colleagues as visits to the emergency room, doctors' offices, or hospital outpatient departments (Woodward et al. 1988). However, these studies used administrative data, cases identified by pediatricians or parental perception that the child had a mental health problem (Goldberg et al. 1984; Woodward et al. 1988), rather than an independent measure of childhood psychiatric disorder. Meltzer and team (2000) also documented heavier use of general practice, accident and emergency hospital outpatient departments, and more inpatient admissions among children with psychiatric disorder in a British-population-based study, although the reason for the contact was not sought.

Amongst children with psychiatric disorders, rates of contact with primary care appear to be increasing. In the United Kingdom Rutter and colleagues (1970) found that only 4% of children with psychiatric disorders in the Isle of Wight study had these problems managed in primary care. In contrast, general practitioners (28% abnormal or borderline on the psychiatric SDQ screening tool; 9% in the normal range) and health visitors (19% and 7% respectively) were commonly consulted by parents of 5913 4-15-year-olds participating in the more recent Health Survey for England (Haines et al. 2002). In a follow-up of 2461 British school-age children over three years, mental-health-related contact with primary care was reported in 8% of the whole sample and 29% of those with a psychiatric disorder at baseline (Ford et al. 2007). Contact with primary care was predicted by poor physical health and poor parental mental health at baseline, and was commoner among girls (Ford et al. 2008). When considered in terms of lifetime use, rates of 13% are reported in the United States and up to 40% in the UK, possibly reflecting differences in service organization (Meltzer et al. 2000; Zahner et al. 1992).

Despite the modest rates of overt presentation of child and adolescent mental health problems in primary care, presenting complaints might primarily reflect educational or social problems (Starfield et al. 1980). This distinction may explain the emphasis on "psychosocial" problems by some researchers (Kelleher et al. 1997). All types of child psychiatric disorders are seen in primary care. However, in preschool children there is a greater than expected proportion of oppositional defiant disorder (Lavigne et al. 1993). Conversely, in school-age children, emotional disorders predominate over conduct disorders (Garralda 2002).

Less is known about the correlates of routine use of primary care by children with specific types of mental health problems. A study of pathways to care for children with pervasive hyperactivity reported that parental perception of hyperactivity as a problem predicted contact with primary care for any reason replicating the findings of earlier authors, while under-recognition by the general practitioner was the major barrier to referral (Sayal et al. 2002; Woodward et al. 1988). These findings were replicated when examining data on children with ADHD participating in the 1999 British Child and Adolescent Mental Health Survey (Sayal et al. 2006a). Lifetime contact with primary care for any reason was predicted by parental recognition of problems and perceived parental burden as well as by parental views that their child had poor general health. In contrast, for children with conduct disorder participating in the same survey, contact with primary care services was associated with comorbid physical or emotional disorders (Vostanis et al. 2003). Other investigators have reported high levels of family stress, maternal psychopathology, somatic symptoms, and adverse life events among children with high levels of psychopathology attending general practice (Garralda and Bailey 1986b; Woodward et al. 1988). The presenting problem is rarely psychological (Garralda and Bailey 1986a; Kramer and Garralda 1998).

Schools and Educational Services

Teachers were the most commonly consulted professionals about mental health by the parents of 5913 4-15-year-olds participating in the Health Survey for England, regardless of the level of psychopathology (Haines et al. 2002). A Finnish general population study of teacher referrals to mental health services over four years among children aged 8-12 at intake reported that only 3% of the sample had been referred, although referral had been considered for a further 3% (Kumpulainen and Rasanen 2002). A follow-up of 2461 British school-age children also suggested that teachers were the most commonly consulted professional about mental issues, contacted by 14% of whole sample, and 41% of those with a disorder at baseline (Ford et al. 2007). In addition, mental-health-related contacts were as common with specialist educational resources as they were with specialist mental health services in this study (5% whole population, 25% of those with psychiatric disorder at baseline). Contact with teachers was predicted by parental recognition that the child had psychopathology, parental psychopathology, and the impact of the psychopathology at baseline and was commoner in younger children. In addition to the impact of psychopsychology on others, and parental psychopathology at baseline, teacher recognition of psychopathology predicted contact with educational specialists at three years (Ford et al. 2008). Thus, it is vital that teachers receive training about the nature of childhood psychiatric disorders, their identification, and the management of minor difficulties. Specialist mental health services should support their colleagues in schools and specialist educational services because the same study suggested that contacts with teachers predict contact with specialist educational provision rather than mental health services. This is particularly applicable for children with ADHD as teachers are well placed to identify children with these difficulties (Sayal et al. 2006b). In a UK survey two-thirds of parents of children with ADHD reported that they had made contact with educational professionals. The main predictors of these contacts were parental recognition of problems and perceived parental burden (Sayal et al. 2006a).

In the Great Smoky Mountain Study contact with education services was associated with symptoms, younger age, and having more highly educated parents (Farmer et al. 1999). A later study found that the correlates of contact with school-based services were the presence of a psychiatric disorder and impairment, parental perceived barriers to accessing help, and psychological impact on the parent (Angold et al. 2002). Feehan and colleagues (1990) reported an interaction between gender, age, and the type of service, so that younger boys were more likely to be in contact with teachers and medical services, but while medical contacts decreased with age for both genders, contacts with teachers regarding girls increased.

Secondary Care Pediatric Services

In the British Child and Adolescent Mental Health Survey 3% of the 2461 school-age children, and 14% of those with a psychiatric disorder at baseline, were in contact with secondary general health care or what in Britain are called pediatric services. In this study, contact with pediatric services was not associated with the impact of the psychopathology, but was predicted by parental recognition, the presence of a neurodevelopmental disorder, large family size, and living in the north of Britain as well as contact with primary health care or teachers (Ford et al. 2008). Few have studied pediatric services but those that have, have reported an association with the presence or impact of psychopathology and it is unclear why the findings from the British child and adolescent mental health surveys should contradict them (Angold et al. 2002; Zahner and Daskalakis 1997). In a sample from the United States contact with general medical services was associated with younger age, having a psychiatric disorder, and psychological impact on the parent (Angold et al. 2002).

Social Services

Mental-health-related contacts with social services and youth justice have rarely been studied, but the three-year follow-up of the British Child and Adolescent Mental Health Survey (1999, Meltzer et al. 2000) reported that 3% of the whole population and 14% of those with impairing psychiatric disorder contacted social services. In a secondary analysis of the lifetime reports of service use among children with a psychiatric disorder in the initial survey, Vostanis and colleagues (2003) reported that children with conduct disorder were more likely to be in contact with social services and education-based services than children with other psychiatric disorders. However, this finding was only partially mirrored in a similar American study (Garland et al. 2001). After adjusting for age and gender, children in contact with mental health, specialist education services, and substance abuse teams were statistically more likely to have a disruptive disorder than children in contact with the juvenile justice or child welfare services. The prevalence of emotional disorders was more evenly distributed across the services and more similar to that reported by community-based studies, but children with separation anxiety, post-traumatic stress disorder, or obsessive compulsive disorder were more likely to be attending mental health services. In another American study, contact with social services was related to younger age, psychiatric disorder, and impairment (Angold et al. 2002). In the three-year follow-up of the British Child and Adolescent Mental Health survey, there was little difference in the level of psychopathology among children in contact with social services who were or were not also seen by specialist mental health services (Guglani, Ford and Rushton 2008). During this study, it became clear that many parents were using social services as a "first line" service to seek help, but that many families did not progress beyond assessment and the opportunity to redirect to mental health services was missed in most cases. Perhaps, as with primary care, the ticket of entry does not signal the mental health problem which social workers then fail to identify as they carry out a service-specific assessment?

CONCLUSIONS

Large numbers of children with impairing psychiatric disorders are in contact with all the public sector services, thus providing an opportunity for identification and intervention. However, several authors report low levels of identification of significant mental health problems among children attending primary care and pediatric services (Dulcan et al. 1990; Garralda and Bailey 1986a; Glazebrook et al. 2003; Kramer and Garralda 1998; Sayal and Taylor 2004).

Both structural and perception-related barriers to care need to be addressed. The former reflect service provision, organization, and availability. Addressing perception-related barriers could help target those most in need but least likely to use services and influence parental views about help-seeking. For children with symptoms or disorders, the effectiveness of strategies to modify parental perception of problems also needs to be investigated. However, health services face considerable challenges in addressing these issues. Repeated cross-sectional studies suggest that rates of service use have increased in recent years (Sourander et al. 2004; Tick et al. 2008). If specialist mental health services are to support their colleagues working with children in other services, then thought is needed about how to deal with the increased demand as many specialist services are already struggling to meet current demand. Possibilities include automating parts of the assessment and treatment process and treating an increasing proportion of children and/or parents in groups (Ford 2008). A recent study revealed that very little group work was reported by parents of children in contact with child and adolescent mental health services (CAMHS) (Ford, Hamilton & Goodman 2005). This is particularly important given the evidence base for interventions for behavioral problems (including ADHD and disruptive behavior disorders) in younger children. The adoption of manualized treatments and protocols with an evidence base might actually speed some children's recovery, allowing more children to be treated by any given number of staff. There is some preliminary evidence of the effectiveness of cognitive behavioral therapy administered over the telephone in adults, and one group is investigating its use with children who have obsessive compulsive disorder (Lovell et al., 2006; Heyman, personal communication). Greater use could be made of telephone, video-conferencing, and e-mail consultations, thus freeing up clinical time and reducing the disruption to families during clinic appointments. Children and parents could complete standardized assessments prior to their first clinic attendance thereby allowing clinicians to focus on problem areas and proceed more quickly to intervention.

In terms of research implications for improving knowledge and developing interventions to reduce barriers to care, theoretical models that draw together the overlapping and multiple help-seeking processes are being developed (Zwaanswijk et al. 2005). Secondary research using existing datasets to investigate international differences in service use could also help to improve our understanding of barriers to care. A greater emphasis on developing resources at population and primary care levels may help bypass some of the current difficulties of stigma related to limited recognition of problems by parents and GPs and access to specialist services. Training and supporting professionals in the recognition and management of child mental health problems are an important public health task. However, all novel methods of working would have to be thoroughly evaluated in terms of effectiveness, acceptability to service users and clinicians, and cost-effectiveness prior to being widely adopted, which in itself would require time and investment (Bower and Gilbody 2005).

REFERENCES

Almqvist, F., Puura, K., Kumpulainen, K. et al. "Psychiatric disorders in 8-9-year-old children based on a diagnostic interview with the parents." *European Child & Adolescent Psychiatry* 8 (1999): Suppl 4, 17-28.

Anderson, J.C., Williams, S., McGee, R. et al. "DSM-III disorders in preadolescent children. Prevalence in a large sample from the general population." *Archives of General Psychiatry* 44 (1987): 69-76.

Angold, A., Erkanli, A., Farmer, E.M. et al. "Psychiatric disorder, impairment, and service use in rural African American and white youth." *Archives of General Psychiatry* 59 (2002): 893-901.

Angold, A., Messer, S.C., Stangl, D. et al. "Perceived parental burden and service use for child and adolescent psychiatric disorders." *American Journal of Public Health* 88 (1998): 75-80.

Bindman, A., & Majeed, A. "Primary care in the United States: Organisation of primary care in the United States." *British Medical Journal* 326 (2003): 631-634.

Bower P. & Gilbody, S. "Stepped care in psychological therapies: Access, effectiveness and efficiency." *British Journal of Psychiatry* 186 (2005): 11-17.

Bowman, F. & Garralda, M.E. "Psychiatric morbidity among children who are frequent attenders in general practice." *British Journal of General Practice* 43 (1993): 6-9.

Boyle, M.H., Cunningham, C.E., Georgiades, K., Cullen, J., Racine, Y. & Pettingill, P. "The Brief Child and Family Phone Interview (BCFPI): 2. Usefulness in screening for child and adolescent psychopathology." *Journal of Child Psychology and Psychiatry* 50 (2009): 424-31.

Boyle, M.H. & Offord, D.R. "Prevalence of childhood disorder, perceived need for help, family dysfunction and resource allocation for child welfare and children's mental health services in Ontario." *Canadian Journal of Behavioural Science* 20 (1988): 374-388.

Boyle, M.H. & Pickles, A. "Influence of maternal depressive symptoms on ratings of childhood behaviour." *Journal of Abnormal Child Psychology* 25 (1997): 399-412.

Briggs-Gowan, M.J., Horwitz, S.M., Schwab-Stone, M.E. et al. "Mental health in pediatric settings: Distribution of disorders and factors related to service use." *Journal of the American Academy of Child & Adolescent Psychiatry* 39 (2000): 841-849.

Burns, B.J., Costello, E.J. & Angold, A. et al. "Childrens mental health service use across service sectors." *Health Affairs (Millwood)* 14 (1995): 147-159.

Bussing, R., Zima, B.T., Belin, T.R. "Differential access to care for children with ADHD in special education programs." *Psychiatric Services* 49 (1998): 1226-1229.

Costello E.J., Burns, B.J., Angold, A. et al. "How can epidemiology improve mental health services for children and adolescents?" *Journal of the American Academy of Child & Adolescent Psychiatry* 32 (1993): 1106-1113.

Costello, E.J., Egger, H. & Angold, A. "10-Year research update review: The epidemiology of child and adolescent psychiatric disorders: 1. Methods and Public Health Burden." *Journal of the American Academy of Child and Adolescent Psychiatry* 44 (2005): 972-986.

Costello, E.J. & Janiszewski, S. "Who gets treated? Factors associated with referral in children with psychiatric disorders." *Acta Psychiatrica Scandinavica* 81 (1990): 523-529.

Cunningham, P.J. & Freiman, M.P. "Determinants of ambulatory mental health service use for school-age children and adolescents." *Health Service Research* 31 (1996): 409-421.

Dulcan, M.K., Costello, E.J., Costello, A.J. et al. "The pediatrician as gatekeeper to mental health care for children: do parents' concerns open the gate?" *Journal of the American Academy of Child & Adolescent Psychiatry* 29 (1990): 453-458.

Farmer, E.M., Burns, B.J., Angold, A. et al. "Impact of child mental health problems on families: relationships with service use." *Journal of Emotional and Behavioral Disorders* 5 (1997): 230-238.

Farmer, E.M., Burns, B.J., Phillips, S.D. et al. "Pathways into and through mental health services for children and adolescents." *Psychiatric Services* 54 (2003): 60-66.

Farmer, E.M., Stangl, D.K., Burns, B.J. et al. "Use, persistence, and intensity: Patterns of care for children's mental health across one year." *Community Mental Health Journal* 35 (1999): 31-46.

Feehan, M., Stanton, W., McGee, R. et al. "Parental help-seeking for behavioural and emotional problems in childhood and adolescence." *Community Health Studies* 14 (1990): 303-309.

Fergusson, D.M., Horwood, J., Lynskey, M.T. et al. "Prevalence and comorbidity of DSM-III-R diagnoses in a birth cohort of 15 year olds." *Journal of the American Academy of Child & Adolescent Psychiatry* 32 (1993): 1127-1134.

Flisher, A.J., Kramer, R.A., Grosser, R.C. et al. "Correlates of unmet need for mental health services by children and adolescents." *Psychological Medicine* 27 (1997): 1145-1154.

Foreman, D., Moreton, S. & Ford, T. "Exploring the clinical utility of the development and well-being assessment (DAWBA) in the detection of hyperactivity and associated disorders in clinical practice." *Journal of Child Psychology and Psychiatry* 50 (2009): 460-470.

Ford, T. "Practitioner review: How can epidemiological surveys help us plan and deliver effective child and adolescent mental health services?" *Journal of Child Psychology and Psychiatry* 49 (2008): 900-914.

Ford, T., Hamilton, H. & Goodman, R. "Service contacts among the children participating in the 1999 British child and adolescent mental health survey and its follow-ups." *Child and Adolescent Mental Health* 10 (2005): 2-9.

Ford, T., Hamilton, H., Meltzer, H. & Goodman, R. "Child mental health is everybody's business; the prevalence of contacts with public sectors services by the types of disorder among British school children in a three-year period." *Child and Adolescent Mental Health* 12 (2007): 13-20.

Ford, T., Hamilton, H., Meltzer, H. & Goodman, R. "Predictors of service use for mental health problems among British school children." *Child and Adolescent Mental Health* 13 (2008): 32-40.

Ford, T., Tingay, K., Wolpert, M. & the CORC Steering Group. "CORC's survey of Routine Outcome Monitoring and the National CAMHS dataset: A response to Johnston and Gower." *Child and Adolescent Mental Health* 11 (2006): 50-52.

Garland, A.F., Hough, R.L., McCabe, K.M., Yeh, M., Wood, P. & Aarons, G. "Prevalence of psychiatric disorders across five sectors of care." *Journal of the American Academy of Child and Adolescent Psychiatry* 40 (2001): 409-418.

Garralda, M.E. "Primary health care psychiatry." In: Taylor, E. & Rutter, M. (eds) *Child and adolescent psychiatry: Modern approaches* (4th edition), pp 1090-1100. Blackwell Press, 2002.

Garralda, M.E. "Accountability of specialist child and adolescent mental health services." *British Journal of Psychiatry* 194(5) (2009): 389-391.

Garralda, M.E. & Bailey, D. "Psychological deviance in children attending general practice." *Psychological Medicine* 16 (1986a): 423-429.

Garralda, M.E. & Bailey, D. "Children with psychiatric disorders in primary care." *Journal of Child Psychology and Psychiatry* 27 (1986b): 611-624.

Garralda, M.E. & Bailey, D. "Child and family factors associated with referral to child psychiatrists." *British Journal of Psychiatry* 153 (1988): 81-89.

Gasquet, L., Ledoux, S., Chavance, M. & Choquest, M. "Consultation of mental health professionals by French adolescents with probable psychiatric problems." *Acta Psychiatrica Scandinavia* 99 (1999): 126-134.

Giel, R., de Arango, M.V., Climent, C.E. et al. "Childhood mental disorders in primary health care: Results of observations in four developing countries. A report from the WHO collaborative Study on Strategies for Extending Mental Health Care." *Pediatrics* 68 (1981): 677-683.

Glazebrook, C., Hollis, C., Heussler, H., Goodman, R. & Coates, L. "Detecting emotional and behavioural problems in paediatric clinics. *Child Care, Health and Development* 29 (2003): 141-149.

Glugani, S., Rushton, A. & Ford, T. "Mental health and educational Difficulties among children in contact with social services." *Child and Family Social Work* 13 (2008): 188-196.

Goodman, R., Ford, T., Corbin, T. & Meltzer, H. "Using the Strengths and Difficulties Questionnaire (SDQ) multi-informant algorithm to screen looked after children for psychiatric disorders." *European Child and Adolescent Psychiatry* 13 supplement 2 (2004): 25-31.

Goodman, A. & Goodman, R. "Strengths and Difficulties Questionnaire as a dimensional measure of mental child health." *Journal of the American Academy of Child and Adolescent Psychiatry* 48 (2009): 400-403.

Goldberg, I.D., Roghmann, K.J., McInerny, T.K. et al. "Mental health problems among children seen in pediatric practice: Prevalence and management." *Pediatrics* 73 (1984): 278-293.

Griest, D.L., Forehand, R., Wells, K.C. et al. "An examination of differences between nonclinic and behavior-problem clinic-referred children and their mothers." *Journal of Abnormal Psychology* 89 (1980): 497-500.

Griest, D., Wells, K.C. & Forehand, R. "An examination of predictors of maternal perceptions of maladjustment in clinic-referred children." *Journal of Abnormal Psychology* 88 (1979): 277-281.

Gunther, N., Slavenburg, B., Feron, F. et al. "Childhood social and early developmental factors associated with mental health service use." *Social Psychiatry and Psychiatric Epidemiology* 38 (2003): 101-108.

Gureje, O., Omigbodun, O.O., Gater, R. et al. "Psychiatric disorders in a paediatric primary care clinic." *British Journal of Psychiatry* 165 (1994): 527-530.

Haines, M.M., McMunn, A. & Nazroo, JY. & Kelly, YJ. "Social and demographic predictors of parental consultation for child and adolescent difficulties." *Journal of Public Health Medicine* 24 (2002): 276-284.

Harrington, R.C., Kerfoot, M. & Verduyn, C. "Developing needs led child and adolescent mental health services: Issues and prospects." *European Child & Adolescent Psychiatry* 8 (1999): 1-10.

Jenkins, R. "Making epidemiology useful: the contribution of epidemiology to government policy. *Acta Psychiatrica Scandinavia* 103 (2001): 2-14.

Jensen, P.S., Bloedau, L., & Davis H. "Children at risk: II. Risk factors and clinic utilization." *Journal of the American Academy of Child & Adolescent Psychiatry*, 29 (1990), 804-812.

Johnstone, C. & Gower, S. "Routine outcome measurement: a survey of UK child and adolescent mental health services." *Child and Adolescent Mental Health* 10 (2005): 133-139.

Kataoka, S.H., Zhang, L. & Wells, K.B. "Unmet need for mental health care among U.S. children: Variation by ethnicity and insurance status." *American Journal of Psychiatry* 59 (2002): 1548-1555.

Kelleher, K.J., Childs, G.E., Wasserman, R.C. et al. "Insurance status and recognition of psychosocial problems. A report from the Pediatric Research in Office Settings and the Ambulatory Sentinel Practice Networks." *Archives of Pediatrics & Adolescent Medicine* 151 (1997): 1109-1115.

Koot, H.M. & Verhulst, F.C. "Prediction of children's referral to mental health and special education services from earlier adjustment." *Journal of Child Psychology and Psychiatry* 33 (1992): 717-729.

Kramer, T. & Garralda, M.E. "Psychiatric disorders in adolescents in primary care." *British Journal of Psychiatry* 173 (1998): 508-513.

Kumpulainen, K. & Rasanen, E. "Symptoms and deviant behaviour among 8 year olds as predictors of referral for psychiatric evaluation by age 12." *Psychiatric Services* 53 (2002): 201-206.

Laitinen-Krispijn, S., Van der Ende, J., Wierdsma, A.I. et al. "Predicting adolescent mental health service use in a prospective record-linkage study." *Journal of the American Academy of Child & Adolescent Psychiatry* 38 (1999): 1073-1080.

Lavigne, J.V., Binns, H.J., Christoffel, K.K. et al. "Behavioral and emotional problems among preschool children in pediatric primary care: Prevalence and pediatricians' recognition." *Pediatrics* 91 (1993): 649-655.

Lavigne, J.V., Binns, H.J., Rosenbaum, D. et al. "Mental health service use among young children receiving pediatric primary care." *Journal of the American Academy of Child and Adolescent Psychiatry* 37 (1998): 1175-1183.

Leaf, P.J., Alegria, M., Cohen, P. et al. "Mental health service use in the community and schools: Results from the four-community MECA Study. Methods for the Epidemiology of Child and Adolescent Mental Disorders Study." *Journal of the American Academy of Child & Adolescent Psychiatry* 35 (1996): 889-897.

Logan, D.E. & King, C.A. "Parental identification of depression and mental health service use amongst depressed adolescents." *Journal of the American Academy of Child & Adolescent Psychiatry* 41 (2002): 296-304.

Lovell, K., Cox, D., Haddock, G., Jones, C., Raines, D., Garvey, R., Roberts, C. & Hadley, S. "Telephone administered cognitive behavioural therapy for obsessive compulsive disorder: Randomised non-inferiority trial." *British Medical Journal* 333 (2006): 883- 888.

Meltzer, H., Gatward, R., Goodman, R. et al. "*Mental health of children and adolescents in Great Britain.*" ONS. London: The Stationery Office, 2000.

Offord, D., Boyle, M., Szatmari, P. et al. "Ontario Child Health Study II. Six-month prevalence of disorder and rates of service utilization." *Archives of General Psychiatry* 44 (1987): 832-836.

Owens, P.L., Hoagwood, K., Horwitz, S.M. et al. "Barriers to children's mental health services." *Journal of the American Academy of Child & Adolescent Psychiatry* 41 (2002): 731-738.

Patton, G.C., Coffey, C., Posterino, M., Carlin, J.B., Wolfe, R. & Bowes, G. "A computerised screening instrument for adolescent depression: Population-based validation and application to a two-phase case-control study." *Social Psychiatry and Psychiatric Epidemiology* 34 (1999): 166-172.

Pavuluri, M.N., Luk, S. & McGee, R. "Help-seeking for behaviour problems by parents of preschool children: A community study." *Journal of the American Academy of Child & Adolescent Psychiatry* 35 (1996): 215-222.

Rutter, M., Tizard, J. & Whitmore, K. *Education, health, and behaviour*. London: Longman, 1970.

Sayal, K. "The role of parental burden in child mental health service use: Longitudinal study." *Journal of the American Academy of Child and Adolescent Psychiatry* 43 (2004): 1328-1333.

Sayal, K. "Annotation: Pathways to care for children with mental health problems." *Journal of Child Psychology and Psychiatry* 47 (2006): 649-659.

Sayal, K., Goodman, R. & Ford, T. "Barriers to the identification of children with Attention Deficit/Hyperactivity Disorder." *Journal of Child Psychology and Psychiatry* 47 (2006a): 744-750.

Sayal, K., Hornsey, H., Warren, S., MacDiarmid, F. & Taylor, E. "Identification of children at risk of ADHD: A school-based intervention." *Social Psychiatry and Psychiatric Epidemiology* 41 (2006b): 806-813.

Sayal, K., Letch, N. & El Abd, S. "Evaluation of screening in children referred for an ADHD assessment." *Child and Adolescent Mental Health* 13 (2008): 41-16.

Sayal, K. & Taylor, E. "Detection of child mental health disorders by general practitioners." *British Journal of General Practice* 54 (2004): 348-352.

Sayal, K., Taylor, E., & Beecham, J. "Parental perception of problems and mental health service use for hyperactivity." *Journal of the American Academy of Child and Adolescent Psychiatry*, 42 (2003), 1410-1414.

Sayal, K., Taylor, E., Beecham, J. & Byrne, P. "Pathways to care in children at risk of attention deficit/hyperactivity disorder." *British Journal of Psychiatry* 181 (2002): 43-48.

Sourander, A., Helstela, L., Ristkari, T. et al. "Child and adolescent mental health service use in Finland." *Social Psychiatry and Psychiatric Epidemiology* 36 (2001): 294-298.

Sourander, A., Santalahti, P., Haavisto, A., Piha, J., IkAheimo, K. & Helenius, H. "Have there been changes in children's psychiatric symptoms and mental health service use? A 10-year comparison from Finland." *Journal of the American Academy of Child and Adolescent Psychiatry* 43 (2004): 1134-1145.

Staghezza-Jaramillo, B., Bird, H.R., Gould, M.S. et al. "Mental health service utilization among Puerto Rican children ages 4 through 16." *Journal of Child & Family Studies* 4 (1995): 399-418.

Starfield, B., Gross, E., Wood, M. et al. "Psychosocial and psychosomatic diagnoses in primary care of children." *Pediatrics* 66 (1980): 159-167.

Sturm, R., Ringel, J.S. & Andreyva, T. "Geographic disparities in children's mental health care." *Pediatrics* 112 (2003): e308-e315.

Teagle, S.E. "Parental problem recognition and child mental health service use." *Mental Health Services Research* 4 (2002): 257-266.

Thomas, C.R. & Holzer, C.E. III. "National distribution of child and adolescent psychiatrists." *Journal of the American Academy of Child and Adolescent Psychiatry* 38 (1999): 9-15.

Tick, N.T., van der Ende, J. & Verhulst FC. "Ten-year increase in service use in the Dutch population." *European Child and Adolescent Psychiatry* 17 (2008): 373-380.

Verhulst, F.C. & van der Ende, J. "Factors associated with child mental health service use in the community." *Journal of the American Academy of Child & Adolescent Psychiatry* 36 (1997): 901-909.

Vostanis, P., Meltzer, H., Goodman, R. et al. "Service utilisation by children with conduct disorders: Findings from the GB National Study." *European Child & Adolescent Psychiatry* 12 (2003): 231-238.

Weisz, J.R. & Weiss, B. "Studying the 'referability' of child clinical problems." *Journal of Consulting & Clinical Psychology* 59 (1991): 266-273.

Woodward, C.A., Boyle, M.H., Offord, D.R. et al. "Ontario Child Health Study: Patterns of ambulatory medical care utilization and their correlates." *Pediatrics* 82 (1988): 425-434.

Wu, P., Hoven, C.W., Bird, H.R. et al. "Depressive and disruptive disorders and mental health service utilization in children and adolescents." *Journal of the American Academy of Child & Adolescent Psychiatry* 38 (1999): 1081-1090.

Yokley, J.M., & Reuter, JM. "The computer assisted child diagnostic system: A research and development project." *Computers in Human Behavior* 5 (1989): 277-295.

Zahner, G.E.P. & Daskalalis, C. "Factors associated with mental health, general health, and school-based service use for child psychopathology." *American Journal of Public Health* 87 (1997): 1440-1448.

Zahner, G.E.P., Pawelkiewicz, W., DeFrancesco, J.J. et al. "Children's mental health service needs and utilization patterns in an urban community: An epidemiological assessment." *Journal of the American Academy of Child & Adolescent Psychiatry* 31 (1992): 951-960.

Zwaanswijk, M., Verhaak, P.F.M., Bensing, J.M. et al. "Help seeking for emotional and behavioural problems in children and adolescents—A review of recent literature." *European Child & Adolescent Psychiatry* 12 (2003): 153-161.

Zwaanswijk, M., Verhaak, P.F.M., Bensing, J.M. et al. "Help-seeking for child psychopathology: Pathways to informal and professional services in the Netherlands." *Journal of the American Academy of Child & Adolescent Psychiatry* 44 (2005): 1292-1300.

2

Family Structure and Children's Mental Health in Western Countries

Rossana Bisceglia, C. Cheung, Emily Swinkin, and Jennifer Jenkins

INTRODUCTION

In the last several decades, the Western family has undergone significant changes in its composition. Census data from Canada indicate that in 2006 65.7% of Canada's 5.6 million children under 14 years of age lived with married parents, a decline from 81.2% in 1986 (Demography Division, Statistics Canada, 2007). Comparable patterns are evident in the United States (U.S. Census Bureau, 2007) and Europe (European Foundation for the Improvement of Living and Working Conditions, 2007).

We begin this chapter by presenting several issues regarding the operationalization and measurement of family structure. We then summarize empirical findings on the link between family structure and children's well-being. Finally, we consider the mechanisms involved in this link, including the factors that protect children from negative outcomes. Throughout the chapter we give consideration to the practice and policy issues that emerge from the findings.

OPERATIONALIZATION OF FAMILY STRUCTURE

There is debate about how to best capture the variability in family structures (e.g., see Apel & Kaukinen, 2008). In general it is agreed that the binary classification of intact versus non-intact is not very useful because it obscures several issues that we know are important for children's well-being. For example, imagine two children where one lives with his biological mother and a step-father who also has a child from a previous relationship, while the second child lives with her biological father and step-mother but no siblings. A binary categorization would classify both of these examples as "non-intact" despite important differences in the biological relatedness between the children, mother, father, and siblings. A further differentiation includes the type of union between parents (i.e., married versus cohabitation).

Two distinctions are important; children's biological relatedness to the parents with whom they live, and the family type. *Nuclear* families include those families where all members share biological relatedness and where parents are in a married relationship. *Cohabiting* families consist of parents that are not married but both are biologically related with all children in the family. *Blended* families include children that share biological relatedness with both parents but only half-biological relatedness with their siblings. Non-intact families include biological single parents (mother or father), *simple step-families* include children living with one biological and one non-biological parent but no step-siblings, and *complex step-families* include children sharing biological relatedness with only one parent but no relation to at least one other child in the home.

CAVEATS AND MEASUREMENT CONSIDERATIONS ON THE ASSOCIATION BETWEEN FAMILY STRUCTURE AND CHILDREN'S FUNCTIONING

The fact that children are not randomly assigned to family types significantly obscures the causal effect of family structure on children's well-being. There is evidence that family structure does not occur at random; rather, parental personal characteristics and early experiences are associated with family structure. For instance, men who become step-fathers tend to have less education, work fewer hours, and to be of younger age than biological fathers (Brown, 2004; Manning & Lichter, 1996). Likewise, relative to married parents, parents that choose cohabitation show lower education and income (Brown, 2004). Hence, differences between children in non-nuclear and nuclear families may be due to selection processes that led to the formation of the family structure in the first place, rather than family type per se. Next, we discuss two types of selection processes: genetic and environmental.

There is evidence that genetics are related to family structure. For instance, divorce is more common among monozygotic twins than dizygotic twins (McGue & Lykken, 1992). These data do not imply that there is a gene for divorce, rather that genetic factors might predispose individuals to certain traits (i.e., personality and behavioral patterns) that increase the risk of divorce. Indeed, personality characteristics (i.e., negative emotionality) account for 30% to 42% of the genetic effect on divorce (Jocklin, McGue, & Lykken, 1996). One way that personality characteristics influence family structure is through the selection of a mate. For instance, individuals with negative personality traits (i.e., antisocial) and problems (i.e., substance abuse, depression) have been shown to select partners with similar difficulties (Champion, Goodall, & Rutter, 1995) thereby further increasing their risk of relationship problems and divorce (Jocklin et al., 1996). Children may resemble their parents with respect to personal characteristics. For instance, parental antisocial behavior is a strong predictor of child conduct problems (Frick & Loney, 2002). Although resemblance may be attributable to genetics and/or environmental experience (which we discuss next), these findings indicate that parental characteristics are associated with *both* the family structure (by means of selection processes) and children's characteristics. Therefore, when attempting to make causal inferences about the effect of family type on child well-being it is important to partial out the effects of personality or other personal characteristics on child well-being. Before we discuss methodologies that allow for this kind of control, we present a second source of influence that might also account for the compromised well-being in children from non-nuclear families: environmental experience.

Children do not only inherit genes from their parents; they also inherit an environmental context which can place children at risk of disturbance (e.g., poverty, living in a high-crime neighborhood (Sampson et al., 1997)), and experiences of harsh parenting (Dodge, Bates, & Pettit, 1990). Exposure to these environmental factors is also not random; rather, it is associated with parental characteristics and family type. For instance, cohabiting families tend to show lower economic resources relative to traditional nuclear homes (Brown, 2002, 2004). Parents from non-nuclear family structures are also more likely to experience various forms of psychopathology. For instance, depression is more common in mothers in cohabiting unions than nuclear family types (Brown, 2004). In turn, parental psychopathology is associated with other factors that increase children's risk of disturbance, such as overt marital conflict and ineffective parenting practices (Johnson, Cohen, Kasen, Smailes, & Brook, 2001). Family structure is also dependent on previous family transitions like divorce; therefore, relative to children from nuclear families, those in non-nuclear family structures may differ in behavior due to the experience of previous stressful experiences (Hao & Xie, 2002). Hence, in addition to the family structure, children are exposed to multiple sources of risks. Causal inferences about the effect of family type on children's well-being must partial out the effect of these various risk factors.

Two methodologies that are particularly useful in partitioning the effects of selection variables from risk factors include Fixed Effects models (see

Hao & Xie, 2002 for a description) and the Children-of-Twins (CoT) design (Heath, Kendler, Eaves, & Markell, 1985); we provide a brief description below.

The CoT is a quasi-experimental design that partitions the effect of risk variables from the effects of selection processes. One comparison that is performed using this design is between the functioning of children of identical twin pairs. For instance, Twin 1 and Twin 2 are identical twin sisters who each have children; the behavior of their children would be compared. If Twin 1 is a single mother but Twin 2 is in a marital relationship, the twins are said to be discordant on single mother status. The comparison of children's functioning between the discordant twin parents allows for the partitioning of the effect of single mother status from other influences. If single mother status matters, we would expect that children of Twin 1 would show greater disturbance than children of Twin 2. Differences in children's behavior can only be attributable to factors that *vary* between the twin parents. Since the twin parents share 100% of their genes and therefore genetics do not vary between them the mothers' genetic influences cannot account for differences in the behavior among the twin's children. Other selection factors that do not vary between the twin parents (e.g., history of own parents' divorce, etc.) also cannot account for disparity in children's behavior. Thus, the effect of single mother status on children's functioning is pulled apart from genetic and other selection processes common to the twin parents. Factors that are specific to the single mother twin should then account for some of the disparity in children's well-being. Alternatively, if children of twins discordant for single mother status show *similar* behaviors, then selection variables common to both twin parents (including genetics) must account for at least some of the association between single mother status and child well-being (for an in-depth description of the CoT design see D'Onofrio et al., 2003).

Longitudinal studies are also helpful in the interpretation of the compromised outcomes of children from non-nuclear homes. Following families and children over time allows researchers to assess children's and family functioning before and after changes in the family structure. The effects of problems and risk factors that predated changes in family structure are entered into the statistical models to control for their influence. Changes in children's behavior over time can be interpreted as being related to *changes* in the family structure and/or in family components (i.e., change in economics following divorce). The importance of taking into account pre-existing functioning is exemplified by research on the effects of divorce which shows that while divorce is associated with poor outcomes, many of the children's problems were present prior to the divorce (e.g., see Aseltine, 1996; Hetherington, 1999).

FAMILY STRUCTURE AND ASSOCIATIONS WITH CHILD AND ADOLESCENT PSYCHOPATHOLOGY

Nuclear, Cohabitating, and Blended Families

The literature on the adjustment of children from traditional nuclear families is unequivocal; children that reside with two biological married parents fare better on a myriad of outcomes than those from non-intact family structures. Brown (2004) found that after controlling for various child characteristics, children from nuclear families scored higher on school engagement and lower on emotional and behavioral problems than those in cohabiting families and non-intact family types. Similar results have been shown for delinquent behavior. In the United States it is estimated that the delinquency rates for children who reside in families without two biological parents is 10% to 15% higher than their peers from cohabiting and blended families (Wells & Rankin, 1991).

Compromised outcomes are found for children raised in cohabiting families and children who are biologically related to both parents but live in a blended family. Adolescents from cohabiting homes show more delinquent and antisocial behavior followed by those from blended families (Apel & Kaukinen, 2008). Children from cohabiting families exhibit more emotional and behavioral problems than those in nuclear homes (Brown, 2004) and often fare similarly to children from single mother families (for children aged 6-11 years) or cohabiting step-families (for adolescents). Despite some inconsistencies (e.g., see Ram & Hou, 2003), similar findings across outcomes such as academic and behavioral outcomes have been found (see Ginther & Pollak, 2004; Hao & Xie, 2002; Hofferth, 2007; Manning & Lamb, 2003). The disadvantage in children from blended and cohabiting families has been linked to disparity in family components; this will be discussed in the final section of this chapter.

Separated/Divorced

In Europe, the percentage of families that divorce has been steadily increasing over the last two decades. For instance, across the 25 countries of the European Union where 9% to 49% of marriages ended in divorce in the 1990s, 2003 saw an increase from 13% to 75% (European Foundation for the Improvement of Living and Working Conditions, 2007). Similar trends have been noted in the United States (U.S. Census Bureau, 2007) and Canada (Demography Division, Statistics Canada, 2007).

In 1991 Amato and Keith conducted a meta-analysis to estimate the effect of parental divorce on children's well-being. The results showed that children from divorced families scored significantly lower on a variety of domains including academic achievement, conduct, psychological adjustment, self-concept, social adjustment, and parent-child relationship.

Despite the findings on the long-lasting and pervasive consequences of divorce, the majority of children who experience parental divorce do not go on to show disturbance over time. Hetherington and Kelly (2002) found that 75% of individuals from divorced parents did not show serious long-term consequences. Amato and Keith's (1991) meta-analysis showed that the effects of divorce tend to be small to modest in magnitude. In a meta-analysis the effect sizes across studies are examined. The effect size refers to the strength of the relationship between variables (e.g., divorce and child depression). There are different kinds of effect sizes (for a description see Amato & Keith, 1991). In the Amato and Keith (1991) meta-analysis negative effect sizes indicated reduced well-being in children from divorced families. Amato and Keith (1991) found a modest mean effect size of -0.13. Similar results were found in an updated meta-analysis (Amato, 2001).

The following family components have been shown to explain some of the increased risk to children: growing up in a family marked by parental difficulties, prolonged exposure to marital conflict, and the need to adjust to various changes following the divorce (e.g., economic instability).

Single Mother and Single Father Families

The last few decades have seen a steady increase in the percentage of children living in lone-parent families in the United States and Canada. In 2007, 26% of American children lived with a single parent (23% lone mothers and 3% lone fathers) compared to 9% in 1960, 20% in 1980, and 27% in 2000 (U.S. Census Bureau, 2007).

Converging evidence from North American and European samples indicates that children from single mother families fare worse than their peers from nuclear families across various domains including increased risk of antisocial behavior, teen pregnancy, and school dropout (Amato, 2000; Breivik & Olweus, 2006; Brown, 2004; Emery, 1999; Hetherington & Stanley-Hagan, 1999; Jablonska & Lindberg, 2007; Simons, 1996).

Existing research on single father families has produced mixed results (e.g., see Clarke-Stewart & Hayward, 1996). However, evidence is being accumulated that children from singlefather families are at considerable risk. In a Norwegian sample, adolescents from single father homes were four times more likely to have used illegal substances and displayed externalizing behaviors than their peers in other non-intact and two-parent intact family types (Breivik & Olweus, 2006). These results are similar to another Norwegian study (Naevdal & Thuen, 2004) and studies from Sweden (e.g., see Jablonska & Lindberg, 2007) and the United States (e.g., see Apel &

Kaukinen, 2008; Demuth & Brown, 2004; Hofferth, 2007). However, some inconsistencies are found depending on the age of the children. Brown (2004) showed that children aged 6-11 years from single father homes were no worse off than their peers from nuclear families with regards to emotional and behavioral problems, and school engagement. However, for adolescents, residing with a single father was associated with increased emotional and behavioral problems and lower school engagement.

Two explanations have been proposed for these findings. One is that single father status may be a marker for serious underlying problems in the child's family experience (e.g., severe maternal problems) that led to the paternal sole custody arrangement (Breivik & Olweus, 2006). To the best of our knowledge no study has empirically examined this hypothesis. The second possibility is that single fathers engage in ineffective parenting (e.g., less monitoring), which is particularly important for adolescents' well-being; we explore this hypothesis further in the subsequent sections of the chapter.

Step-Parent Families

Reduced well-being is also seen for children in step-families relative to nuclear families (Amato & Rivera, 1999; Dunn et al., 1998; Hanson, McLanahan, & Thomson, 1996; Hetherington & Clingempeel, 1992; Thomson, Hanson, & McLanahan, 1994). The effect size of these associations across 12 studies was about one-third of a standard deviation (Amato & Keith, 1991).

Recent studies suggest that the gender and biological relatedness of the custodial parent are important for children's adjustment in step-parent families. Hoffman (2006) found that after controlling for various children and family factors, adolescents from step-father families continued to show more problems relative to two-biological-parent families, and step-mother families. Comparable findings are evident for delinquency (e.g., see Demuth & Brown, 2004) and academic outcomes (e.g., see Astone & McLanahan, 1991; Hofferth, 2007). Conversely, where the custodial parent is the biological mother adolescents from step-families show only marginally higher rates of delinquency than children from two-biological-parent families (Demuth & Brown, 2004; but see O'Connor, Dunn, Jenkins, Pickering, & Rasbash, 2001 for inconsistencies).

There is mixed evidence with respect to whether children from step-parent families fare better or worse than those in single mother families. Some note worse adjustment for children from step-families (e.g., see Amato & Keith, 1991); others find the opposite effects, with children from single parent families faring better than those from step-parent families (Hao & Xie, 2002), while others note no differences (Ram & Hou, 2003).

Foster, Adoptive, and Next-of-Kin Homes

Foster care refers to living arrangement for children whose biological parents are unable to provide care. Compared to children from nuclear families, children in foster care display maladaptive outcomes including higher levels of externalizing and internalizing behaviors (Hoffman, 2006; Keil & Price, 2006; Lawrence, Carlson, & Egeland, 2006), poor academic performance (Sun, 2003), elevated levels of stress (Dozier et al., 2006), and poor socio-emotional adjustment (Lewis, Dozier, Ackerman, & Sepulveda-Kozakowski, 2007; Tarren-Sweeney & Hazell, 2006).

Children in next-of-kin homes (where a relative is the caregiver) fare better on academic, behavioral, and socio-emotional adjustment, than those in foster care (Holtan, Ronning, Handegård, & Sourander, 2005; Keller et al., 2001); but see De Robertis and Litrownik (2004) for inconsistent findings. There are some indications that although children who are placed under the supervision of their grandparents report more emotional and behavioral difficulties (Smith & Palmieri, 2007) and lower academic achievement (Solomon & Marx, 1995) than children in nuclear families, there is some evidence that they show similar or better outcomes when compared to children from single parent families (Solomon & Marx, 1995). In the subsequent section we review the factors that account for the reduced well-being in children living in out-of-home care.

Gay and Lesbian Families

Census data from the United States in 2002 indicate that there were approximately 600,000 lesbian and gay couples (Simmons, O'Connell, & United States Bureau of the Census, 2003). Since research has not yet examined developmental outcomes of children raised by single gay fathers or gay male couples, our comments pertain to the association between children outcomes and lesbian parents. On the basis of cross-sectional studies, children who reside with lesbian parents do not fare worse than children raised by heterosexual parents on cognitive, socio-emotional, or behavioral functioning (including delinquency and substance use), or in scholastic achievement (e.g., see Bos, van Balen, & van den Boom, 2007; Flaks, Ficher, Masterpasqua, & Joseph, 1995; Telingator & Patterson, 2008). Preliminary longitudinal research (e.g., see Golombok et al., 2003) suggests the same.

COMPONENTS OF FAMILY STRUCTURE
RELATED TO CHILD PSYCHOPATHOLOGY

In the previous section we saw that children from non-nuclear family organizations (except for lesbian parents) fare worse than those from nuclear homes. We also noted that children in cohabiting and single parent families, on average, show higher rates of disturbance than their peers from other non-intact family structures. How and why does family structure relate to children's well-being? Mediation models describe the mediating processes that account for the relationship between a predictor variable (i.e., family structure) and children's functioning. When a mediator is in the statistical model it partially or completely attenuates the relationship between the predictor variable and the child's functioning (Baron & Kenny, 1986).

Research on the effects of family type on children's well-being has identified several family components that are important for children's adjustment. These components are economic resources and parental functioning, interparental conflict, non-resident father involvement, length of time spent in a family structure, the number of family transitions, and the timing of family change. Next we summarize what is known about the role of these components in explaining how and why family structure relates to children's well-being.

Economic Resources and Parental Functioning

Family economic standing is an important correlate of family structure. Since nuclear families show greater economic advantage than other family structures, it has been hypothesized that the disparity in economic resources accounts for the reduced well-being in children from non-nuclear homes. Lower family income may constrain parents' provision of essential resources for their children (i.e., adequate food and housing) that foster healthy child development (Hanson, McLanahan, & Thomson, 1997; Hill et al., 2001). The association between children's reduced well-being and low family income is well established (e.g., see Hobcraft, 2004).

Family economics are also consequential for parental emotional well-being and parenting competence (Conger & Donnellan, 2007). Parents from non-nuclear family structures fare worse on mental health functioning. For example, divorced mothers report more depressive symptoms and withdrawal than married mothers (Wood, Repetti, & Roesch, 2004). Parents in step-families show similar patterns (e.g., see Brown, 2000; Demo & Acock, 1996; Foley et al., 2004). Disparity is also seen in parenting practices. For instance, parents from non-nuclear homes (including divorced) show lower levels of warmth, support, and supervision of their children (e.g., see Buchanan, Maccoby, & Dornbusch, 1996; Hetherington & Clingempeel, 1992; Hetherington & Stanley-Hagan, 1999; McLanahan & Sandefur, 1994).

Numerous studies have demonstrated that, on average, after accounting for family economics and parental functioning, the association between family structure and children's well-being is reduced but still remains statistically significant. This pattern of results has been found for a range of outcomes including emotional and behavioral problems, antisocial behavior, delinquency, educational outcomes, and cognitive ability (e.g., see Apel & Kaukinen, 2008; Manning & Lamb, 2003). A comparable pattern of findings are noted for divorced families and foster/grandparent families (e.g., see Amato, 1986; Amato & Gilbreth, 1999; Apel & Kaukinen, 2008; Martinez & Forgatch, 2002; Smith, Palmieri, Hancock, & Richardson, 2008; Videon, 2002).

Interparental Conflict

As noted previously, children from divorced families show compromised outcomes across various domains. Longitudinal evidence indicates that some proportion of children's reduced well-being is accounted for by "pre-divorce" factors including interparental conflict (Cherlin, Furstenberg, Chase-Lansdale, & Kiernan, 1991). The notion that interparental conflict relates to poor child outcomes is widely accepted among researchers (Long, Slater, Forehand, & Fauber, 1988). Two perspectives on the influence of interparental conflict have predominated.

First, it has been proposed that interparental conflict accounts for children's adjustment problems rather than divorce per se. If this view is correct, then children from high conflict families should show similar problems to those shown by children from divorced families. Many studies support this perspective. For instance, Camara, Resnick, Hetherington, and Arasteh (1988) found that marital conflict completely accounted for the relationship between marital status (divorce versus intact) across five domains of children's well-being. Comparable results are found elsewhere (e.g., see Amato & Keith, 1991; Juby & Farrington, 2001). Longitudinal evidence also indicates that after controlling for parent and child characteristics children whose highly conflicted parents separated showed better adjustment in adulthood than those whose parents remained married (Amato, Loomis, & Booth, 1995). These findings indicate that conflict among parents is a risk factor for children in both divorced and intact families.

Second, child adjustment problems are inversely related to post-divorce conflict. Post-divorce conflict usually involves disputes about child access and custody and financial support. Better child adjustment is related to lower levels of parental conflict and greater post-divorce cooperation (e.g., see Johnston, González, & Campbell, 1987; Long et al., 1988). Studies have also shown that child-focused conflict (e.g., child custody disputes) is particularly harmful to children (e.g., see Johnston et al., 1987; Jenkins, Simpson et al., 2005) with long-lasting consequences (Johnston, Kline, & Tschann, 1989). These findings suggest that the combination of shared child custody and continued interparental conflict among divorced parents increases children's exposure to conflict thereby reducing their well-being.

Research on the adverse effects of post-divorce conflict raises the question of how to best promote low conflict parental separation. Evidence for the positive effects of mediation in reducing adversarial parental separation is accumulating. In a longitudinal randomized control trial, Emery and colleagues (2001) found that mediation kept most couples out of court (i.e., 80% of mediation couples stayed out of court versus 25% of a traditional litigation group). Moreover, follow-up two years later showed that children whose parents were involved in mediation reported more contact with the non-resident parent. Also, the custodial parent positively evaluated the non-resident parent's behavior in caring for the children and managing shared custody. These findings suggest that mediation was beneficial in promoting cooperation between the parents during and after separation.

Non-Resident Father Involvement

Previously, we saw that the frequency of parental divorce is steadily increasing across Europe, Canada, and the United States. Hence, there are an increasing number of fathers who live in different households than their children. Studies that have examined the significance of fathers' presence in the child's life have focused on three components: (1) economic support provided by the non-resident father, (2) the frequency of contact, and (3) the quality of the father-child relationship.

Economic Support

Amato and Gilbreth's (1999) meta-analysis indicated that children's adaptive outcomes were related to non-resident fathers' payment of child support. The effect sizes, although variable, remained strong across the various decades. Others have documented comparable findings (e.g., see King, 1994a, 1994b; McLanahan & Sandefur, 1994) with some tentative evidence suggesting that, relative to other forms of financial support, the non-resident fathers' economic support may be the source of income most strongly related to child well-being (Seltzer & Bianchi, 1988). Some have also suggested that paying child support may be a marker for the presence of a good quality father-child relationship hence resulting in more involvement and support (e.g., see Pryor & Rodgers, 2001).

Frequency of Contact and Quality of Father-Child Relationship

Studies that have examined the relationship between fathers' frequency of contact and children's well-being have noted inconsistent findings, with some showing positive associations (e.g., see Dunn, Cheng, O'Connor, & Bridges, 2004), while others find weak or no relationships (King, 1994a).

In fact, the effect sizes for frequency of father contact on children's well-being are small (Amato & Gilbreth, 1999).

Relationship quality is an important aspect of this association. Better quality non-custodial father-child relationships are associated with better child outcomes (Lamb, 1999) across multiple dimensions (Amato & Gilbreth, 1999). These studies do not have a design that can inform the direction of causality between fathers' involvement and children's well-being. That is, does lack of father involvement lead to poor child well-being (father effect on child), or do fathers of children who are better adjusted find it easier and more rewarding to remain involved in their children's lives (child effect on father)? Hawkins, Amato, and King (2007) compared two cross-lagged models to differentiate between child effects on fathers and father effects on children. Evidence for the child effects perspective was found. Adolescents' externalizing and internalizing behavior at Wave 1 was significantly associated with fathers' behavior at Wave 2. None of the cross-lagged paths for fathering measures at Wave 1 were associated with adolescents' well-being at Wave 2. These findings indicate that over time children's problematic behavior may result in fathers' absence. Hence, programs geared to maintaining high levels of post-divorce father involvement may need to consider ways in which fathers can be helped to respond to difficult child behavior such that the relationship is not undermined.

Length of Time Spent in a Family Structure, the Number of Transitions, and the Timing of Family Change

In the previous section we saw that non-nuclear family structure is associated with family components that increase children's risk of psychopathology. Longer duration of time spent in a non-nuclear family structure may result in prolonged exposure to these risks. Previously we also saw that children's living arrangements have become more diverse and complex. These changes have resulted in children experiencing more transitions and instability in family organization. For example, a child may be born to a single, never-married mother, who then marries and subsequently divorces. Stress theory suggests that changes in the family structure may cause stress in children's lives due to the need to readapt to modification in family dynamics and roles (Hill et al., 2001). Hence, the number of transitions may be more consequential to children than family structure per se. Last, the child's life stage at the time that a family transition occurs has been proposed as an additional influence on children's well being. Two views have been suggested; one, that younger children may be more sensitive to family transition due to their limited cognitive resources, dependency on parents, and lack of external support systems (Hetherington, Camara, & Featherman, 1983), and two, for those families that adapt well to family change, children that experience the family transition early in development might be able to initiate the recovery process sooner than children who experience the change later in life (Garmezy, 1983; Heard, 2007).

Heard (2007) found that the length of time spent in a cohabiting home predicted children's school behavior. Each year that children lived in a co-habiting mother–step-father family type the odds of expulsion/suspension in the following year increased by 12%. The duration effect remained statistically significant even after controlling for the effect of previous step-father transitions. Therefore, the effects of cohabiting family structure were distinct from those of previous step-father change (Heard, 2007).

Furthermore, Heard (2007) found that after controlling for child, parental, and family characteristics (e.g., cognitive ability, education, etc.) a greater number of early mother transitions (prior to age 6) increased adolescents' odds of school suspension/expulsion by 70% compared to later mother transitions (after age 7) or early father transitions. In contrast, father changes increased the odds of school discipline problems (by 10%) only if they occurred later in development (after age 7). The author proposes several reasons for the conditional relationship between timing of parent change and parent gender. In early childhood mothers' involvement may be more significant as they provide daily structure and order (i.e., school readiness, supervision with homework). Early mother transitions may disrupt these routines. The influence of fathers may become pronounced later in childhood when children have grown older and refer to role models for appropriate decision making (e.g., selection of romantic partners (Parke, 1996)).

Sibling Relationships

It is also important to consider the roles played by siblings in diverse family types. This is an area that has been very under-studied. The degree of biological relationship shared by a sibling dyad explains the degree of affection and antagonism in their relationship. Unrelated siblings are less close and affectionate with one another than full siblings (Jenkins et al., submitted). They are also less negative and rivalrous when compared to full siblings (Jenkins, Dunn, et al., 2005). This pattern is also evident in step-parents; they show lower levels of negativity and positivity towards their children when compared with biological parents (Hetherington 1999). Given that sibling relationship quality has been found to be important for children's mental health and that relationship quality differs in families in which all children are not full siblings, it will be important to consider the role that sibling relationship quality plays in mediating the association between family type and children's well-being in future studies.

AUGMENTATION OF RISK AND PROTECTIVE FACTORS

An important finding that has come out of risk research is that risks do not operate in isolation. This finding relates to the study of family structure and children's outcomes given that, as noted above, environmental risks such as poverty and negative parent-child relationships occur more often in diverse family types than nuclear families. Also, as we reported previously, although these family components explain some of the relationship between family type and children's well-being, other processes are also operating. The combination of multiple risks and the role of protective factors in the lives of children who are raised in non-nuclear family structures are important for understanding the diversity of children's outcomes.

Augmentation of Risk

Factors that increase children's rate or level of disturbance are called risk factors. Risk research indicates that risks "cluster" such that experiencing a few risks increases the odds of exposure to further risk (Hobcraft, 2004). Children's rates of disturbance have been examined as a function of the number of risks present in their lives. Generally this is done by adding the number of risks to which a child is exposed to. For instance, a child born to teenage mother who suffers from severe depression would have a count of two risks. Rutter and colleagues (1975) found that the level of psychiatric disorder amongst children experiencing a single risk factor was the same as children experiencing no risks. Children experiencing two risks showed a fourfold increase in rates of disturbance, while children experiencing four risks showed a 20-fold increase in disturbance. Hence, risks potentiate one another or they multiply the detrimental effect on children's well-being. This means, however, that a reduction in one or two risk factors should also reduce the probability of disturbance, since the removal of one factor might reduce the potentiating effect of other factors. This kind of research is helpful in identifying groups of families that might be at increased risk for child disturbance and has direct implications for policy interventions in terms of where efforts and resources should be targeted so that children's exposure to multiple risks is reduced.

Cavanagh, Schiller, and Riegle-Crumb (2006) examined the association between number of family transitions and children's negative/disruptive behaviors with peers. The most problematic behaviors were seen when multiple family transitions occurred in *combination* with (a) single mother status, (b) moderate increases in maternal depression, and (c) low income-to-needs ratios. Hence, intervention efforts targeted at highly unstable families should pay particular attention to single mother families,

families with limited financial resources, and even moderate levels of maternal depression.

Protective Effects

A resiliency framework (Jenkins, 2008) provides an additional perspective on how multiple factors combine. From this perspective, positive aspects of children's lives are said to combine with risk factors thereby protecting children from the effects of the risk, and reducing the odds of child disturbance. This has been termed the "study of protective effects."

One type of protective factor, and the one that we concentrate on here, (see Luthar, 1993 for other types of protective effects) is associated with disturbance among children in high risk environments, but not children's well-being in low risk environments. This pattern of protective effect is assessed by examining the statistical interaction between a risk and a protective factor. If the interaction term is significant, this indicates that the effect of the protective factor is different across high and low levels of risk.

In the previous section we saw that children from single father families tend to fare worse on problem behaviors than their peers in other non-nuclear family organizations. Cookston (1999) examined the association between supervision levels, family structure, and adolescents' delinquency and substance abuse. Single fathers showed the *lowest* levels of supervision of their children, relative to single mothers and two-parent families. The effect of monitoring on children's behavior varied as a function of the child's gender. For girls, lower levels of problem behaviors were similarly related to moderate and high levels of supervision. For males, however, only high levels of supervision were associated with lower problematic behavior, while the relation with moderate supervision approximated that of low supervision. Since single father family structure is associated with higher delinquency and substance abuse for adolescents, these findings suggest that intervention and prevention efforts geared at single father families should emphasize fathers' active and high levels of monitoring of their adolescent children.

CONCLUSIONS

Children showing the lowest levels of mental health problems are those whose parents are married (same or opposite sex) and remain together through the course of their childhood. Cohabiting, single, step, and blended family status have all been found to be associated with decreased well-being in children. This is explained both by the biological and personality characteristics of the parents that predate the family structure, as well as the child's experience of living in the family structure (e.g., the quality of the child's relationships with custodial and non-custodial parents, and the economics of the family). The way in which risk and protective factors combine, and operate contingently, is also an important component in understanding adjustment differences between children. As diversity in family types is becoming more common, it is important to expand research work in this area. Future studies would benefit from the inclusion of multiple siblings per family with an investigation of the role of the sibling relationship in explaining children's outcomes in diverse family types. Most of the studies in this area have relied on survey methodology. Finally, it will be of value to include high quality observational and longitudinal data that allow the examination of the reciprocal influences of parents, children, and siblings in diverse family structures.

Acknowledgments

The authors are grateful to Aarti Kumar for her contribution to this chapter.

REFERENCES

Amato, P. R. (1986). Marital conflict, the parent-child relationship and child self-esteem. *Family Relations, 35*(3), 403-410.

Amato, P. R. (2000). The consequences of divorce for adults and children. *Journal of Marriage & the Family, 62*(4), 1269-1287.

Amato, P. R. (2001). Children of divorce in the 1990's: An update of the Amato and Keith (1991) meta-analysis. *Journal of Family Psychology, 15*(3), 355-370.

Amato, P. R., & Gilbreth, J. G. (1999). Nonresident fathers and children's well-being: A meta-analysis. *Journal of Marriage & the Family, 61*(3), 557-573.

Amato, P. R., & Keith, B. (1991). Parental divorce and the well-being of children: A meta-analysis. *Psychological Bulletin, 110*(1), 26-46.

Amato, P. R., Loomis, L. S., & Booth, A. (1995). Parental divorce, marital conflict, and offspring well-being during early adulthood. *Social Forces, 73*(3), 895-915.

Amato, P. R., & Rivera, F. (1999). Parental involvement and children's behavior problems. *Journal of Marriage and the Family, 61*(2), 375-384.

Apel, R., & Kaukinen, C. (2008). On the relationship between family structure and antisocial behavior: Parental cohabitation and blended households. *Criminology, 46*(1), 35-70.

Aseltine, R. H., Jr. (1996). Pathways linking parental divorce with adolescent depression. *Journal of Health and Social Behavior, 37*(2), 133-148.

Astone, N. M., & McLanahan, S. S. (1991). Family structure, parental practices and high school completion. *American Sociological Review, 56*(3), 309-320.

Baron, R. M., & Kenny, D. A. (1986). The moderator-mediator variable distinction in social psychological research: Conceptual, strategic, and statistical considerations. *Journal of Personality and Social Psychology, 51*(6), 1173-1182.

Bos, H. M. W., van Balen, F., & van den Boom, D. C. (2007). Child adjustment and parenting in planned lesbian-parent families. *American Journal of Orthopsychiatry, 77*(1), 38-48.

Breivik, K., & Olweus, D. (2006). Adolescents' adjustment in four post-divorce family structures: Single mother, stepfather, joint physical custody and single father families. *Journal of Divorce & Remarriage, 44*(3/4), 99-124.

Brown, S. L. (2000). The effect of union type on psychological well-being: Depression among cohabitors versus marrieds. *Journal of Health and Social Behavior, 41*(3), 241-255.

Brown, S. L. (2002). *Child well-being in cohabiting families.* In A. Booth & A. C. Crouter (Eds.), *Just living together: Implications of cohabitation for children, families and social policy* (pp. 173-187). Mahwah, NJ: Lawrence Erlbaum Associates Publishers.

Brown, S. L. (2004). Family structure and child well-being: The significance of parental cohabitation. *Journal of Marriage and Family, 66*(2), 351-367.

Buchanan, C. M., Maccoby, E. E., & Dornbusch, S. M. (1996). *Adolescents after divorce.* Cambridge, MA: Harvard University Press.

Camara, K. A., Resnick, G., Hetherington, E. M., & Arasteh, J. D. (1988). Interparental conflict and cooperation: Factors moderating children's post-divorce adjustment. In E. M. Hetherington and J. D. Arasteh (Eds.), *Impact of divorce, single parenting, and step-parenting on children.* (pp. 169-195). Hillsdale, NJ: Lawrence Erlbaum Associates, Inc.

Cavanagh, S. E., Schiller, K. S., & Riegle-Crumb, C. (2006). Marital transitions, parenting, and schooling: Exploring the link between family-structure history and adolescents' academic status. *Sociology of Education, 79*(4), 329-354.

Champion, L. A., Goodall, G., & Rutter, M. (1995). Behaviour problems in childhood and stressors in early adult life: I. A 20 year follow-up of London school children. *Psychological Medicine, 25*(2), 231-246.

Cherlin, A. J., Furstenberg, F. F., Chase-Lansdale, P. L., & Kiernan, K. E. (1991). Longitudinal studies of effects of divorce on children in Great Britain and the United States. *Science, 252*(5011), 1386-1389.

Clarke-Stewart, K. A., & Hayward, C. (1996). Advantages of father custody and contact for the psychological well-being of school-age children. *Journal of Applied Developmental Psychology, 17*(2), 239-270.

Conger, R. D., & Donnellan, M. B. (2007). An interactionist perspective on the socioeconomic context of human development. *Annual Review of Psychology, 58,* 175-199.

Cookston, J. T. (1999). Parental supervision and family structure: Effects on adolescent problem behaviors. *Journal of Divorce & Remarriage, 32*(1-2), 107-122.

D'Onofrio, B. M., Turkheimer, E. N., Eaves, L. J., Corey, L. A., Berg, K., Solaas, M. H., et al. (2003). The role of the Children of Twins design in elucidating causal relations between parent characteristics and child outcomes. *Journal of Child Psychology and Psychiatry, 44*(8), 1130-1144.

Demo, D. H., & Acock, A. C. (1996). Singlehood, marriage, and remarriage: The effects of family structure and family relationships on mothers' well-being. *Journal of Family Issues, 17*(3), 388-407.

Demography Division, Statistics Canada. (2007). *Family portrait: Continuity and change in Canadian families and households in 2006*. (Statistics Canada – Catalogue no. 97-553). Ottawa, ON: Statistics Canada.

Demuth, S., & Brown, S. L. (2004). Family structure, family processes, and adolescent delinquency: The significance of parental absence versus parental gender. *Journal of Research in Crime and Delinquency, 41*(1), 58-81.

De Robertis, M.T., & Litrownik, A. J. (2004). The experience of foster care: Relationship between foster parent disciplinary approaches and aggression in a sample of young foster children. *Child Maltreatment, 1*, 92-102.

Dodge, K. A., Bates, J. E., & Pettit, G. S. (1990). Mechanisms in the cycle of violence. *Science, 250*(4988), 1678-1683.

Dozier, M., Manni, M., Gordon, M. K., Peloso, E., Gunnar, M. R., Stovall-McClough, K. C., et al. (2006). Foster children's diurnal production of cortisol: An exploratory study. *Child Maltreatment, 11*(2), 189-197.

Dunn, J., Cheng, H., O'Connor, T. G., & Bridges, L. (2004). Children's perspectives on their relationships with their nonresident fathers: Influences, outcomes and implications. *Journal of Child Psychology and Psychiatry and Allied Disciplines, 45*(3), 553-566.

Dunn, J., Deater-Deckard, K., Pickering, K., O'Connor, T. G., & Golding, J. (1998). Children's adjustment and prosocial behaviour in step-, single-parent, and non-stepfamily settings: Findings from a community study. *Journal of Child Psychology and Psychiatry, 39*(8), 1083-1095.

Emery, R. E. (1999). *Marriage, divorce, and children's adjustment* (2nd ed.). Thousand Oaks, CA: Sage Publications, Inc.

Emery, R. E., Laumann-Billings, L., Waldron, M. C., Sbarra, D. A., & Dillon, P. (2001). Child custody mediation and litigation: Custody, contact, and co-parenting 12 years after initial dispute resolution. *Journal of Consulting and Clinical Psychology, 69*(2), 323-332.

European Foundation for the Improvement of Living and Working Conditions. (2007). *Monitoring quality of life in Europe: Divorce rate*. Retrieved May 10, 2009, from http://www.eurofound.europa.eu/areas/qualityoflife/eurlife/index.php?template=3&radioindic=54&idDomain=5.

Flaks, D. K., Ficher, I., Masterpasqua, F., & Joseph, G. (1995). Lesbians choosing motherhood: A comparative study of lesbian and heterosexual parents and their children. *Developmental Psychology, 31*(1), 105-114.

Foley, D. L., Pickles, A., Rutter, M., Gardner, C. O., Maes, H. H., Silberg, J. L., et al. (2004). Risks for conduct disorder symptoms associated with parental alcoholism in stepfather families versus intact families from a community sample. *Journal of Child Psychology and Psychiatry, 45*(4), 687-696.

Frick, P. J., & Loney, B. R. (2002). Understanding the association between parent and child antisocial behavior. In R. J. McMahon & R. D. Peters (Eds.), *The effects of parental dysfunction on children* (pp. 105-126). New York: Kluwer Academic/Plenum Publishers.

Garmezy, N. (1983). Stressors of childhood. In N. Garmezy & M. Rutter (Eds.), *Stress, coping, and development in children* (pp. 43–84). New York: McGraw-Hill.

Ginther, D. K., & Pollak, R. A. (2004). Family structure and children's educational outcomes: Blended families, stylized facts, and descriptive regressions. *Demography, 41*(4), 671-697.

Golombok, S., Perry, B., Burston, A., Murray, C., Mooney-Somers, J., Stevens, M., et al. (2003). Children with lesbian parents: A community study. *Developmental Psychology, 39*(11), 20-33.

Hanson, T. L., McLanahan, S. S., & Thomson, E. (1996). Double jeopardy: Parental conflict and stepfamily outcomes for children. *Journal of Marriage & the Family, 58*(1), 141-154.

Hanson, T. L., McLanahan, S., & Thomson, E. (1997). Economic resources, parental practices, and children's well-being. In G. J. Duncan & J Brooks-Gunn (Eds.), *Consequences of growing up poor* (pp. 190-238). New York: Russell Sage Foundation.

Hao, L., & Xie, G. (2002). The complexity and endogeneity of family structure in explaining children's misbehavior. *Social Science Research, 31*(1), 1-28.

Hawkins, D. N., Amato, P. R., & King, V. (2007). Nonresident father involvement and adolescent well-being: Father effects or child effects? *American Sociological Review, 72*(6), 990-1010.

Heard, H. E. (2007). Fathers, mothers, and family structure: Family trajectories, parent gender, and adolescent schooling. *Journal of Marriage and Family, 69(2),* 435-450.

Heath, A. C., Kendler, K. S., Eaves, L. J., & Markell, D. (1985). The resolution of cultural and biological inheritance: Informativeness of different relationships. *Behavior Genetics, 15*(5), 439-465.

Hetherington, E. M. (1999). Should we stay together for the sake of the children? In E. M. Hetherington (Ed.), *Coping with divorce, single parenting, and remarriage: A risk and resiliency perspective.* Mahway, NJ: Earlbaum Press.

Hetherington, E. M., Camara, K. A., & Featherman, D. L. (1983). Achievement and intellectual functioning of children in one-parent households. In J. T. Spence (Ed.), *Achievement and achievement motives: Psychological and sociological approaches* (pp. 205–284). San Francisco: W. H. Freeman.

Hetherington, E. M., & Clingempeel, W. G. (1992). Coping with marital transitions: A family systems perspective. *Monographs of the Society for Research in Child Development, 57*(2-3), 1-242.

Hetherington, E. M., & Kelly, J. (2002). *For better or for worse: Divorce reconsidered.* New York: W W Norton & Co.

Hetherington, E. M., & Stanley-Hagan, M. (1999). The adjustment of children with divorced parents: A risk and resiliency perspective. *Journal of Child Psychology and Psychiatry, 40*(1), 129-140.

Hill, J., Pickles, A., Burnside, E., Byatt, M., Rollinson, L., Davis, R., et al. (2001). Child sexual abuse, poor parental care and adult depression: Evidence for different mechanisms. *British Journal of Psychiatry, 179*, 104-109.

Hobcraft, J. (2004). Parental, childhood, and early adult legacies in the emergence of adult social exclusion: Evidence on what matters from a British cohort. In P. L. Chase-Lansdale, K. Kiernan, & R. J. Friedman (Eds.), *Human development across lives and generations: The potential for change* (pp. 63-92). New York: Cambridge University Press.

Hofferth, S. L. (2007). Improving data collection on fathers: Comments on methods and measurement papers, National Fatherhood Forum. *Applied Developmental Science, 11*(4), 247-248.

Hoffman, D. A. (2006). The future of ADR practice: Three hopes, three fears, and three predictions. *Negotiation Journal, 22*(4), 467-473.

Hoffman, J. P. (2006). Family structure, community context, and adolescent problem behaviors. *Journal of Youth and Adolescence, 35*(6), 867-880.

Holtan, A., Ronning, J. A., Handegård, B. H., & Sourander, A. (2005). A comparison of mental health problems in kinship and nonkinship foster care. *European Child & Adolescent Psychiatry, 14*(4), 200-207.

Jablonska, B., & Lindberg, L. (Writer) (2007). Risk behaviours, victimisation and mental distress among adolescents in different family structures. *Social Psychiatry and Psychiatric Epidemiology, 42*(8), 656-663.

Jenkins, J. M. (2008). Psychosocial adversity and resilience. In M. Rutter, D. Bishop, D. Pine, S. Scott, J. Stevenson, E. A. Taylor, & A. Thapar (Eds.) *Rutter's handbook of child and adolescent psychiatry* (pp. 377-391). Oxford, UK: Blackwell.

Jenkins, J. M., Dunn, J., O'Connor, T. G., Rasbash, J., & Behnke, P. (2005). Change in maternal perception of sibling negativity: Within- and between-family influences. *Journal of Family Psychology, 19*, 533-541.

Jenkins, J. M., Rasbash, J., Gass, K, & Dunn, J. (Submitted). The multilevel dynamics of sibling relationships: Influences over time.

Jenkins, J. M., Simpson, A., Dunn, J., Rasbash, J., & O'Conner, T. G. (2005). The mutual influence of marital conflict and children's behavior problems: Shared and non-shared family risks. *Child Development, 76*, 24-39.

Jocklin, V., McGue, M., & Lykken, D. T. (1996). Personality and divorce: A genetic analysis. *Journal of Personality and Social Psychology, 71*(2), 288-299.

Johnson, J. G., Cohen, P., Kasen, S., Smailes, E., & Brook, J. S. (2001). Association of maladaptive parental behavior with psychiatric disorder among parents and their offspring. *Archives of General Psychiatry, 58*(5), 453-460.

Johnston, J. R., Gonzǎlez, R., & Campbell, L. E. (1987). Ongoing postdivorce conflict and child disturbance. *Journal of Abnormal Child Psychology, 15*(4), 493-509.

Johnston, J. R., Kline, M., & Tschann, J. M. (1989). Ongoing post-divorce conflict: Effects on children of joint custody and frequent access. *American Journal of Orthopsychiatry, 59*(4), 576-592.

Juby, H., & Farrington, D. P. (2001). Disentangling the link between disrupted families and delinquency. *British Journal of Criminology, 41*(1), 22-40.

Keil, V., & Price, J. M. (2006). Externalizing behavior disorders in child welfare settings: Definition, prevalence, and implications for assessment and treatment. *Children and Youth Services Review, 28*(7), 761-779.

Keller, T. E., Wetherbee, K., LeProhn, N. S., Payne, V., Sim, K., & Lamont, E. R. (2001). Competencies and problem behaviors of children in family foster care: Variations by kinship placement status and race. *Children and Youth Services Review, 23*(12), 915-940.

King, V. (1994a). Nonresident father involvement and child well-being: Can dads make a difference? *Journal of Family Issues, 15*(1), 78-96.

King, V. (1994b). Variation in the consequences of nonresident father involvement for children's well-being. *Journal of Marriage and Family, 56*(4), 963-972.

Lamb, M. E. (1999). Noncustodial fathers and their impact on the children of divorce. In R. A. Thompson & P. R. Amato (Eds.), *The post-divorce family: Children, parenting, and society* (pp. 105-125). Thousand Oaks, CA: Sage Publications.

Lawrence, C. R., Carlson, E. A., & Egeland, B. (2006). The impact of foster care on development. *Development and Psychopathology, 18*(1), 57-76.

Lewis, E. E., Dozier, M., Ackerman, J., & Sepulveda-Kozakowski, S. (2007). The effect of placement instability on adopted children's inhibitory control abilities and oppositional behavior. *Developmental Psychology, 43*(6), 1415-1427.

Long, N., Slater, E., Forehand, R., & Fauber, R. (1988). Continued high or reduced interparental conflict following divorce: Relation to young adolescent adjustment. *Journal of Consulting and Clinical Psychology, 56*(3), 467-469.

Luthar, S. S. (1993). Annotation: Methodological and conceptual issues in research on childhood resilience. *Journal of Child Psychology and Psychiatry, 34*, 441-453.

Manning, W. D., & Lamb, K. A. (2003). Adolescent well-being in cohabiting, married, and single-parent families. *Journal of Marriage and Family, 65*(4), 876-893.

Manning, W. D., & Lichter, D. T. (1996). Parental cohabitation and children's economic well-being. *Journal of Marriage and Family, 58*(4), 998-1010.

Martinez, C. R., Jr., & Forgatch, M. S. (2002). Adjusting to change: Linking family structure transitions with parenting and boys' adjustment, *Journal of Family Psychology, 16*(2), 107-117.

McGue, M., & Lykken, D. T. (1992). Genetic influence on risk of divorce. *Psychological Science, 3*(6), 368.

McLanahan, S., & Sandefur, G. (1994). *Growing up with a single parent. What hurts, what helps.* Cambridge, MA: Harvard University press.

Naevdal, F., & Thuen, F. (2004). Residence arrangements and well-being: A study of Norwegian adolescents. *Scandinavian Journal of Psychology, 45*(5), 363-371.

O'Connor, T. G., Dunn, J., Jenkins, J. M., Pickering, K., & Rasbash, J. (2001). Family settings and children's adjustment: Differential adjustment within and across families. *British Journal of Psychiatry, 179*, 110-115.

Parke, R. D. (1996). *Fatherhood.* Cambridge, MA: Harvard University Press.

Popenoe, D., & Whitehead, B.D. (2009). *The state of our unions 2008: The social health of marriage in America.* Piscataway, NJ: The National Marriage Project at Rutgers University.

Pryor, J., & Rodgers, B. (2001). *Children in changing families: Life after parental separation.* Malden, MA: Blackwell Publishing.

Ram, B., & Hou, F. (2003). Changes in family structure and child outcomes: Roles of economic and familial resources. *Policy Studies Journal, 31*(3), 309-330.

Rutter, M., Cox, A., Templing, C., et al. (1975). Attainment and adjustment in two geographical areas. 1. The prevalence of psychiatric disorders. *British Journal of Psychiatry, 126*, 493-509.

Sampson, P. D., Kerr, B., Olson, H. C., Streissguth, A. P., Hunt, E., Barr, H. M., et al. (1997). The effects of prenatal alcohol exposure on adolescent cognitive processing: A speed-accuracy tradeoff. *Intelligence, 24*(2), 329-353.

Seltzer, J. A., & Bianchi, S. M. (1988). Children's contact with absent parents. *Journal of Marriage and Family, 50*(3), 663-677.

Simmons, T., & O'Connell, M. (2003). *Married couple and unmarried-partner households: 2000.* Washington, DC: United States Bureau of the Census.

Simons, R. L. (1996). *Understanding differences between divorced and intact families: Stress, interaction, and child outcome.* Thousand Oaks, CA: Sage Publications.

Smith, G. C., & Palmieri, P. A. (2007). Risk of psychological difficulties among children raised by custodial grandparents. *Psychiatric Services, 58*, 1303-1310.

Smith, G. C., Palmieri, P. A., Hancock, G. R., & Richardson, R. A. (2008). Custodial grandmothers' psychological distress, dysfunctional parenting, and grandchildren's adjustment. *The International Journal of Aging and Human Development, 67(4)*, 327-357.

Solomon, J. C., & Marx, J. (1995). "To grandmother's house we go": Health and school adjustment of children raised solely by grandparents. *The Gerontologist, 35(3)*, 386-394.

Sun, Y. (2003). The well-being of adolescents in households with no biological parents. *Journal of Marriage and Family, 65(4)*, 894-909.

Tarren-Sweeney, M., & Hazell, P. (2006). Mental health of children in foster and kinship care in New South Wales, Australia. *Journal of Paediatrics and Child Health, 42(3)*, 89-97.

Telingator, C. J., & Patterson, C. (2008). Children and adolescents of lesbian and gay parents. *Journal of the American Academy of Child & Adolescent Psychiatry, 47(12)*, 1364-1368.

Thomson, E., Hanson, T. L., & McLanahan, S. S. (1994). Family structure and child well-being: Economic resources vs. parental behaviors. *Social Forces, 73(1)*, 221-242.

Tripp De Robertis, M., & Litrownik, A. J. (2004). The experience of foster care: Relationship between foster parent disciplinary approaches and aggression in a sample of young foster children. *Child Maltreatment, 9(1)*, 92-102.

U.S. Census Bureau. (2007). *Current population survey: 2007 annual social and economic supplement.* Washington, DC: U.S. Government Printing Office.

Videon, T. M. (2002). The effects of parent-adolescent relationships and parental separation on adolescent well-being. *Journal of Marriage and Family, 64(2)*, 489-503.

Wells, L. E., & Rankin, J. H. (1991). Families and delinquency: A meta-analysis of the impact of broken homes. *Social Problems, 38(1)*, 71-93.

Wood, J. J., Repetti, R. L., & Roesch, S. C. (2004). Divorce and children's adjustment problems at home and school: The role of depressive/withdrawn parenting. *Child Psychiatry & Human Development, 35(2)*, 121-142.

3

One-Child Policy and Child Mental Health

Yi Zheng

INTRODUCTION OF THE ONE-CHILD POLICY

China is a developing country holding almost a quarter of the world's total population; a country with the world's biggest population puts a strain on scarce land, water, and energy resources. We could imagine, in such a country, population would be a constant challenge to coordinated and sustainable development; indeed it is. And it has been one of the most critical factors influencing the overall economic and social development of China. The huge ever growing population will not only be a burden to economic development and the prosperity of the country but it will also raise social problems and have a disastrous effect on the limited natural resources and an already delicate environment.

Between 1949 and 1970, improvements in quality of life and better access to health care led to a remarkable population boom in China. Within three decades the birthrate rose from 33 per thousand to 38 per thousand while mortality dropped from 18 per thousand to 8 per thousand. Consequently, the population increased from 500 million in 1947 to 800 million in 1970, coming close to 1 billion by the end of 1980. According to predictions, if the birthrate remained at the 1978 level of 2.3 per woman, the population will reach 2.1 billion by 2080. The disastrous aftermath of "The Great Leap Forward" and the great famine of 1958-1961 made it evident that economic development and natural resources could not sustain such population growth. It was in the hope of striking a balance between population and economy, society, natural resources, and environment that enforced rules to restrict family size were introduced in the

49

1970s and the One-Child Policy (also known as the Family Plan Policy) was launched in 1979.

Control of fertility was voluntary in China until 1970 when the Chinese government began limiting each couple to a maximum of two children. During the Cultural Revolution (1966-1976) this policy was loosely enforced in many areas. The government promulgated the One-Child Policy in 1978, after Deng Xiaoping's rise to power. Since then, the policy has been more strictly enforced. These regulations include restrictions on family size, late marriage and childbearing, and the spacing of children (in cases in which second children are permitted). The State Family Planning Bureau sets the overall targets and policy direction. Family planning committees at provincial and county levels devise local strategies for implementation.

The integrated policy on population and development implemented holistic reform, and the introduction of policies and a family planning program since the 1970s has resulted in China's historic transcendence from poverty to basic subsistence and now to a well-off society in the general sense. This is an historic transition in China's population reproduction pattern, and created two miracles in China: rapid economic development and overall human development. The accomplishments China has achieved in its population and family planning program have mitigated population pressure on resources and the environment, promoted economic development and social progress, and contributed significantly to stabilization of the world population (Bing 2009).

Before the One-Child Policy China had always had a large family culture with families of multiple generations and many members living together. In the year 1949, China had about 400-500 million people. Guided by the theory of "the more people, the stronger we are," people were encouraged to have as many children as they could. In the following 30 years it was regarded the greatest honor to have many children in one's family, which was also in accordance with traditional Chinese family values. However, by the time of Deng Xiaoping's tenure the government started to focus more on developing the economy instead of the population. At that time, China was already way ahead of what would have been an affordable population—with about 1 billion inhabitants. So birth control and slowing down population growth were urgently called for; and it was under these circumstances that the One-Child Policy was introduced.

From there on, China's giant social engineering project has drawn worldwide attention. Described by some as the "boldest experiment in population control in the history of the world," China's One-Child Policy remains a widely debated topic 30 years after its inception. The policy has engendered wide concern and discussion because of its far-reaching political, economic, social, and cultural implications. Others have expressed concerns that this policy would result in generations of Chinese singletons who would become "little emperors" after growing up with high doses of parental attention and indulgence not experienced by previous generations (Greenhalgh 2008).

MAIN ACHIEVEMENTS OF THE ONE-CHILD POLICY PROGRAM IN CHINA

China is the most populous developing country in the world. According to the *Statistical Bulletin of the People's Republic of China* at the end of 2008 China had a population of over 1 billion, and the vast territories of 9.6 million square kilometers were inhabited by 56 nationality groups (National Bureau of Statistics 2009).

China's population makes up 21% of the world's total, but its arable land is only 7% of the world's total. This very fact means there is a severe conflict between the country's huge population base, and the growth momentum that comes with it, and socioeconomic development, utilization of natural resources, and environmental protection. The family planning program has brought the excessive growth of population under control, promoting coordinated development between population and economy, society, environment, and resources. At the same time, it has also improved people's standard of living, ensuring them better living and working conditions, and provided more chance of education and better health care for the children (Hesketh, Lu, & Xing 2005; National Poulation and Family Planning Commission 2006; Zheng et al. 2004).

Curbing Excessive Population Growth and Maintaining a Low and Stable Fertility Rate

With an underdeveloped economy, China has succeeded in controlling excessive population growth and achieved an historic change from a reproductive pattern of a high birth rate, low mortality rate, and high natural increase rate to one of a low birth rate, low mortality rate, and low natural increase rate. The average life expectancy has risen from 68 years at the end of the 1970s to 73 years at present, the infant and under-5-years mortality rate have reduced to 14.9 per thousand and 24 per thousand respectively, and maternal mortality rates to 34.2 per 100,000.

When the One-Child Policy was introduced, the government set a target population of 1.2 billion by the year 2000. The census of 2000 put the population at 1.27 billion. "Because China has worked hard over the last 30 years, we have 400 million fewer people," said Zhang Weiqing, minister in charge of the National Population and Family Planning Commission, earlier in 2008. According to official statistics, the One-Child Policy has helped prevent 400 million births—about the size of the U.S. and Mexican populations combined—and aided China's rapid economic development.

The total fertility rate, which is defined as the mean number of children born per woman, decreased from 2.9 in 1979 to 1.7 in 2004, with a rate of 1.3 in urban areas and just under 2.0 in rural areas. This trend has created a distinct demographic pattern of urban families with predominantly one child and rural families with predominantly two children.

REINFORCING SERVICES AND GUIDANCE AND IMPROVING REPRODUCTIVE HEALTH LEVEL

The key to the family planning program is upgrading people's reproductive health level by providing safe, effective, high quality, and appropriate services and disseminating knowledge. After years of effort, both the maternal mortality rate and infant mortality rate have been reduced significantly and the average life expectancy has increased.

In China, contraceptive drugs, devices, and family planning surgical operations are provided free to people of childbearing age. Family planning services stress contraception, informed choice, and counseling and guidance so that clients can make an informed choice of contraceptive method on their own; induced abortion is not used as an officially endorsed means of family planning. The Population and Family Planning Law explicitly states that non-medically necessary sex identification of fetus and selective abortions are prohibited.

China boasts a five-tier family planning network at national, provincial, prefectural, county, and township levels. By 2003, the national population and family service network covered all urban and rural areas with over 2500 county level technical service units, 140,000 technical service staff, and nearly 1 million grassroots service providers and volunteers. Additionally, the national population and family planning network is supplemented by 3200 maternal and child health (MCH) hospitals provided by the Ministry of Health, with about 500,000 MCH workers. The service network covering both urban and rural areas provides services such as health counseling for women of all ages, prevention and treatment of gynecological disease, diagnosis and treatment of infertility, and education on STDs/AIDS prevention.

In order to provide better services to people living in the poor and remote areas, the central government allocated 480 million RMB Yuan and local governments allocated 120 million RMB Yuan to make mobile service vans available for 2,404 counties. These vans are equipped with instruments for treating gynecological diseases, breast scanners, gynecological examination tables, and other facilities for first aid as well as sterilizers and power generators. Initiation of this activity has helped alleviate the inherent difficulties in delivering services to people in remote areas and has been well received by the locals.

DEVELOPING HUMAN RESOURCES, STRENGTHENING CAPACITY BUILDING, AND IMPROVING SERVICE NETWORKS

In the process of advocating family planning and promoting reproductive health an effective operational network that serves the needs of people at the grassroots level has been formed. In the past decade, over 100 universities and colleges all over the country started undergraduate courses on population and family planning and over ten universities including Beijing University, the People's University of China, and the Harbin Medical University started to offer master's and doctorate courses on subjects related to population and family planning. As a result, large numbers of highly qualified professionals have been trained for the family planning program. Service providers at grassroots levels must attend standardized training, pass examinations, and have their qualifications verified before they are allowed to provide services. The education structure for family planning workers has undergone great change. The proportion of family planning workers with college and higher education increased from 14.1% in 1995 to 30.7% in 2003. Compared to 1995, family planning workers have now become younger, better educated, and more professional.

Demography and family-planning-related medical research has witnessed great development and experts and researchers are playing important roles in the population and family planning policy-making and implementation process. The two Expert Committees of the State Family Planning Commission hold cross-disciplinary discussion meetings and workshops on a regular and frequent basis. Expert databanks have also been set up at various local levels. There are 27 family planning scientific research institutes in the country that are devoted to basic research on reproductive health and contraception and development of safe, effective, and easy-to-use contraceptive drugs, devices, and methods.

Improving the Quality of the Population, Reinforcing Nationwide Primary Education

China has increased the average per capita education attainment of the population aged 15 and above from 4.5 years to 8.5 years in 2007, and achieved 99.3% coverage nationwide with regard to universal access to the nine years of compulsory education. The rural poor population has been reduced from 250 million to 40.1 million, which helped accelerate the global poverty alleviation process. China's rank on the Human Development Index (HDI) rose from no. 105 in 1990 to no. 81 in 2007.

Children in China, especially those living in rural areas, have more access to education due to the nation's implementation of the family planning policy. Statistics from the educational authority of Henan, the province with the largest population in the country, shows that the number of school-age children has been decreasing since 1996. The number of primary school students in the province is expected to drop from 11.3 million in 2000 to 8.3 million in 2005. In the past, 70 to 80 students packed into one classroom was not an uncommon sight in Henan.

Analysts have said that the dramatic cut in the number of newborns has made it possible for the nation to improve its educational services. According to the figures collected in the nation's fifth census, 85% of the province's population had received at least a primary level of schooling in 2000, 16% higher than in 1990. Nationwide, 85% of Chinese people had received the nine-year compulsory education by 2000, while some 99.1% of school-aged children were enrolled.

Implemented in the 1970s, the family planning policy, which advocates a one-child family, has effectively curbed the nation's rapid population growth. In the late 1990s, China began to witness a low birth rate, low mortality rate, and low population growth rate.

In rural China where the family planning policy was hard to implement because most farmers habitually wanted to have as many children as possible, changes are now taking place. Most farmers now prefer one well-educated child to many poorly educated children. The size of a family perhaps does not matter as much as the nation's future development hinges more upon science and technology.

Many children living in rural areas couldn't complete primary school when there were too many children in one family relying on support from their parents. But after 30 years of implementation of the One-Child Policy many rural families are now expecting their only child to receive a higher education instead of wanting to have more children. Many parents in rural China are also willing to invest more in their child's education, which is a great change compared to the past. Attitudes are shifting and this has also contributed to the improvement in educational status of Chinese children today.

As rural China's education service constantly improves and farmers' education awareness gets stronger, experts believe that more talented people will be cultivated and the prosperity of China is just around the corner.

CONTINUOUSLY EXPANDING INTERNATIONAL EXCHANGES AND COOPERATION

The issue of population and development is a global strategic concern and a common challenge confronted by all humankind. The situation of population and development in China has an important bearing on the stabilization of the world's population, enhancement of safety, peace, and development. Therefore, the Chinese government attaches great importance to international exchanges and cooperation, which greatly help China draw on the successful experiences of the international population and development programs to improve the family planning program of China. At the same time, it also promotes south-south collaboration between developing countries.

China takes an active part in international activities in the population and development area. China attended the Asia-Pacific Population and Development Conference in Bali, Indonesia, in 1992; the International Conference on Population and Development in Cairo, Egypt, in 1994; the UN special meeting on reviewing implementation of the ICPD Programme of Action in 1999; and the Asia-Pacific Population Conference in Bangkok, Thailand, in 2002, as well as a range of other international and regional conferences on population and development. China was involved in the drafting of documents at all those conferences. China also participated in the Fourth World Conference on Women. China has been consistently following the program of actions and principles set by these international conferences and has taken action to implement them.

In 1977 China became a member of the Partners in Population and Development (PPD) and plays an important role in it. In 2000, China successfully hosted the sixth annual board meeting, and in 2002 H.E. Mr. Weiqing Zhang, minister of NPFPC, was elected chairman of the PPD. In 2001 China officially joined the World Family Organization and has been actively involved in its activities. Today China serves as a member of its executive board and vice chair of the Asia-Pacific region.

The National Population and Family Planning Commission has conducted inter-governmental exchanges and cooperation with over 30 countries in the world and established cooperative relationships with 22 international governmental organizations, foundations, and non-governmental organizations. These wide-ranging cooperative programs involve reproductive health/family planning, mother and child health care, reproductive health for adolescents, emergency contraception, male participation, prevention and treatment of STDs/AIDS, women's development, and poverty alleviation. The PRC/UNFPA RH/FP project has created successful innovations in protecting civil rights, providing quality services, improving women's reproductive health, caring for adolescents' needs for reproductive health, promoting gender equality, preventing HIV/AIDS, and reducing maternal and infant mortality. These innovations are being expanded throughout the country. Collaboration with the World Health Organization (WHO) has helped China improve its family planning research network and the level of science and technology, and advance the reproductive health promotion program featuring QoC in family planning, reproductive tract infections (RTI) intervention, and birth defect intervention. The RH/FP quality of care project supported by the Ford Foundation has had a positive effect on promoting informed choice in contraceptive methods and the standardization of RTI prevention, diagnosis, and treatment; setting up and improving the management and evaluation system under the QoC system; exploring new working mechanisms and models for the circumstances of the emerging socialist market economic system; disseminating and advocating training for HIV/AIDS prevention; and encouraying change in social gender perspective and analysis. The Integrated Project, with the support of IPPF and in collaboration with the Japanese Organization for International Cooperation in Family Planning (JOICFP), has advocated thinking of ways to integrate FP (family planning) with health education and increase trust between FP staff and clients, and has helped change the ways of thinking and methods of working. Currently the project has been expanded to 42 counties across all 31 provinces including Tibet.

COMPREHENSIVELY ADDRESSING POPULATION ISSUES IN CHINA

The General Implementation Method of the Policy (Lin 2003; McLoughlin 2005)

Strategies for implementing the One-Child Policy at the local level are devised by birth-planning committees at provincial and county levels via a practical system of rewards and penalties, including financial incentives for compliance, and significant fines, confiscation of property, and dismissal from work for noncompliance.

It is important to note that enforcement of the single child policy is generally strict only among urban residents and government employees. In rural areas, where resistance to the policy is substantially higher, the policy is typically understood to mean "two children per couple" especially if the first child is female. A third child can be allowed among some ethnic minorities and in remote, under-populated areas. Because of the local implementation, there are wide regional variations in adherence to the policy. Exceptions are also made in certain circumstances, for example in families in which the first child dies or has a disability, or when both parents work in high risk occupations, or are themselves singletons.

While the government has emphasized conservation of resources, concerns for the environment, and the hazards of overpopulation in promoting the One-Child Policy, local officials who implement and enforce the policy have taken the Chinese approach of focusing on practical benefits. The message conveyed to the ordinary citizen is that having a single child is a way to improve their standard of living and is a quick path to modernization.

The coercive way in which the One-Child Policy is implemented has been criticized and questioned from the start. Women may be forced to make use of recommended contraception methods without choice. In recent years, with the opening up of Chinese society, globalization, and the growing migrating population, it has become harder to implement the One-Child Policy in the old-fashioned way, through economic incentives and penalties. New problems arise, for instance people who are well off are willing to "pay" for a second child. And it is harder for the family plan worker to track down migrating couples trying not to comply with the policy.

Amid the controversy, China continues to look ahead at ways of improving its population policies. The National Population and Family Planning Commission of China (NPFPC) is planning programs and advances in the quality of both social and reproductive health services. Already in many of China's provinces, the requirement to obtain prior government permission to have a child, known as birth permits, has been lifted. The NPFPC also has plans to study state population development and social support programs to help rural families practice family planning ("fewer births, faster affluence").

According to guidelines from the National Population and Family Planning Commission of China, establishing the guiding principles of "People First" and "Overall Development of Human Beings" is now the goal of family planning work. More emphasis is now placed on overall human development and the top priority now is human. In carrying out the One-Child Policy the government will guarantee the right of clients to informed choice of contraceptive methods, encourage public participation in family planning programs, and ensure access to quality family planning services for all people, especially those in remote locations.

In 1995 the State Family Planning Commission started a pilot project of "quality of care" in 11 counties (cities) in China. After initial success in the eastern part of China, where the economy is relatively more developed, it was expanded to the central and western parts of China since 2000. Currently, the project is being carried out in over 800 counties all over China. In 2002, a contest for Advanced County (city, district) in Quality of Care was launched. The "quality of care" program centers on human needs for reproductive health. A key element is the provision of technical services.

Human rights are emphasized more. In the course of promoting family planning special attention has been paid to protecting the ten basic rights of clients, namely, the right to information, right to have access to services, right to choice, right to safety, right to privacy, right to secrecy, right to dignity, right to comfort, right to continued use of services, and right to express.

Informed choices are promoted. People of childbearing age can inquire about different contraceptive methods and select the method most suitable to them. After several years of work the variety of contraceptive methods has become more diversified.

In 2000 the State Family Planning Commission decided to launch pilot work on reforming the family planning program. The aim of the project was to introduce a new working mechanism known as "administration by law, self-management by villagers (urban residents), quality of services, policy-driven and integrated solution," in order to broaden the reform that has already achieved preliminary success.

ONE-CHILD POLICY AND GENDER (LINGLI 2009)

One of the challenges in implementing the One-Child Policy lies in the clash with deep-rooted beliefs and traditions, most notably parents' preference for a male child. Under the traditional patrilineal descent system in China, sons bear the responsibility of looking after the elders and, therefore, are viewed as a form of old-age insurance by parents. Overcoming the traditional preference for male children has become a priority for the government.

Critics say the policy has led to forced abortions and a dangerously imbalanced sex ratio due to a traditional preference for male heirs, which has prompted countless families to abort female fetuses in the hope of getting boys. Experts have said the gender imbalance resulting from sex-selective abortions and other practices could have dangerous social consequences due to anticipated shortages of marriageable young women.

The sex ratio at birth, defined as the proportion of male live births to female live births, ranges from 1.03 to 1.07 in industrialized countries. Government statistics show that since the onset of the One-Child Policy there has been a steady increase in the reported sex ratio from 1.06 in 1979 to 1.11 in 1988 to 1.17 in 2001. There are marked and well-documented local differences, with ratios of up to 1.3 in rural Anhui, Guangdong, and Qinghai provinces.

The Chinese government has declared that the One-Child Policy is to remain for at least another decade, and is usually represented by well-to-do nuclear families with a beaming girl sandwiched between young parents.

There are ubiqituous advertisements promoting the One-Child Policy. More practically minded advertisements promote the value of girls, claiming that women are apt to take better care of their parents than men. Although preference for a male child is by no means a thing of the past, these days most urban Chinese are reluctant to admit to such preference; it has come to be viewed as backward and unenlightened.

In 2008 in Shanghai, one of the better developed cities in China, according to the city's family planning committee the male-biased gender imbalance declined for the first time in eight years. The ratio for the city's most stable population was 106.5 boys to 100 girls in 2008, 1.2 points lower than in 2007. But the biggest change among the three indicators tracked by the Shanghai Population and Family Planning Commission was among migrants who have been in the city less than six months. That rate fell from 123.4 boys to every 100 girls in 2007 to 121.9 to 100 in 2008.

The Shanghai government has instituted several policies, including education, subsidies, and more training opportunities for girls, to help reverse the gender imbalance that could cause problems when the children grow up and try to find a spouse. The moves were designed primarily to encourage migrants from rural areas to have daughters.

The city also tightened inspections to close down underground medical clinics that perform gender checks on fetuses, which are illegal, and perform unlicensed abortions. The practice in Shanghai may shed some light on the solution of the now skewed sex ratio, which might in time lead to severe social unstablity.

The State Family Planning Commission is actively addressing the imbalanced sex ratio at birth by implementing the pilot "Girl Care" project. China has also made it illegal to discriminate against women who give birth to baby girls and has prohibited sex-selective abortions after ultrasound.

The proportion of girls receiving various levels of education has been increasing, and consequently, the overall educational level of women has been improved. Since the 1990s, the school attendance rate for girls has reached over 97%, and the illiteracy rate for women has reduced from 90% in 1949 to about 14% in 2002.

The proportion of women employees in the total workforce rose from 45.7% in 1995 to 46.0% in 2000. Women enjoy a relatively high and stable employment rate and the structure of employment has become more rational.

There are also some indications that the traditional preference for boys may be shifting. In the National Family Planning and Reproductive Health Survey, 37% of women (predominantly young, urban women) claimed to have no preference for one sex over the other, whereas 45% said the ideal family consisted of one boy and one girl. In fact, slightly more women expressed a preference for one girl (5.9%) than for one boy (5.6%).

ONE-CHILD POLICY AND AN AGING POPULATION (WORLD BANK HEALTH NUTRITION AND POPULATION DIVISION 2008)

The rapid decrease in the birthrate, combined with a stable or improving life expectancy, has led to an increasing proportion of elderly people and an increase in the ratio between elderly parents and adult children. In China, the proportion of the population over the age of 65 years was 5% in 1982 and now stands at 7.5% but is expected to rise to more than 15% by 2025. The aging population is increasing and those aged 65 and above made up 7.83% of the population in 2001 up from 5.8% in 1990. Although these figures are lower than those in most industrialized countries (especially Japan, where the proportion of people over the age of 65 years is 20%), a lack of adequate pension coverage in China means that financial dependence on offspring is still necessary for approximately 70% of elderly people. Pension coverage is available only to those employed in the government sector and in large companies. In China, this problem has been named the "4:2:1" phenomenon, meaning that increasing numbers of couples will be solely responsible for the care of one child and four parents. China may face considerable problems because a smaller workforce made of only-children is forced to support a large, aging population.

The pressure on employment has become greater and an increasingly aging population means more resources will have to be allocated to support them (old dependency ratio grew from 8.75% in 1990 to 11.25% in 2001). The fact that most of the aged population lives in rural areas where the social security system is not well established adds to the complexity of the problem.

In response to these problems, various changes and even reforms in the social security system are needed. In 2005, the government began giving US$150 annual pensions to older couples with a daughter as a reward for complying with the policy and as an incentive to others to have just one girl child. In 2009 nearly 30 million retired people throughout the country were covered by the basic retirement insurance scheme, and there were some 1,000 social welfare institutions run by the government and around 40,000 community-run old folk's homes.

The State Family Planing Commision has a plan for setting up and improving the basic insurance system for the elderly in cities and towns, while mainly adhering to family-based insurance for the elderly in rural areas. Meanwhile, the commission will further upgrade the social assistance as well as the "five-guarantee" supply mechanism (focusing on guaranteeing food, clothing, housing, medicare, and burial services) and gradually establish an insurance system combining the country, society, family, and individual to promote an holistic system and the quality of life of old people.

CHILD DEVELOPMENT AND
ONE-CHILD POLICY (BAO ET AL. 1995; ZHENG 2007)

The past three decades saw great social and economic reform in China. These changes are substantial and extensive in that they not only affect the way people live; they also have had great impact on the way people think. These unprecedented changes have brought with them many social phenomena that have not been experienced before, among which is the One-Child Policy.

Since the end of 1970s China's One-Child Policy has created a generation of "only" children that now numbers 90 million. A society which had always had a large family culture found itself caught off-guard and rather at a loss when the first generation of only-children and the 4:2:1 family structure came into being.

In 1985 an article published by an American magazine referred to this generation of only-children as "little emperors," and great debate about the issue of education and development of only-children has ensued ever since. With economic growth Chinese families find themselves in a new era with changes in family structure and the way in which parents and grandparents treat their "little emperors." The only-child receives parental attention and indulgence that was not experienced by any preceding generations. Parents and grandparents are willing to do whatever they can to meet any need these "little emperors" have because they are the precious only-children.

This social phenomenon has raised awareness and concern for society, and in particular the issues of education and the development of only-children have become so important that some refer to it as a "time bomb" whose potential detrimental effects will be seen in 40 or 50 years time, when the only-child generation takes on a pivotal role in society.

Extensive research has been done in China aiming to describe current functioning of the only-child and his/her pattern of development (Guotai et al. 1999; Linyan 1993; Yuyan 1987). The shortcomings of being an only-child can be summarized as follows:

- *Excesssive dependence on parents, family, and environment.* This mainly results from the excessive attention and care provided by parents and family to the child during his/her development.
- *Self-centered.* This also stems from the central position the child has in the family. Also, parents tend to teach their children to be self-centered through being overprotective.
- *Unsocial and petulant.* The lack of siblings and playmates may contribute to this trait in only-children. They tend to have less opportunity than other children to play and share with peers. Having become used to getting everything they demand it would be difficult for these children to deal with adversity. They can also be more emotionally fragile.

We have outlined only-children's undesirable traits which may derive from the way parents raise and educate them. In the education of only-children parents will tend to be

- Indulgent and overprotective.
- Have high expectations, which can lead to too much pressure on the children.
- Extensive studies also show that only-children are likely to be subject to more pressure from their parents who have high expectations, which

may have an adverse effect on the child's development (Fang et al. 2006; Zheng et al. 2001).

- Overdependent on schools and knowledge-based education; too much stress is put on the intellectual development of the children. The importance of a balanced personality and intregrity of character can often be overlooked. As a matter of fact, there have been various educational programs aimed at different age groups, focusing mainly on intellectual ability and enhancing children's knowledge about children, but this kind of program can create a group of children who later turn out to be uncooperative, lacking in communication skills, and poorly adapted socially (Wang 2001; Xu & Feng 2008).

As the old saying goes, every coin has two sides. Previous research from outside China has shown that only-children tend to achieve better than other children because they have had full access to resources and their education has received more attention from the parents. For example, a 1987 quantitative review of 141 studies on 16 different personality traits found, in contrast with the earlier comments, no evidence of maladjustment in only-children and these children were not very different from children with siblings. The main exception was the finding that only-children had higher achievement motivation. A second analysis revealed that only-children, firstborns, and children with only one sibling scored higher on tests of verbal ability than later-borns and children with multiple siblings. These advantages will apply to the only-child situation in China. More resources, more time, and more parental attention are devoted to the only-child. A freer environment is provided for the children to learn and grow; this is in favor of cultivating more creative minds. From a societal point of view, with fewer children born, more resources are allocated to each one. Nationwide, 85% of Chinese people had received the nine-year compulsory education by 2000, while some 99.1% of school-aged children were enrolled.

While in the city parents are busy taking their children to various math, English, and music classes many children of rural couples are left with their grandparents or other relatives without seeing their parents for long periods, sometimes years, because their parents are the so-called migrating workers who leave to find better work opportunities in the city. The significant disparity between urban and rural areas in relation to child education and development reflects a general social problem on a larger scale in China.

Challenges and dilemmas are often the price of social progress. When facing a situation for which no precedent exists problems will surely arise. Every problem in child education and development is a snapshot of problems in social development. No single policy or event should be blamed or could take the blame for current problems; rather, the awareness of the whole society should be raised and all of society should join forces to find a solution as is the case in China now. The government and related organizations are aware of the situation and the public is also taking an active part in looking for solutions. Most importantly, education is not only about the children; parents and teachers should be better informed about the uniqueness of the only-child situation and should be equipped with scientific knowledge about child development and education rather than with only blind indulgence and love.

The first generation of only-children is now reaching its 20th and 30th birthdays. Universities and workforces are filled with only-children, and some of them are to have their own child soon. The degree to which any problems associated with their development and education will affect their ability to take up their role as independent social individuals still waits to be seen.

ONE-CHILD POLICY AND CHILD MENTAL HEALTH

China has worked hard to stick to the One-Child Policy using means of persuasion, coercion, and encouragement and has achieved much. However, problems come hand in hand with success. At the center of the debate is the problem of an aging population and a skewed sex ratio at birth. As the first "only-child" generation was born and raised in the 1980s more and more people are concerned with the way these children were raised. The 4:2:1 family pattern that ensues from the policy is also seen as a potential problem for this generation. The problem has raised great social awareness and many studies have been conducted since 1984 concerning these issues.

In 1984, a research study conducted by the Psychological Research Institute of the Chinese Academy of Sciences involving children aged 5-7 years old in 6 kindergartens in Beijing with 138 only-children and 127 children with siblings compared on personality traits. Behaviors in four categories (independence, supportive, aggressive, and empathic behavior) were the subject of the research. The results show that in all three age groups, there were few differences in empathic, supportive, and aggressive behaviors; children with siblings scored slightly higher. In the 5-year-old group, notable differences were shown between only-child and child with sibling groups in relation to independence with only-children being less independent ($p<0.05$) (Chuanwen et al. 1984).

Another study lead by Tseng and colleagues (1988) studied the impact of China's one-child-per-couple family planning policy on child development in 697 preschool children in the city of Nanjing and two rural areas surrounding Nanjing. A home-visit questionnaire survey, including a Chinese version of Achenbach's Child Behavior Checklist, was used. The behavior problem profiles of only-children and those who had siblings were compared revealing a significant difference between girls who were only-children and those who had siblings. Girls who were only-children tended to have slightly higher scores on the depression, mood, and temper domains. But otherwise only-children were not inferior in adaptability compared to children with siblings.

In 1996 the Chinese Adolescent Research Center conducted a study covering 12 major cities with 3284 children and their parents (Chinese One Child Personality Research Group 1998). The results showed that children from one-child families seemed to develop without major problems, but with some slight shortcomings in aspects such as creativity, independence, and financial management when compared with those from multi-sibling families.

More recently studies concerning children's overall health status and suicidal risks were carried out in Zhejiang province by T. Hesketh and colleagues (2002). A cross-sectional survey using self-completion questionnaires was carried out in six middle schools (predominant age range 13-17 years) in urban and rural settings in Zhejiang province in eastern China. Results were available from 1,576 completed questionnaires. One-third of the students had suffered symptoms of severe depression, with 16% admitting to suicide ideation and 9% to actually having attempted suicide. Factors independently associated with severe depression were female gender, poor self-reported academic performance, and rural residence. Similar factors were associated with suicide ideation and attempted suicide. Depression was less common in only-children. Patterns of help-seeking showed reliance on friends and parents with very low levels of professional help-seeking (around 1%) and 30% not having sought help from any source for psychological problems.

Another cross-sectional survey was carried out in middle schools (predominant age 12-16 years) in three distinct socioeconomic areas of Zhejiang province in eastern China and using self-completion questionnaires, anthropometry, and hemoglobin measurement (Hesketh, Qu, & Tomkins 2003). Data was obtained for 4197 participants. Significant differences were found between only-children and those with siblings on a number of key indicators. However, after adjusting for area, sex, and parental education levels, only two significant predictors remained; children with siblings were more likely to be bullied (OR 1.5, 95%CI: 1.1–2.0; $p=0.006$) and less likely to confide in their parents (OR 0.6, 95% CI: 0.3–0.8; $p=0.009$). There were no significant differences in the key parameters between first and second born children.

Many parents are used to attaching importance to the body, knowledge, and intelligence of their children with comparative neglect of psychosocial development, ability, and personality traits. The development of personality begins from embryo. Life experiences will impact significantly not only growth but also future personality, intelligence, and social adaptability. A well-integrated experience will help bring up a well-functioning personality.

Zheng and colleagues conducted several studies on the developing personality and psychological problems of the only-child. For example, examination of 911 singletons in Beijing aged 6 to 12 years showed that prevalence of social adaption problems was 23%, similar to the average in developed countries. American children of similar age scored better on "independence" while the Chinese participants showed lower levels of "aggressiveness" (Zheng & Chen 2001).

A six-year study ("Multicentre Controlled Trial of Early Systemic Intervention on Psychosocial Development in Children without Siblings") not only focused on the personality and psychological problems of the only-child but also on the effect of an early intervention (Chen et al. 2006). The research aimed to explore the effect of early systemic intervention on psychosocial development in only-children; 315 only-children aged 0-6 years were chosen at random from 9 cities in China and received an intervention determined by developmental stage. Another 300 children were recruited as controls matched by age, sex, and family background. The standard instruments used to assess the effects of the intervention were the Personality Tendency Scale for Children, Achenbach Children Behavior Checklist, Chinese Binet Intelligent Test, Adaptive Behavior Scales, and a Temperament Questionnaire. The behavior problems of the intervention group were significantly lower than those of the control group ($p<0.01$). The psychosocial development, mean IQ, temperament, and adaptability of the intervention group were also significantly better than the control group ($p< 0.05$ or 0.01).

Children's adjustment can clearly be studied in a scientific way (Chen et al. 2006). One such study was to become a momentous scientific research item of the National Family Planning Committee of China. The intervention program in this study was established by a special committee. The participants were selected from ten provinces or cities and were representative. The aim was to prove and analyze the validity and characteristics of the intervention program, as well as explore the new model for promoting the adjustment of only-children. The parent training program developed by an authoritative committee, including 17 specialists, has proven to be highly successful and many trials have used this intervention technique.

The studies show that early systemic intervention does benefit the psychosocial development of only-children. The age chosen (from birth to 6 years of age) is the golden period for the development of a healthy personality. The results show that the earlier the intervention the better. It is important to realize that the so-called "only-child" is a "normal" child brought up in a special environment. It is to be expected that parental education and parenting programs will influence child development in these circumstances as in many other areas of developmental psychopathology.

In March 2008 the Chinese government declared that the One-Child Policy is here to stay for at least for another decade, although there may be minor changes. For example, the majority of cities can permit couples who are themselves from an only-child family or parents who lost their child in the Sichuan earthquake to have two children. This suggests that the Chinese government is resolute in controlling China's population but wants the policy to be humanitarian. Thus, at least another generation of only-children is to be born. We need to make a serious effort towards the education of parents and towards early intervention for only-children to maximize the opportunities of a well-functioning and educated generation.

PROMOTION OF ALL-AROUND HUMAN DEVELOPMENT (BIN 2009; ROSENBERG 2009)

As indicated above, in 2008, an official announced that the One-Child Policy will remain for at least another decade with only minor modifications (Rosenberg 2009). In the coming decades, China's population and development program will enter a new historical period. On the premise of stabilizing a low fertility rate, China will achieve a gradual transition from a low population growth rate to zero growth, and the total population, after reaching its peak, will slowly decrease.

By 2010 the total population of the country (excluding Hong Kong, Macao, and Taiwan) will reach 1.4 billion. People's lives will be more prosperous, the health of the newborn population will be substantially improved, and the sex ratio at birth will become normal. People of reproductive age will be able to enjoy the basic reproductive health services and an informed choice of contraceptive method will be universally practiced. Great efforts will be made to solve problems brought on by an aging population and a basic social security system that covers the whole society will be established.

By the mid-21st century, the population of China will peak at 1.6 billion. After that, it will start to decline slowly. The health and educational level of the population will be improved considerably. Senior middle school and university education will be popularized. A complete social security system will be established. Population distribution and employment structure will become more rational and urbanization will increase significantly. People will live a prosperous life with the per capita income reaching the level of medium-developed countries. Society will be more civilized and a balance will be struck between population and economy, society, natural resources, and environment.

These are the government announced goals of the birth control policy and family planning. Though the policy is to stay problems in population size, quality, and structure make China's population issue unprecedentedly complex. Resource shortages and developmental imbalances will continue to exist for a long time and much remains to be done in reforming and innovating the family planning program.

The National Population and Family Planning Commission of China promised that they would continue efforts to stabilize the low fertility level and improve the current family planning policy based on what is a changing situation. This is the primary task for China's population and family planning program at present and for a period to come. Through integrated use of education, science and technology, and economic, legal, and administrative means, they will aim to develop a long-term, effective mechanism in the area of population and family planning. They are also guaranteed to improve the legal system concerning family planning and to intensify the publicity and education about the One-Child Policy and related subjects through financial investment.

The main challenge now is the promotion of Family Planning with Quality Services for Reproductive Health, to improve the overall quality of the entire people of the nation. In order to improve quality of life for newborn babies, it is essential to improve the health of women and children by promoting maternal and child health care. Knowledge on child bearing and rearing should be publicized and supported by pre-marital medical check-ups, antenatal diagnosis, genetic counseling, prevention and treatment of newborn babies' diseases, and other preventive services. Pregnancy and prenatal care should be improved and hospitalized delivery and breast-feeding encouraged. In this way, maternity and child health care can be improved and birth defects reduced.

Protecting the rights of the elderly is also an important task since the demographical makeup of the country is shifting and more elderly people are in need of protection. The elderly support system should be established and improved. The old-age welfare service system should be based on the family, supported by the community welfare service, and supplemented by social welfare organizations. A basic insurance system for the elderly will be set up and improved in cities and towns, while mainly adhering to family-based insurance of the elderly in the rural areas. Meanwhile, social assistance as well as the "five-guarantee" supply mechanism focused on guaranteeing food, clothing, housing, medicare, and a burial service should be further upgraded; and an insurance system encompassing the country, society, family, and individual should be gradually established so as to promote the quality of life of the older generation.

Strengthening people's awareness of the integrated development of population, resources, and environment is also a top priority for decision makers. Although the One-Child Policy has slowed down population growth, due to its already large existing population growth remains a threat to the environment and natural resources within China. But fortunately awareness about environmental protection and sustainable development has been raised and the government is taking pains to make progress.

As for child development, education, and mental health, recently the work on early education has been brought under the responsibility of all tiers of Population and Family Planning work. It has also been listed at all levels of the government's people-benefit project. It is the responsibility of the Population and Family Planning's social management and public service network to provide families with consultation guidance. Many cities have put into place policies to strengthen the education of children; for example, Shanghai is taking steps to promote preschool education for children under 3 years old.

SUMMARY

In response to challenges China is trying its best to promote all-around human development, improving birth quality as well as controlling birth quantity, to construct a healthy society and protect the rights of women, children, and the elders, and to cultivate a generation of children with both good knowledge and integrity of character.

REFERENCES

Bao, X., Zheng, Y., et al. *Behavior of Newborn Baby and Education of 0-3 Years Old.* Beijing: Chinese Adolescent and Child Publishing Company, 1995: 240-278.

Bin, L., Minister for China's National Population and Family Planning Commission on *Item 4 General Debate on National Experience* at the 42nd Session of the UN Commission on Population and Development. New York, 31 March 2009

Bing, L., Comprehensively Addressing Population Issues for Promotion of All-round Human Development. *China Population: Introduction Book of China's National Population and Family Planning Commission,* 2009: 1-3

Chen X.S., Zheng Y. et al. Multicentre study of early systemic intervention on psychosocial development in nonsibling children. *Chinese Journal of Behavioral Medical Science* 15 (2006): 1126-1128.

Chinese One Child Personality Research Group. The Survey of the Personality and Education in Urban Chinese Non-sibling Children. *Chinese Journal Education Research* 10 (1998): 254-256.

Chuanwen, W., Cunren, F., & Guobin L. A comparative study on certain differences in individuality and sex-based differences between 5 to 7-year old onlies and nononlies. *Acta Psychologica Sinica* 4 (1984): 360-362.

Fang, S-F., Jing, C-X., & Wang, L-L. Relationship between psychological problems in middle school students and parental rearing behaviours. *Journal of Applied Clinical Pediatrics* 17 (2006): 34-36.

Greenhalgh, S. *Just One Child: Science and Policy in Deng's China.* Berkeley: University of California Press, 2008.

Guotai, T., Jinghua, Q., Wenxing, Z., et al. Longitudinal study of psychological development of single and non-single child in family: A 10-year follow-up study in Nanjing. *Chinese Mental Health* 4 (1999): 210-212.

Hesketh, T., Ding, Q. J., & Jenkins, R. Suicide ideation in Chinese adolescents. *Social Psychiatry and Psychiatric Epidemiology* 37 (2002): 230-235.

Hesketh T., Lu L., Xing Z.W. The effect of China's one-child family policy after 25 years. *New England Journal of Medicine* 353 (2005): 1171-1176.

Hesketh, T., Qu, J.D., & Tomkins, A. Health effects of family size: Cross sectional survey in Chinese adolescents. *Archives of Disease in Childhood* 88 (2003): 467-471.

Lin B. Fertility desires of women of childbearing age and influencing factors. In *Theses Collection of 2001 National Family Planning and Reproductive Health Survey.* Beijing: China Population Publishing House, 2003: 57-65.

Lingli, X. "It's a Girl" is more likely to be heard in Shanghai. *Shanghai Daily:* April 8, 2009.

Linyan, S. The mental health problems of only children in Hunnan province. *Chinese Journal of Nervous and Mental Disease* 5 (1993): 262-265.

National Bureau of Statistics. Chinese Population in 2008. *Statistical Bulletin of the People's Republic of China:* February 26, 2009.

National Population and Family Planning Commission of P.R. China. *Main Achievements of Population and Family Planning Program of China.* December 7, 2006: www.npfpc.gov.cn.

McLoughlin, C. The coming-of-age of China's single-child policy. *Psychology in the Schools* 42(3) (2005); 305-313.

Rosenberg, M. *One Child Policy in China Designed to Limit Population Growth.* By About.com: Geography. April 12, 2009.

Tseng W.S., Kuotai T., Hsu J. et al. Family planning and child mental health in China: The Nanjing Survey. *American Journal of Psychiatry* 145(11) (1988): 1396–1403.

Wang, X.-P. The status quo of mentality health of singleton undergraduate and countermeasure. *Journal of Nanjing Institute of Physical Education* 4 (2001): 61-62.

World Bank Health Nutrition and Population Division. *Development data.* 2008.

Xu, C-X., and Feng, X-T. Review of research on female college students in one-child family. *Population and Development* 6 (2008): 23-26.

Yuyan, M. A comparative study of the characteristics of behaviours between the only-child and the non-only-child. *Acta Psychologica Sinica* 2 (1987): 195-198.

Zheng, G. et al. Family planning and the value of children in China. Ongoing themes in psychology and culture. *Proceedings of the 16th International Congress of the International Association for Crosscultural Psychology.* Yogyakarta, Indonesia: Yogyakarta University Press, 2004: 381-398.

Zheng, L.X., Peng, J.W., Xi, Y.J. Comparative study of parental rearing patters between single and non-single child in family. *Chinese Journal of Child Health Care* 3 (2001): 9-11.

Zheng, Y. *The Guidelines of Education for One Child in Family.* Reference Book of China's National Population and Family Planning Commission, 2007

Zheng, Y. & Chen X.S. Analysis of social adaptive behavior and correlative factors in Chinese children. *Chinese Journal of Health Education* 17 (2001): 392-396.

4

Industrialization

Its Impact on Child and Adolescent Mental Health

Cornelio G. Banaag, Jr.

INTRODUCTION

Industrialization involves the process by which manufacturing industries develop within predominantly agricultural societies, affecting a shift in the development of a country to a predominantly industrial economy. Industrialization has been happening over the centuries. But the rapidity of its growth in the last half century is unprecedented in developing countries. It has received much appeal because of the historical economic success in those countries that have completed the shift from agricultural to predominantly industrial. Developing countries, like the Philippines and Indonesia, have looked up to industrialization as the key strategy to mitigate the burden of poverty among their people. Industrialized countries have created more jobs, increased the country's wealth measured in gross domestic product (GDP), increased technology and inventions in transportation, communication, and agricultural products. Industrialization has greatly increased the production of goods worldwide and the exchange of goods within countries and between countries. The children in industrialized countries are healthier and better educated. On the other hand, industrialization has brought negative effects that are now well recognized. These include the tremendous and rapid growth of population in major cities and towns, the growth of inequalities (political, social, and economic), the growth of slum areas in cities, unregulated and poor working conditions in factories, and increased environmental pollution leading to health hazards and climatic change.

Industrialization has also brought with it the interrelated, overlapping phenomena of globalization, rapid urbanization, migration, and revolutionary growth of communication technology and mass media; all of them creating profound social changes that affect human development and security, with the impact possibly greatest on children and youth.

Several trends that correlated with industrialization have been well documented in the literature since the 1970s (Coleman 1996; Sardon 2000; Shanahan 2000). Among these are demographic changes in family structure and family dynamics including decline and postponement of parenting, increase in divorce and marriage annulment, single parent families, cohabitation, births outside marriage, and an increase in female labor force participation (Gauthier 2002). These trends have been observed in all industrialized countries although with different degrees of magnitude. These demographic changes serve as challenges to the growth and development of children and youth.

Growth and Development of Children and Industrialization

The growth and development of children proceeds well as long as certain universal and unchanging requirements are met. First of all children's material needs for food, clothing, and shelter must be met because without them children may not even survive. Children must be protected from their own immature state and from the hazards of their environment. Such protection will allow children to survive and grow. They need an affectionate system of nurturing that will allow their innate capacities to bloom; human capacities like loving, communicating, establishing relationships, hoping, and dreaming. Such a system of nurturing must help children learn the limits of acceptable behavior thereby helping them develop self-control and self-mastery. Children also need new experiences; thus they need peers to play with and schools to teach them about their world and about themselves. They need a family that is capable of meeting their basic needs for the long term. They need responsible adults who will not only provide for, protect, and nurture them but will also transmit certain values that will allow them to live with some harmony in the society where they are developing. They need an environment that is safe, relatively stable, and fairly predictable. Whatever changes happen to the family and the environment will have profound effects, for better or worse, on the growth and development of children. The profound social, economic, political, and environmental changes brought about by rapid industrialization, globalization, urbanization, communication technology, and mass media will understandably influence the growth, development, and mental health of children and youth. The mental health of children cannot be separated from the mental health of their parents or other adult caregivers and from the influence of their physical and social environment.

GLOBALIZATION

Globalization is a process that opens countries to many influences from beyond their borders. Such processes necessarily will reduce the primacy of local and national economic, political, and social institutions, thus affecting the everyday environment in which children grow up and interact with the rest of society (Kaufman et al. 2004). Global trade and financial activity have risen to a scale never seen before. In many developing countries, massive investments flowed into export industries. However, these investments were built on foreign debts and therefore were vulnerable to currency crises. Countries that were forced to devaluate their currencies found themselves burdened with foreign debts compounded by flow of capital from these countries. Such financial crises hit many countries in Asia in 1997. Many developing countries continue to battle high levels of poverty. The current environment of global recession has also made matters worse for many countries. No discussion of the economic effects of global change can ignore the reality of the growing inequality within and between countries. While poverty is falling in many countries, inequality continues to rise. In many countries the poor get poorer and the rich get richer. In other countries where some gains against poverty have been made, the poor get richer but the rich get richer at a faster rate. These growing social, political, and economic inequalities have resulted in pervasive poverty. Fifty percent (50%) of the world's children continue to live under conditions of abject poverty; 80% of these children live in developing countries (UNCTAD 2006).

The Effects of Poverty

The effects of poverty can be seen in gross measures of children's and parents' well-being. Using such measures the World Bank reports striking examples; life expectancy in Sub-Saharan Africa is 50 years; in Japan it is almost 80. Mortality among children below age 5 in South Asian countries exceeds 170 deaths per thousand; in Sweden it is below 10 per thousand. More than 110 million children in low income nations lack access to primary education; close to universal enrollment is the norm in industrialized countries (World Bank 1990, cited by Kaufman et al. 2004). It is difficult to measure the damage to the mind of young children and youth living in poverty in the midst of wealth around them, feeling excluded, marginalized with severely limited opportunities to grow well and to move out of the culture of poverty. Thus, poverty has become transgenerational. Pervasive poverty in many developing countries has bred civil unrest, domestic wars, political and social instability, material and spiritual corruption from top to bottom. Children of poor families learn corruption early as a means to survival. Millions of children around the world miss out on childhood because of poverty. They become vulnerable to exploitation, abuse, violence, and discrimination.

So massive is the problem of poverty that in 2000 the United Nations adopted the Millennium Declaration consisting of eight Millennium Development Goals (MDGs) that will be met with at least 50% success by year 2015. The Millennium Declaration, supported by 189 UN member states, reflects the global commitment to improving the lot of humanity in the new century. All the Millennium Development Goals have direct or indirect bearing on the physical and mental well-being of the world's children and youth. Among the most important of the MDGs is the eradication of poverty and hunger. Very few of the developing countries are anywhere near the target. The prospect of hitting the target is especially dim given the current global financial crisis.

Child Labor

One immense problem spawned by pervasive poverty is child labor. It is as pervasive as poverty, found in all parts of the world, and has been growing as a very striking issue in developing countries. The International Labor Organization (ILO), the monitoring and regulatory international body on matters of labor, defines child labor as children under 18 engaged in harmful occupation or work activities in the labor market or in their own household interfering with their education or posing a threat to their health. It is notable that the definition of child labor is linked to education and health, two markers that reflect a country's investment in its children. Higher educational achievement and good physical health translate to a sense of competence, good self-esteem, more marketable skills, greater capacity for independence, and a general sense of well-being.

ILO estimates that there are close to 250 million child laborers across the globe (IPEC 2002). Seventy-three million working children are less than 10 years old. No country appears to be exempted. In developed industrialized countries there are 2.5 million child laborers. Another 2.5 million are found in transitional economies. The children are forced to work to help support their families. It is estimated that working children contribute up to 20-25% of the family income. The largest group of working children, aged 14 years and under, are found in the Asia Pacific region. Most working children are found in the informal sector of the economy where there are no legal or regulatory protections. Children are easily hired because they receive wages below the minimum standards without social and health benefits. Many are engaged in hazardous working conditions inimical to life and health, not to mention mental health: pyrotechnique factories, mining areas, deep sea diving, sweatshops like garment factories where children (mostly girls) are kept inside 24 hours a day seven days a week, never seeing sunlight. Some are also engaged in prostitution and pornography; these are the children who are bonded in veritable slavery and often caught up in human trafficking. These are mostly adolescent females recruited from provinces, promised a job as domestic helpers or waitresses in restaurants but end up in prostitution and pornography. They are shipped from the provinces to major cities in the same country and other countries.

A very moving documentary made in the Philippines took shots of young children at work in real time at the real site of work. One segment shows young teenage boys with small frames unloading backbreaking weights of cement from a newly anchored ship. At work's end, they look tired but jovial, drinking alcohol and smoking cigarettes, joking around, talking of their dreams that they admit would never happen. Another segment shows pre-teenage boys and girls, working in a sugar plantation under the noon day sun, looking tired, eyes lacking luster, nonresponsive to interview. Many clearly looked depressed. These boys and girls are essentially bonded workers. Their work helps pay for the debts incurred by their parents from landlords during the long wait for harvest when there is no work.

A study by Federman and Levine (2002) examined how education intersected with child labor in a large developing country at a period of rapid industrialization and economic growth. The study examined the relationship between industrialization, school enrollment, labor force participation, and household responsibilities for youth. The study was done both at the household level (individual families) and at the district level (a district is larger than counties in the United States but smaller than states). Federman and Levine cited the concern of some authors that industrialization may, in fact, reduce enrollment by drawing youth into factory work or by increasing need for youth to help at home while their parents work in factories. The results of the study demonstrated that growth in industrial employment at the district level correlated with higher school enrollment and lower youth labor force participation for teens aged 13-15 years. However, for teens aged 16-17 years enrollment remained modest. Thus, it is likely that non-enrollment in the age group 16-17 represents a social problem or a cultural expectation that children help family income when they hit this age. There was also a gender bias demonstrated by the study. The predominantly male employment in manufacturing correlated positively with higher male youth enrollment. At the household level having an adult female employed in manufacturing predicted lower school enrollment for female youth. Two possible explanations were given. First, responsibilities at home may increase for female youth when mothers work. Second, having an adult female employed in manufacturing may increase the possibility that younger females will also work in factory jobs.

School Enrollment

Among other effects the structural and social changes brought about by industrialization and globalization mediate higher school enrollment. The study by Federman and Levine (2002) showed that regions with strong manufacturing growth had elements that would encourage school enrollment: more household-level consumption (reflecting increased income), better roads (making school more accessible with decreased travel cost), higher school density (increased number of private and government schools per 1000 students), and higher urbanization (partly brought about by migration pulled by the opportunities for employment in industrialized areas). Yet dropout rates remain high in the secondary schools in industrializing countries like the Philippines. Obviously the phenomenon of child labor is driven not by poverty alone. Complex familial and cultural reasons continue to push child labor in many low income and middle income countries.

URBANIZATION

Urbanization involves the physical transition of rural areas into urban areas as a result of population growth partly due to migration. More and more people will leave villages and move to cities and towns that have become industrialized because of the perceived benefits in living in these places. This movement of people results in rapid urban growth. The WHO World Urbanization Prospects Report (2005) estimates that by 2030 the urban population will comprise approximately 60% of the global population. The UN-Habitat Annual Report (2008) estimates that 93% of urban growth will happen in Asia and Africa. Some countries in Asia have already exceeded the 2030 prediction. In the Philippines, for example, 65% of the population now lives in urban areas. Migration to cities is fuelled by the search for employment or better paying jobs, a better quality of life in terms of health and education, a greater diversity of entertainment and lifestyle options. Rapid migration may be influenced by the portrayal of urban life by the media or the success stories of relatives and friends who have already moved to the cities.

Positive Aspects of Urbanization

Like industrialization, urbanization has an upside and a downside. The positive view looks at urbanization as a natural result of modernization and industrialization and of bringing beneficial effects to society. In urban areas, family income is much higher than in rural areas. In China the average household income in the cities is almost three times higher than that in rural areas (Bloom and Khanna 2007). Quality of life in the cities is much better in terms of basic services like transportation, communication, sanitation, water supply, waste management. The educational system is also more effective. There is a greater pool of well-educated people who can teach in schools and universities. School enrollment is greater in the urban areas, and female literacy is 35% higher. In terms of health, there is a larger supply of health care providers, and greater specialization in medical centers. Thus, the urban population generally enjoys a better health status than their rural relatives. Because housing is expensive and child care while parents work is costly the birth rate is relatively low. Couples tend to plan their family more effectively, making use of reproductive health services that are easily accessible. With fewer children, parents are able to pay more attention to their needs. Families spend more quality time together resulting in overall better upbringing of children.

Negative Aspects of Urbanization

The negative view of urbanization recognizes that many major cities in the world grew without adequate planning. As a result, living conditions are adverse, undercutting many of the benefits brought by industrialization. Overcrowding, traffic congestion, environmental pollution, and contamination compromise the health status of urban dwellers, especially among the very poor. Urban poverty continues to rise despite increases in income. In many developing countries the rate of growth of the urban poor exceeds the rate of growth of the urban population (Bloom and Khanna 2007), taxing the adequacy of basic services in the community (notably waste management, water and sanitation facilities, recreational space and facilities). Because of the costly housing, slums of the urban poor develop in the margins of the major cities, along the banks of waterways, on dangerous land sites, or on any unguarded vacant areas. With makeshift shanties of light material packed together in limited areas, inadequate water and sanitation, no system of waste disposal except nearby rivers, inadequate food supply, and no space for children's activities except the streets, slum areas make for hazardous living conditions any season of the year.

The UN (2008) estimates the number of people living in slums had reached one billion in 2007 and could reach 1.39 billion by 2020. There are large variations among regions. Asia has the highest number of city dwellers living in slums.

Bartlett (1999) describes how children's needs are routinely ignored or misunderstood by urban development planners and policy makers. Such neglect brings a very high cost for the children in terms of ill health, injury, premature death, and impaired physical, mental, and social development. Provision of water, sanitation, and housing fails to address the main requirements for child health. In many poor areas water is available but not piped to the homes. Sometimes it takes 30 minutes per trip to get water from a communal standpipe or well. Often it is the children who make the trips and carry heavy loads causing damage to the neck, head, and spine as well as causing a serious drain on the energy of under-nourished children. The time required to fetch water can be sufficient to prevent school attendance. Stored water in the house presents with dangers of contamination like when thirsty children scoop water with their hands or use buckets left on the ground. Household conditions marked by overcrowding and poor ventilation encourage spread of infection. Children suffer the two global leading causes of burden of disease: lower respiratory infection and diarrheal diseases. In low income countries the third leading cause of burden of disease is HIV/AIDS, which continues to inflict suffering on young children (WHO 2004).

The unremitting poverty in many urban centers of the world has bred special groups of children UNICEF has called "children in need of special protection." Among these overlapping groups are street children, abused children (physical and sexual), children in conflict with the law, substance abusing children and youth, children with disabilities (including psychological/psychiatric disabilities), and children engaged in labor. These children are growing in numbers in the urban centers of the world, especially in the developing countries. It is easy to blame the rising inequalities brought by rapid industrialization and globalization for the growing horde of children in need of special protection. Admittedly these phenomena are too complex to be blamed on poverty alone.

Disappearance of a Safe Geographical Space

One disturbing development in urban centers is the disappearance of safe geographic space where children meet and chat and play face-to-face. For many children, especially among the middle class, this safe geographic space is taken over, for better or worse, by cyber-space in the form of social networks sites, chat rooms, and blogs. Children of the urban poor are not altogether excluded. They save their meager school allowance or whatever earnings they make on the streets, or they skip school, to visit the proliferating cyber-cafes to play games or chat and connect with others in a virtual world.

The disappearing physical space has implications in terms of the significance of play for child development. Given the opportunity, children will choose to play "to engage passionately with the world around them through exploration, manipulation, physical exuberance, experimentation and pretense, either alone or with others" (Bartlett 1999). Child mental health professionals know well the important role of play in child development.

Through play children learn to master their environments and their emotions. They learn the rules of games sometimes even before they really learn the rules in the family and in society. They learn the value of friendships and a social network, and the means of resolving conflicts with their peers. For many, play becomes a substitute for expressing the thoughts and feelings they cannot yet express in words. Can cyber-space capture these nuanced face-to-face transactions that happen when children play in real geographic space?

The Effects of Play

Play is a basic human drive fundamental to human development. Interestingly, the young of lower animal species also engage in playfulness. Neuroscience now suggests that changes in the brain occur as a result of play, and that both social behavior and the capacity to learn are affected. On the way to adolescence and adulthood so much pruning of neurons and synaptic connections takes place. Connections that are not being used are pruned. The simple rule is "use it or lose it." The enormous potential for learning is activated by the child's play, assuring that the proper connections in the brain are not pruned. Play in turn is encouraged by a rich and stimulating environment. Children do not need expensive formal toys; they are very creative and resourceful in drawing excitement from their surroundings. They tend to prefer spontaneous play activities offered by the school playground, or the streets and alleys and vacant lots. Even the poorest households and neighborhoods can be a rich environment given the imaginativeness of children. But such environments may not always be safe and may in fact be high risk for unintentional injuries. All that the children need is safe space. What happens then when safe space is gone, when the sidewalks and the playgrounds are gone?

Effects on Children's Emotional and Social Well-Being

The quality of housing and community space affects not only the physical health and learning abilities of children but also their emotional and social well-being. The overcrowded home environment of the urban poor is a significant source of stress for young people. Overcrowding has been related in many research studies in the past to increased stress. Research with working-class children in India has linked chronic overcrowding to behavioral difficulties in school, poor academic achievement, elevated blood pressure, and impaired relationships with parents (Bartlett 1999). Overwork, fatigue and anxiety from work, and frustrations from overcrowding and poor living conditions trigger tensions at home especially among the adult male members of the household. Such tensions are often released against the weakest members of the household, the children and women who easily become victims of violence and abuse. Not infrequently mothers are the ones who abuse their children in the name of corporal punishment. In many urban poor communities vandalism, violence, alcohol and drug use, and criminal behavior are common responses from older children and adolescents to their boredom due to lack of recreational facilities. Moreover, they feel excluded from the relative affluence they see in large shopping centers and residential areas of middle and upper class people. Their experience of economic and social inequality begins to hurt as they reach adolescence.

A study of an innovative program in the United States ("Move to Opportunity") found that in families who were helped to move from high poverty neighborhoods to neighborhoods with low levels of poverty, the parents reported significantly less mental stress than parents who remained in the high poverty areas (Leventhal and Brooks-Gunn 2003). Boys who moved to neighborhoods with less poverty also scored better on several measures of mental health. The researchers found no significant group differences for girls, raising speculation that the girls may have been somehow more sheltered from the effects of the high poverty neighborhood. Parents who moved to low poverty neighborhood reported less physical and social disorder (e.g., trash, graffiti, public drinking, abandoned buildings, public drug use and dealing) and more satisfaction with their neighborhood compared to the group that stayed in the high poverty area. While the move appeared to have had beneficial effects on mental health, it had no effect on parental employment, welfare receipt, or income. The benefits of moving to low poverty neighborhood may therefore be attributed to reduced community violence and disorder or improved community resources: better schools, health services, housing, parks, and sports facilities.

MIGRATION

Migration has become an essential part of economic development everywhere. More people are now moving more frequently and farther than ever before in search of better economic opportunities and a better life. Poverty, climate change, famine, war, persecution, and the strong desire to explore have always pushed people to move. Today when both relative and absolute poverty is becoming more severe in many countries, and with the growing inequalities between the rich and the poor, people are being pushed in greater numbers to seek work elsewhere. At the same time rich countries are actively recruiting people from other parts of the world to meet their emerging labor needs. Easier travel, access to information about distant places, the mass media constantly flashing images of what life could be like in other places, and opportunities for improving living standards—all of these factors have fuelled the dramatically increased international and national movements of individuals and families. Because of these factors migration is not likely to stop any time soon. Indeed, there is reason to believe that in years to come migration, both rural to urban and across countries, will continue to grow. Internal rural-to-urban migration has resulted in rapid urbanization seen in major cities and towns around the world. There are serious implications of this growing migration for those who move and for those left behind, especially the children who are left behind.

Migration is always difficult, no matter where the destination, no matter whether it is forced or voluntary. It involves uprooting, leaving some family members behind, and breaking with social customs and values that give a sense of identity and continuity. For many it means leaving loved ones without guarantee of good work or successful resettlement, leaving home and family knowing the chances of success may be limited at best. This is particularly true of the growing number of people moving clandestinely across borders, being smuggled or trafficked and being placed in situations that threaten life as well as physical and psychological health (Carballo 2007)

Migration presents both opportunities and challenges for societies, communities, families, and individuals. Migration alters the structure of families. Experience has shown that children are affected by migration in different ways. Many children are left behind by parents who migrate for reasons of work. Parents who migrate to resettle in another country generally bring their children along, although some leave the children in their country of origin under the care of relatives. Living in a family with at least one parent (sometimes both parents) away for long periods has become part of normal experience for many children in developing countries. Some children migrate independently of parents and adults. These children are sometimes referred to as "unaccompanied minors."

Effects on Mental Health

The literature on migration mostly shows that the process is stressful and may present with potentially negative impacts on mental health. Migrants experience a series of losses: loss of home, separation from family and friends, loss of a sense of belonging, loss of identity, loss of social support networks while in the process of settling in the host country. As they settle they feel a sense of isolation from the mainstream life in the host country. For some it takes a generation to finally feel at home. The children of families who migrate to industrialized countries may initially experience marginalization and discrimination in the country of settlement, but they generally adapt faster to the dominant culture and learn the language faster. They become the interpreter of the new culture for their parents, which affects the dynamics and balance of power in the family. The children's new acquired power diminishes the parent's authority and control over them. Most migrant children flourish and contribute positively to their new communities (Innocenti 2005).

Children who migrate independently of their parents or adult guardians are in many ways similar to adult migrants seeking new social and economic opportunities. Many of them are young teenagers coming from countries with a history of political instability and persecution such as the boat people in Southeast Asia in the 1970s and 1980s. Many of these "unaccompanied minors" are placed as foster children with families or with nongovernmental organizations (NGOs) in the host countries. Many of them work as domestic workers or engage in different entry level jobs that do not require complex skills. Many send remittances to their families but still manage to save combining work with school or training. There is little information to facilitate comparison of the benefits against the many costs and risks these migrant young people face.

This author had worked with the refugee camps in Southeast Asia in the 1980s as consultant to a Philippine-based international humanitarian NGO (Community and Family Services International) and experienced working with many "unaccompanied minors." Years later, while teaching in a university medical school in the United States, the author had the opportunity to follow-up at close range many of these young migrants who had turned into young adults and settled on the east and west coast of the country. Their stories are inspiring stories of resiliency and survival. They embraced fully the opportunities offered by their country of settlement. They did very well in school and higher education. Some have become doctors, dentists, and engineers. At least two, personally known to this author, work with U.S. Homeland Security. All are now raising their own families (see also chapter by Henderson et al. in this book).

Migrant Workers

A major global issue of current concern is the growing number of migrant workers coming from many developing countries in Asia and bound for the Middle East, Western European countries, and the rich neighboring countries and regions in Asia (e.g., Japan, South Korea, Singapore, Malaysia, China, Hong Kong, Taiwan). These migrant workers come from India, Sri Lanka, Bangladesh, Pakistan, the Philippines, Thailand, and Indonesia. They seem to share a common pattern of experience: driven by the need for better income, sending money home to support families, suffering indignities/abuses in the host country, and over time increasingly becoming alienated from the loved ones they support. The Philippines is a good case study of the phenomenon of overseas migrant workers. In the Philippines workers who have migrated abroad are known as "OFWs" (Overseas Filipino

Workers). They are regarded as the "modern heroes" of the country. Their remittances, amounting to billions of U.S. dollars yearly, make up the largest single source of foreign exchange, hard currency that alleviates the pressure on the Central Bank of the country and helps the country stay afloat despite the current global financial crisis.

There are 11 million "OFWs" around the globe making up about 11% of the total population of the country (Llorente 2008). They nurse the sick in London, teach in schools in New Jersey, drive fuel tanks in Saudi Arabia, navigate cruise ships and serve in cargo ships across the Pacific Ocean, serve *sake* to Japanese businessmen in Tokyo, take charge of domestic chores in Italy, and take care of little children as nannies in Singapore. While there are executives in mid-management ranks in multinationals and doctors and nurses in hospitals around the world, the great majority of OFWs are construction workers, domestic helpers, drivers, entertainers, dancers, caregivers, and nannies. One out of five Filipinos directly depends on money sent home by OFWs. In some towns, about half the families receive regular overseas remittances from fathers, husbands, wives, mothers, sons, and daughters.

The remittances have elevated the standard of living of families left at home. Families have been able to send children to better schools and gain access to good private health care services. Some families have been able to move to better houses in low poverty neighborhoods. The money also increases the family's consumption of material goods.

The first wave of Asian migrant workers was predominantly male. In recent years, however, Asian women have become the fastest growing component of international migrant workers (Raghavan 2002). In the case of the Philippines, women now account for 60% of legal migrant workers, and constitute about 94% of those in Asia. More than half of the women workers are mothers who leave their children behind.

Social Cost and Migrant Workers?

There is substantial evidence of the suffering and sacrifice borne by those who are forced to work overseas. Mothers and fathers bear much pain separating from their children and from one another. Children and young teenagers are left with grandparents or other relatives and in a few instances with neighbors who are paid to take care of the children. Some families do not survive the long separation, as evidenced by an epidemic of broken families, high dropout rates from school on the part of the children, adolescent pregnancy, and high rates of drug use. In many recipient families a culture of dependency insidiously develops, replacing the drive to be self-sufficient. A generation of children and relatives get used to waiting for the next mail or for the next text message on the mobile phone announcing that once again there is money in the bank. Some male OFWs express fears of going back home after many years of working overseas. They feel they have nothing to return to but broken homes, joblessness, and children who hardly know them. Children have desktops, laptops, computer game consoles, Game Boys, and iPods but they do not have a father or a mother or both. Affectively they express sadness and miss their parents, but cognitively they feel greater satisfaction with their lives when parents work overseas.

A Philippine NGO for migrant workers and returnees provides support to OFW families organizing youth summer camps for the children left behind. In a workshop the youth participants were asked: "Would you prefer your father to come home for good?" The majority of the youth participants actually wanted their fathers to continue working abroad. Their reasons included "there's more food on the table," "(when father) stays long at home there is a drastic cut in my allowance," "when they (fathers) are home, they just go out with their friends drinking," "they appear like strangers in the house." Sadly the children viewed their fathers as simply financiers and providers for the family (Nicodemus 1997).

A study conducted by the author (Banaag et al. 2005) on children left behind by overseas contract workers showed that children learn adaptive and maladaptive mechanisms when confronted with their loneliness and lack of parental guidance. Among the maladaptive behaviors are an excessive fascination with consumer goods and antisocial behavior problems when relating to family members and with peers. There was also a trend towards increased psychiatric disorders that included conduct disorder, major depression, anxiety disorder, dysthymia, and substance use.

Effects on Parenting

Medina (2001) took note of increasing solo parenting partly brought about by labor migration. She cited the problems of "weekend parenting" (when a parent who works in the city would visit her children in the village only on weekends once or twice a month) and "long-distance parenting" (when parents call from long distances, send text messages on the mobile phone, or leave voice messages). Parenting in this manner has weakened parental authority and control over their children. Contemporary communication technology has allowed overseas workers to narrow the long physical distance, but the psychological distance created by long-distance parenting over long periods of time remains difficult to narrow.

COMMUNICATION TECHNOLOGY AND MASS MEDIA

Children today are growing up in a world of revolutionary information technology, communication, and mass media. Children are surrounded by radio, television, DVDs, VCRs, mobile phones, personal computers, access to the Internet, chat rooms, social network sites, YouTube, blogs, IM (Instant Messenger), webcams, Skype, game consoles, and other technologies. Children endlessly play electronic games, online and offline, to the point of true addiction for some. The rapid proliferation of interactive and digital technologies in the past decades has transformed children's everyday routines causing both excitement and worry among parents, educators, and policy makers. Parents are thrilled as they watch their four-year-old boy adroitly moving the mouse of his laptop searching for and playing his favorite cartoon games. They are delighted as they hear him read the texts on the screen (he has learned to read the alphabet and numbers with software programs) and hear him talk to the characters. Will they still be thrilled when he is 15 and plays six hours straight on his electronic games staying up till three or four in the morning?

Access to technology and various media varies substantially from country to country and from region to region, but the spread of cyber-cafes in the cities and towns in developing countries has increased the access to new technologies and media even for the children of the poor. There can be little doubt that mass media and digital immersion affects children's cognitive, emotional, and social development. To understand exactly how the new technologies affect child development is a daunting task.

Television is probably the most ubiquitous of the visual mass media for entertainment and information. Even in many developing countries it is rapidly catching up with or outstripping the radio in its reach. A study supported by UNICEF found that seven out of ten households around the world have televisions sets (Lamb 1997). Although the television penetration into homes and lives of children is extensive, intensity of exposure is quite variable depending on the number of TV sets per 1000 residents, the number of broadcast channels, and the number of satellite per pay cable channels. Some countries like the United States have 817 TV sets per 1000 residents, 345 broadcast channels, and 387 satellite channels. Cambodia, on the other hand, has 8 TV sets per 1000 residents, 2 broadcast channels, and no satellite channels. The survey was conducted in 1997; the figures are likely to be different by now. A UNESCO study (Groebel 1998) finds television viewing to be common place and extensive in countries in Asia, Latin America, Europe, and Africa. Television has become an important and powerful presence in the lives of many children.

Adverse Effects of Television

The spread of television around the globe has raised many concerns, some of particular relevance to children and youth. Wilcox (2004) underscored three issues that tend to dominate policy discussions related to children's television programs; the need for educational programming, the threat of over-commercialization in children's television, and the potential harmful effects of violent programs and sexually explicit content. Of all the issues related to children's television viewing none has drawn more public concern and scholarly interest than the issue of violence. Researchers around the world do not unanimously agree that TV violence is a threat to the mental health and well-being of children. However, the majority of scholars believe that exposure to media violence can potentially harm children in several ways. Wilcox (2007) reviewed recent research on media violence. He reiterated the conclusion that there are three primary types of effects on children's viewing violent television programs. First, there is ample evidence to support the contention that children learn aggressive behaviors and attitudes from viewing violence on TV. Children who are heavily exposed to TV violence are more likely to see violence as a reasonable means to solve disputes. Second, those children who view high levels of TV violence are more likely to develop anxiety over what they perceive as the "mean world." They develop exaggerated fears of becoming a victim of violence. Finally, children who view a lot of violence on TV are more likely to be desensitized to violence. It is important to recognize that not all violent content results in negative effects on the viewer's attitudes, affect, and behavior. Wilcox (2004) cited the work of a group of researchers at the University of California at Santa Barbara (see Wilson et al. 1998) that contextualized violence on TV programs. Based on their review of the research, the Santa Barbara group created a composite index to describe the characteristics of programs that place young viewers at greater risk from the harmful effects of media violence. This composite index includes five factors: (1) whether the perpetrator is *attractive,* (2) whether the violence is *justified,* (3) whether the violence is *rewarded or punished* immediately after it occurs, (4) whether *harm and pain* is shown, and (5) whether the portrayal is likely to be perceived as *realistic.* Based on this composite index, the researchers found that nearly 20% of all TV programs containing violence are high risk. More importantly, 50% of these high risk programs targeted children, and nearly all of these programs (92%) intended for children were animations. Cartoons designed for young children, it appears, have attractive heroes who engage in violence that is portrayed as justified, is often rewarded or rarely punished, and results in minimal harm to the victims. Many adults and critics dismiss concerns about cartoon violence, not mindful of the developmental nature of young children, especially those below seven years of age, who frequently cannot "discount" cartoon violence in their minds. Although the Santa Barbara researchers reported on violence in TV programming in the U.S., it can have consequences due to the distribution of U.S. television programs to many parts of the world. Television programming has clearly been globalized.

Impact of Information Technology

Like with television, much research has been done on the impact of digital communication and information technology on child development and mental health, although the research literature in this area remains fragmented and somewhat inconclusive. The computer, like the TV, has become the focus of concern for parents because of perceived potential harm to their children. The concern is proportional to the increasing reports of gaming addiction coming from different parts of the world. Parents get upset when the hours spent playing electronic games or chatting on social network sites compete with time spent for homework and for other school and family activities. This situation has created an almost universal focus of tension between parents and children.

As a tool for communication, the computer, like the mobile phone, mitigates the space and time constraints of interpersonal communication. With a mobile phone, text messages, and the Internet (e-mail, IM, webcam, or chat rooms), communication is instantaneous. This technology is of special benefit for parents who work overseas and the children they leave behind. It has enabled "long distance" parenting to happen in real time. It has also allowed loved ones to remain connected and for business transactions to happen instantly. Modern technology has built a world of connectedness.

Modern technology also allows children to be active participants and collaborators, rather than passive recipients, in their own learning. In an effort to understand the value and use of technology in fostering child development and well-being, a group of researchers in the U.S. identified and synthesized literature reviews and meta-analyses that focused on the positive effects of technology on children (Atkinson et al. 2001). The researchers reviewed 119 relevant materials and came to the conclusion that empirical research supports the positive impact of educational technology on academic performance and on specific cognitive and social/emotional elements. Among the articles cited was the work by Pierce (1994) that reviewed the literature related to the use of technology with children aged five years and below, including children with disabilities. The technologies included in Pierce's article were television, interactive videos, computers, and software used as part of the curriculum for young children. The research evidence supported the positive impact of computer use on several developmental domains. Several studies reviewed by Pierce demonstrated that computer use helped children develop higher thought processes from concrete to the beginning of symbolic representational thought. Via the computer, preschool children with and without disabilities had greater language production measured by the number of words spoken per minute than when they were participating in other learning activities. In terms of social and emotional development, the children preferred cooperative learning by working in pairs or small groups, improving their interpersonal relationships.

Research cited by Pierce also underscored the special benefits of computer assisted learning for children with disabilities. Conducted largely with hearing impaired and deaf children, research has shown that technology benefited the children in several domains: social skills, peer acceptance, social interaction, reading and writing skills, and communication through sign language. The technology helped the children feel some control over their environment with computer games serving as a point for joint attention and social interaction because the children used the materials in a collaborative way, thus improving their social skills.

Simply using technological applications was not sufficient to achieve developmental gains. Pierce cited several factors that enhanced the positive effect of technology: type of teaching strategy, type of learning activity, features of the instructional design, parental involvement, and establishing clear guidelines and support for social interactions and integration in the school settings.

Research on Information Technology and Child Development

Summarizing the effectiveness of technology used in education, based on an extensive review of the literature, Atkinson and colleagues (2001) cite the following benefits:

All studies reviewed supported the effectiveness of educational technology in child development cognitively, emotionally, and socially.

Focusing on student achievements measured by standardized test scores showed, on average, students in elementary and high schools who used computer based instructions scored significantly higher than students in the control group without computers.

Research among young children showed positive impact on the children's cognitive abilities such as memory, concentration, spatial and logical problem solving, creativity, artistic abilities, verbal and nonverbal language skills, and early mathematic skills.

Research with secondary and high school students has shown positive impact on reading, writing quality, mathematics (analytical skills and problem solving), computer programming (logical thinking, metacognitive processes).

Research also consistently found learning through technology was intrinsically appealing to the children. It promoted positive self-concept, self-esteem, the ability to collaborate, and improved interpersonal skills. Students were more motivated and showed more positive attitudes towards learning.

Contrary to the often repeated concern that technology use will isolate children, research showed that computer use encouraged collaborative learning and access to online peers, experts, and learning communities, thereby reducing social isolation.

Admittedly, Atkinson and colleagues focused on the positive effects of new technology as applied and incorporated in classroom curricula. Outside of formal learning settings, a heated debate continues on the impact of video games on children.

Effects of Information Technology on Child Behavior

Public concerns and scholarly studies revolve around the impact of violent video games on children and the potential danger of addiction. Like in the case of television, opinions are divided on the impact of violent games. Many experts agree that excessive exposure to violent games may make some children more likely to behave in aggressive and harmful ways towards others, or become less sensitive to the pain and suffering of others. Some believe that violence in video games may actually be more potentially harmful than violence in television. "First person" games in which the player sees himself as the shooter can desensitize the player to violence. These types of games are actually used in military training (Gallagher n.d.).

The issue of gaming addiction continues to be a common cause of alarm for parents. In an interview, Gallagher expressed concern about the potential for addiction in relation to video games because these games have high levels of quick gratification and the player is almost constantly being rewarded. Some behaviors commonly associated with addiction include excessive preoccupation with playing the games to the point of sleep deprivation, disruption to daily life, playing to escape problems or bad feeling, and withdrawal from family/friends/school. There is no universal agreement on the profile of a child or adolescent who is at risk of becoming addicted to video games.

Often lost in the debate over violence and addiction to video games is the scholarly work on the cognitive benefits associated with video games (Green and Bavelier 2006). Games put a premium on hand-eye coordination and reaction time. Many games require players to respond exceptionally fast to new "enemies" that pop out of nowhere and need to be eliminated quickly. Experiments that compared players and non-players showed that players have significantly better spatial and sensory motor skills, much improved eye-hand coordination, faster reaction times, and enhanced overall attention capacity. They can effectively maintain focus on a central item and still keep their peripheral attention on the alert.

Taken as a whole, technologies like television, computers, mobile phones, and video games have created a digital culture where children and youth move with greater facility than their parents and other adults. As a consequence, there is a greater disconnect between parents and children today. Elkind (2003) points out the common features of this digital culture. First, it is a speed-dominated culture, fast and getting faster. Young people become impatient and frustrated if they don't get instant responses from online sites that may be thousands of miles away. Second, it is a screen culture, from the movie screen to television screen to computer screen, and now to the downsized mobile phone screen. Young people spend a great portion of their time reading from a screen. Book reading is a less common experience. Third, it is an information culture. Children and youth have immediate access to information without moving out of their homes or a cyber-cafe. There is no need to travel to libraries that scholars of another age had to do in order to research any area of study. Finally, it is a communication culture. The Internet and mobile phones have made communication with peers and loved ones an instant connection. Growing up in this technological culture affects children's language, and perception of reality. The availability of mobile phones, social network sites, chat rooms, and IM has made immediate access to friends possible, and may have simply worsened the divide between parents and children.

CONCLUSIONS

The world struggles in trying to balance the positive and the negative effects of industrialization, globalization, urbanization, and the unparalleled growth of technology. Children are growing up in a world of technology increasingly unfamiliar to their parents. The traditional culture of children is fast disappearing. Children have less time and less space for unstructured play and outdoor games. Children of middle class families are surrounded by many man-made toys. Their digital games are so engaging and addicting that they do not enjoy the world of spontaneous play that allows their imagination to bloom. While the culture of childhood is fast changing, the nature of children remains the same. They still need to be protected from their immature state and the hazards of their rapidly changing environment. While they enjoy the products of new technology, they should be protected from their harmful effects, like pornographic sites and violent programming in television and digital games. They still need nurturing guiding relationships with parents who can help them grow up feeling good about themselves. It is more important than ever before that parents continue to reach out and connect with their children. It is incumbent on child advocates to put children's concerns on the political and economic agenda of the country. It is essential that national governments provide the necessary policies and institutions that will ensure that children grow into physically and mentally healthy adults.

REFERENCES

Andrews, A.B. "Children and Family Lite." In N. Kaufman & I. Rizzini (Eds.), *Globalization and Children*. New York: Kluwer Academic Publisher, 2004.

Atkinson, N.L., Silsby, J., Gold, R.S., Koeple, P.T., Chokshi, A.N., and Gutierrez, L.S. *Technology and development a ten-year review of reviews.* Public Health Informatics Research Laboratory. USA, 2001.

Banaag, C., Quirejero, M., and Balderrama, N. "Long term effects of separation on children of overseas contract workers." *The Philippine Journal of Psychiatry* 29 (2005): 21-26.

Bartlett, S. "Children's experience of the physical environment in poor urban settlements and the implication for policy planning and practice." *Environment & Urbanization* 11(2) (1999): 63-73.

Bloom, D., & Khanna, T. "Urban Revolution." Finance and Development 44(3) (2007): 9-14.

Carballo, M. *The challenge of immigration and health.* International Center for Migration and Health. 2007. www.icmh.ch.

Coleman, D. *Europe's Population in the 1990s.* Oxford: Oxford University Press, 1996.

Durkheim, E. *Suicide: A study in sociology.* Glencoe, IL: Free Press, 1951.

Elkind, D. *Technology's impact on child growth and development.* www.cio.com, September 22, 2003.

Federman, M., and Levine, D. *The effects of industrialization on school enrollment and child labor.* 2002. http://www.fordschool.umich.edu/edts/pdfs.

Gallagher, R. *Video Games: Cons and Pros.* NYU Child Study Center. http://www.education.com/reference/article/Ref_Video_Games_Cons/.

Gauthier, A. "Family policies in industrialized countries: Is there a convergence?" *Population* 57 (2002): 447-474.

Green, S.C., and Bevalier, D. "The cognitive neuroscience of video games." In L. Humphreys & P. Messaris (Eds.), *Digital Media: Transformations in Human Communication.* New York: Peter Lang Publishing, 2006.

Groebel, J. "The UNESCO global study on media violence." In U. Carlsson & C. von Feilitzen (Eds.), *Children and Media Violence.* Sweden: Coronet Books, 1998.

IPEC. *Every child counts: New global estimates on child labor.* International Labor Organization, 2002 http://www.ilo.org/ipecinfo/product/viewProduct.do?productId=742.

Kaufman, N., Rizzini, I., Wilson, K., and Bush, M. "The impact of global economic, political, and social transformation on the lives of children." In N. Kaufman and I. Rizzini (Eds.), *Globalization and Children.* New York: Kluwer Academic Publishers, 2004.

Lamb, R. *The bigger picture: Audio-visual survey and recommendation.* New York: United Nations Children's Fund, 1997.

Leventhal, T., and Brooks-Gunn, J. "Moving to Opportunity: An experimental study of neighborhood effects on mental health." *American Journal of Public Health* 93(9) (2003): 1576-1582.

Llorente, S. *A futuristic look into the Filipino diasporo: Trends, issues, and implications.* In the *Journal of Filipino Studies*, an electronic journal (2009): http://journaloffilipinostudies.csuestbay.edu/html/llorente.html.

Medina, B. *The Filipino Family.* Manila: University of the Philippines Press, 2001.

Nicodemus, M.F. '*Separated by opportunity: The impact of overseas migration of Filipino Families,* presented at the Filipino Migrant Conference, Athens, November 1997 www.philsol.nl/F-OFFamily-nov97.htm.

Pierce, P.L. *Technology integration into early childhood curricula: Where we've been, where we are, where we should go."* Chapel Hill, NC: Center for Literacy and Disability Studies, 1994.

Raghavan, C. *Asian female migrant workers require protection.* Third World Network, November 2002. www.twnside.org.sg/title/ilo1-cn.htm.

Sardon, J-P. "Recent changes in the demographic situation of the developed countries." *Population* 12 (2000): 293.

Shanahan, M.J. "Pathways to a adulthood in changing societies: Variability and mechanism in life course perspective." *Annual Review of Sociology* 12 (2000): 667-692.

UN-Habitat. *Annual Report 2008.* www.unhabitat.org/pmss/getPage. asp?page=bookView&book=2634.

UNICEF. *Migration and Children.* Innocenti Research Centre. www.unicef-irc.org/ knowledge_pages/resource_pages/migration/index.html.

WHO. *The global burden of disease.* 2004 Update.

WHO. *World urbanization prospects.* 2005.

Wilson, B.J., Kunkel, D., Linz, D., Potter, W. J., Donnerstein, E., Smith, S.L., Blumessthal, E., and Berry, M. "Violence in television programming overall: University of California, Santa Barbara Study." *National Television Violence Study (Vol. 2).* Thousand Oaks, CA: Sage, 1998.

5

Child Refugee Mental Health

Schuyler W. Henderson, Charles Baily, and Stevan Weine

INTRODUCTION

In this chapter we review mental health and psychosocial approaches to child refugees using a narrative perspective to explore how these approaches are not only models for practice or investigation, but are themselves stories about what children go through as refugees and how we might be able to help them. These stories compete with many others for attention, including those that come out of politics and socioeconomic development, and in our opinion need to be more compelling and more open if they are going to be heard and help build care and preventive services for child refugees.

We will consider how utilizing a narrative framework to address core issues in mental health and psychosocial services for child refugees may help to improve upon our current best models. The most prominent and contentious recent narrative about suffering in child refugees has been developed around the paradigm of trauma and traumatic stress. This centers on the clinical diagnosis of post-traumatic stress disorder (PTSD), and has produced a body of literature and myriad clinical services that have indeed helped countless children make sense of and work through the consequences of trauma, but it is also a limited narrative in that sufferers are regarded as disordered and impaired and are usually expected to participate in individualized clinic-based care. Furthermore, this narrative has been critiqued for its limitations—its cultural limitations, its public health limitations, its human rights limitations—and for the adverse effects of having a narrative that worked. The over-generalization of a model to include those who do not fit its parameters and the over-dedication of resources that are channelled into individual approaches all too often neglect, for example, the community and family dimensions of child refugees which have been better addressed through other psychosocial frameworks.

Our goal here is not simply to treat mental disorders in child refugees, but to reclaim the social and psychological landscape of childhood for those impacted by political violence and/or forced migration. This means listening not just to the stories people tell about themselves, but the stories that we tell about childhood, the stories that come from and constitute the world of the child—children's stories, but also the stories of parents, grand-parents, other family members, teachers, clergy, professional and lay help-ers. As we hope to show here, it also means listening to the stories we tell when we design psychosocial interventions and research studies. These sto-ries form the basis for the possibility of the social construction (or recon-struction) of childhood.

We believe that the clinical goals of psychosocial interventions are to help children, families, and communities restore the world of childhood; to navigate the politically, socially, and psychologically dangerous waters of being a "refugee"; and to rearticulate what has been torn apart. The ethical goal of a narrative approach is to openly receive, understand, manage, and/ or resolve competing and conflicting narratives, be they stories of develop-ment, resilience, vulnerability, trauma, parenting, schooling, the future, or stories that surprise us because we never knew of them before. In our opin-ion, attending to these ethical dimensions can enhance our capacity to build mental health and psychosocial interventions that are more respon-sive to restoring the very human bonds that are under attack in political violence: family bonds, cultural bonds, the social milieus that humans thrive in, and the narrative milieus that allow people to live in a relation-ship to the past in their history and to the future in their hopes.

CONTESTING THE CHILD REFUGEE

The narrative approach has roots in the precepts of Mikhail Bakhtin and dialogism; people do not have a single story but rather multiple stories they draw upon, create together, contest and change, depending on the stories that are being told around them and which they help craft (Bakhtin 1984; Emerson 1997; Morson and Emerson 1991; Weine 2006). Regarding child refugees and their families, this approach may start with questions that elicit political stories (e.g., how do some people become refugees?), social stories (e.g., who were we as a people before we became refugees and how has that changed?), psychological stories (e.g., what sort of person have I become?); the approach will also elicit parents' stories (e.g., how can I teach my children about the values that have helped our family and community to survive?), and children's stories (e.g., who can I trust in a world that has let me down?). Psychosocial narratives fit into, compete with, and sometimes contradict other narratives including political ones (some of which are deftly laid out by the United Nations High Commission for Refugees 2007a) and social ones (e.g., what is expected of refugee youth and their host communities when they are resettled?). A narrative approach not only pays close attention to these stories but believes that there is great power in them; a narrative approach tries to understand what work is being done by multiple narratives interacting with one another, towards what ends, and whether there are ways that we can make them work better in this case to help child refugees.

Artists can have great skill at representing these multiple narratives of trauma and resilience (Weine 2006). Thus, we find it helpful to begin with a brief vignette—a work of comic fiction. In the summer of 2008 Garry Trudeau's Pulitzer Prize winning comic strip *Doonesbury* dealt with an issue that had been mostly overlooked in much of the media: Iraqi refugees (World Vision 2007).

The cartoon (Trudeau 2008) featured one of Doonesbury's long-standing characters, a journalist named Roland Burton Hedley III, interviewing an Iraqi family who had fled to Syria. Hedley persistently reframes the family's exile as their own choice and finds every opportunity to question their support for the American military project in Iraq. As Hedley offers his heavily editorialized report, focusing on what he imagines is the flourishing of the 15-year-old daughter's newfound hope after the American surge, she is in the background trying to get his attention. She eventually excuses herself to leave for work—as a prostitute. This cartoon is telling three very important stories of immediate relevance to pediatric mental health in refugee populations.

Working as a Prostitute

First, children who are displaced because of political violence are not simply passive witnesses to or victims of political violence accidentally caught in the crossfire. Trudeau's punchline highlights an under-reported and under-represented aspect of contemporary political violence, the way in which children are incorporated into the pervasive political violence directed specifically at children. This ranges from sexual exploitation of children in conflict situations (see, for example, United Nations webpage: http://www. un.org/children/conflict/english/sexualviolence.html) and in refugee camps, including by humanitarian workers (United Nations High Commission for Refugees [UNHCR] 2002), to attacks on the cultural and social institutions of childhood. For example, the United Nations has reported on systematic and deliberate attacks on schoolchildren, teachers, and school buildings in Afghanistan, Iraq, and Thailand (United Nations 2009). Furthermore, children are not passive agents in a world that is collapsing around them.

One of the most visible and, indeed, narrativized ways in which children become active participants in the violence is when they are recruited into armed groups around the world including in Colombia, the Democratic Republic of Congo, Sudan, Uganda, Chad, Sri Lanka, and Nepal (e.g., Betancourt 2008). The notion that children are accidental victims of the wars and political violence occurring around them is one that is preserved in many narratives of political violence—including in much journalism, where this violence is under-reported or mis-reported.

The world of childhood is directly and purposely attacked but psychosocial interventions for refugee children can address their real world needs in a context that recognizes how children are directly targeted, exploited, and incorporated into the violence; failing to do so risks irrelevance. Children are active participants in this world, which may have specific clinical ramifications: for example, those who are involved in the violence as child soldiers may be at increased risk of more severe mental health consequences (Korht et al. 2008); but this also has narrative consequences because these children have stories to tell about how, when, and why they have become incorporated into the violence.

"Refugee"

The use of quotation marks around "refugee" indicates Roland Hedley's skepticism about the political, legal, and social status of this family. People fleeing their native lands as refugees are perpetually subject to questions of credibility and legitimacy, often living in a legal limbo where they may be expected to "prove" such things as a fear of persecution (UNHCR 1998). In other words, their life stories are viewed as suspect; inconsistencies, which are part of any narrative, are not only interpreted as possible lies but can have disastrous legal consequences including rejected asylum.

It is worth recalling the familiar definition of "refugee" offered initially by the United Nations in its Convention and Protocol Relating to the Status of Refugees, in 1951; in its current form it reads:

> A person who is outside his or her country of nationality or habitual residence; has a well-founded fear of persecution because of his or her race, religion, nationality, membership of a particular social group or political opinion; and is unable or unwilling to avail himself or herself of the protection of that country, or to return there, for fear of persecution. (UNHCR 1951)

And yet there is much to be desired in this formulation which tells a particular story about how and why people become refugees; criticisms have ranged from the philosophical to the practical, political, and ethical (e.g., Shacknove 1985). This particular definition, for example, might leave out those who are internally displaced due to famine, hurricanes, and political strife but cannot cross a border. Furthermore, much political violence is enacted through economic inequalities, and yet "economic migrants" are explicitly excluded from the determinant of "refugee" (UNHCR 2007b).

The narrative framework guiding psychosocial interventions can account for the political uncertainty and social marginalization accompanying refugee status while ensuring a cautious approach to the legal and political dimensions of this status. Organizations that provide psychological services without any legal and social context are likely to be unappealing and underwhelming, not just because they do not match the "needs" of some populations, but because they will not fit into their current narratives about who they are, what they want to achieve, and how they want to re-organize their lives. On the other hand, when organizations focus on providing affidavits and psychological/medical-legal advice without providing broader services, the organizations are integrating themselves into the socio-legal machinery without meeting family and community needs; as anybody who has done affidavits knows it is far easier to describe psychological suffering for a court than it is to help that person find community resources for support and relief after the interview is completed.

What She Now Has in Abundance Is Hope

We like stories to have happy endings. We want to find the moral in the story, the "one good thing," the uplifting note that leaves us smiling. In thinking about a narrative framework for mental health and psychosocial services we can be very careful about where and how we find "hope." The irony in Hedley's formulation, of course, is that a child without food and without schooling would have a hard time clinging to "hope."

In the cartoon, the reporter offers the abstract concept of "hope" in place of such necessities as food and schooling. Narratives around political violence tend to justify or romanticize the destruction, violence, and suffering with grand themes, such as "freedom" and "independence." Mental health researchers, amongst others, have shown the yawning chasm between the rhetoric used to justify political violence and the realities of suffering in daily lives (e.g., Weine 1999). This is not simply a quasi-ethical problem involving neutrality, logistical collaboration with perpetrating organizations, or the like; this is about negotiating the uncomfortable tension between psychosocial features of living, i.e., from "mental health" to living in hope, in freedom, or autonomously, and the disruption of life itself that occurs with political violence. The larger concepts we use to organize our lives—culture, society, family, childhood, etc.—are implicated in the political violence and the impulse is to shy away from these and to prioritize or romanticize life itself; it is pragmatic to address the basic needs of refugees with shelter and food, but failing to attend to them as people, i.e., as social, cultural, and psychological agents, is to perpetuate the violence against them.

SCOPE OF THE PROBLEM

A cartoon can be tremendously insightful into the experiences of refugee children and highlight often neglected aspects of their stories. Another way of telling the story of refugees around the world is to draw upon global statistics to show how vast the problem of displacement is in the world today. The United Nations High Commission for Refugees identified 31.7 million "people of concern" in 2007, a broad designation that includes, but is not limited to, refugees, asylum seekers, internally displaced persons (IDPs) protected or assisted by UNHCR, and stateless persons. Of this 31.7 million, there were an estimated 11.4 million refugees (UNHCR 2007c). While media depictions may suggest that refugees are flooding into the West the vast majority (82%, or 9.2 million refugees) are located in the developing world. During 2007 the United States of America resettled 48,300 people; Canada resettled 11,300; Australia resettled 9,600; and Sweden resettled 1,800. The two largest populations of refugees during 2007 were Afghans (accounting for 3 million refugees) and Iraqis (accounting for 2.3 million refugees).

Of the 31.7 million "people of concern" in 2007, approximately half (49%) of the refugees were female, which appeared to be a fairly stable distribution across the world. The age distribution, however, changes by geography. In Africa and Asia, children and adolescents often make up the majority, accounting for over half the population (in some areas, reaching 55%). Older populations were found in Europe, particularly amongst Bosnian and Kosovar populations, where there was a larger proportion of elderly "people of concern." But overall, approximately half of the refugees in the world are children (United Nations Children's Fund 2006).

We can look at these numbers and tell a fairly compelling story; all over the world there are a great many children and families who have lost their homes, jobs, friends, and schools, who are living in states of legal and political limbo, and who may have been exposed to violence, loss, and exploitation.

Within this context, another broad narrative approach can be organized around time and phases. Fazel and Stein propose that children who are forced to flee persecution face three periods, each of which poses its own risks: during the conflict in the country of origin, in their journey from their homes, and in resettlement (Fazel and Stein 2002). Similarly, Lustig and colleagues (2004a) describe the stages of preflight, flight, and resettlement. This way of organizing the story elucidates how refugee children are likely to be exposed to stressors at each stage. For example, during the preflight phase, children are often caught up in social and political conflict as a result of civil war or other forms of institutional violence, and may witness or engage in violence, not infrequently experiencing threats or persecution either directly or to their loved ones (Sourander 1998). In the flight phase, children may spend months traveling to their destination country, either with their families or alone. With the tightening of immigration controls, increasingly children are being entrusted to smugglers thus exposing them to potential abuse and exploitation and possibly life-threatening conditions (Fazel and Stein 2002). The resettlement phase in the destination country carries with it its own set of stressors, such as acculturation issues and stigma within the local culture. It is worth remembering that immigration itself is a challenging experience and has been associated with increased rates of psychopathology (Bhugra and Minas 2007). This has been studied extensively, if haphazardly, from research in Europe on increased rates of psychosis in immigrant populations (McKenzie et al. 2008) to broader studies of anxiety and depression and other mental health disorders in immigrants across the globe. On the other hand, the association between immigration and psychopathology has been challenged. A number of studies of Mexicans in the United States have proposed a "migration of the fittest" and "healthy migrant" effect (e.g., Escobar 1998; Vega and Lopez 2001) to explain the paradoxical finding that despite socioeconomic disadvantages Mexican immigrants in fact have significantly fewer mental health problems than people of Mexican descent born in the United States. We will return to narratives of resettlement towards the end of the chapter.

Based on these large populations and comprehensive stories of persecution and flight it is possible to organize narratives around risk factors, describing the various experiences that could make a child prone to suffering or unable to cope. There are a large number of risks that can be situated within these broader narratives, usually formulated as risk factors for psychopathology or psychosocial impairments (Fazel and Stein 2003; Lustig et al. 2004). Environmental factors include displacement from home, exposure to violence (i.e., war, murder, rape, assaults, kidnapping), poverty, and starvation. Sociocultural factors include cultural displacement and isolation, acculturative stresses, and the challenge of diaspora (re-organizing communities, new conflicts in resettlement, and so on). Psychological risk factors include the number of transitions, possibility of further resettlements, refoulement (von Lersner et al., 2008), uncertainty about future, disruptions in daily life, and barriers to service access (including legal, mental health, medical, and other supportive services). The child's own risk factors will depend upon his or her developmental history and will include losing out on educational opportunities, the number and type of traumatic events, psychiatric comorbidity, learning difficulty, disability, mental retardation, and physical health. Parental factors include orphaning, loss of family, PTSD/depression in mother/parents, unemployment, hopelessness, distress and dysfunction in parents, and generational conflicts/expectations. Although Gilligan (2009) is correct to point out that the concept of vulnerability can be contested in a number of ways, such as by questioning whether the notion of childhood itself is cross-culturally valid and how determinations of vulnerability by powerful political interests open up the opportunity for interventions that are not without political, economic, or social consequences, there is ample evidence theoretically and empirically informed that some children when faced with the onslaught of what are termed "risk factors" suffer on account of their vulnerability.

Each one of these narrative frameworks (the global statistics, the narrative of flight, the narrative of risk) contributes to a broad understanding of where children are and what they might be going through. Given these narratives of tribulation and risk, we expect to find narratives of suffering.

NARRATIVES OF SUFFERING

A central issue to address in understanding the mental health and psychosocial consequences of becoming a refugee for children and adolescents, and for developing mental health and psychosocial programs for children and adolescents, is the nature of the suffering that youth experience. Political violence and displacement, losing one's family, community, and cultural integrity, isolation and segregation, victimization, and trauma can all create or worsen human suffering. The suffering can be manifested in clinically visible ways, i.e., in mental illness, substance abuse, or misery, and it can be manifested socially; in loss of one's place in society (as with unemployment or religious discrimination), in the perpetuation of violence, and in the disintegration of familial and community bonds.

The distinction that has been drawn between individual suffering and social suffering is an important one insofar as it draws our attention to the multiple ways in which human suffering can be experienced and reminds us of the social bonds that both sustain us and, when they are attacked, make us vulnerable. The distinction becomes muddied, however, when we realize that the two are not incompatible and can indeed overlay one another (Zarowsky 2004). The interrelatedness of the individual and the social is always present in the world of child refugees but is prioritized and framed differently by mental health and psychosocial responses.

Mental Health Perspectives

Within the narrative of suffering, one approach is to explain some of the suffering in terms of mental disorders. Epidemiological research into psychopathology in refugee populations has suggested increased risk of emotional distress, post-traumatic stress disorder, depressive disorders, anxiety disorders, and somatic disorders (see Lustig et al. 2004, for a review). Many of the studies that have been conducted have significant limitations, which are usually acknowledged by the authors (though decried as "weaknesses" by some commentators) and are often ethical and cultural compromises that allow the research to be conducted transparently, a point astutely made by Novins about First Nation Canadians (Novins 2009). These limitations include small sample sizes; minimal or no randomization; limited use of controls; and limited blinding. The studies take place in different countries, with different populations, and different age groups; with children, adolescents, and families in different stages of resettlement there is little basis for generalizing the results. The studies also tend to use heterogeneous treatment modalities, outcome measures, and instruments. Nevertheless, the studies do tell a story.

In a review, Fazel and colleagues (2005) identified five studies with 260 refugee children and found a range of PTSD prevalence rates from 7-17%. Papageorgiou and colleagues (2000) examined 95 Bosnian children in a study notable in that more than a quarter of the children (28%) had lost a parent, and the father was absent or injured in 27% of the cases. Almost half of the children in the sample (47%) scored within the clinical range on the Depression Self-Rating Scale for Children, and approximately a quarter had significant scores on the Revised Children's Manifest Anxiety Scale (27%) and on the Impact of Event Scale (28%).

These studies suggest that one way of looking at suffering is to identify children with depression and post-traumatic symptoms; similar studies using the same premises can offer insights into other contexts. In a small study in Greece, the authors compared immigrant children and families to local Greek controls; they did not find an increase in psychiatric diagnoses or service utilization, although they did find an increase in what they termed "psychosocial diagnoses," related to their finding that "immigrant families had significantly worse economic situations, lower status jobs, worse housing and were usually uninsured" (Anagnostopoulos et al. 2004). Two studies paid close attention to the roles of family in pediatric refugee mental health. Tousignant and coresearches (1999) sampled 203 adolescents from 35 countries in Quebec, finding increased rates of psychopathology (21% compared to 11% in a survey of adolescents in the same province), and, in particular, increased rates of anxiety (13% with overanxious disorder). Of particular interest, they also observed that long-term paternal unemployment in the first year of settlement was associated with psychopathology in the adolescents, and family structure (single mother status) was associated with psychopathology in the boys. Thabet and colleagues looked at 100 families, with 200 parents and 197 children aged 9-18 years, and found not only that being exposed to war trauma impacted both parents' and children's mental health, but that their emotional responses appeared to be interrelated (Thabet et al. 2008).

Despite the insights that studies such as the aforementioned provide, the "mental health" approach has been critiqued from a number of different angles. We will briefly provide a précis of some of these critiques of the mental health narrative. Many have asked whether mental disorders are sufficiently universal to apply across cultures, and especially the extent to which these categories are social constructs (Summerfield 2001; Summerfield 2008); this question has been adapted to critique research technologies casting doubt on whether the instruments used to detect mental disorders are valid for any particular population (Gilligan 2009). Another critique is that even if these diagnoses do have cross-cultural validity, the process is not sensitive and specific enough; large numbers of refugees are given a diagnosis, the diagnosis may not be enduring, and the diagnosis may not even speak to particular needs at any particular time. Furthermore, much suffering that is identified may be considered a normal response to the abnormal situation of being a refugee, and a particular label will hardly be helpful. Yet another concern is that the search for mental disorders is a type of labeling; it may result in stigma, confusion (regarding, for example, translation or the permanence of the diagnosis), and pathologizing refugee populations. Given the way in which immigrants and refugees have been characterized as carriers of disease across time (Fairchild 2003), psychiatric illness is added to the list of pathogens being carried across borders.

These problems are all amplified for children and adolescents. Though there is a growing and sophisticated body of research that has created insightful and useful models of childhood emotional suffering the empirical and scientific basis is not as well established as for adults, which means that confidence in generalizations and applicability is limited when adapting these models for children and adolescents in such particular circumstances. While "development" too often seems to end with the end of childhood, as if development ceases when one becomes an "adult" (this is, in fact, only one narrative of development whose end-point is adulthood), it is nevertheless clear that the centrality of "development" to children and adolescents means that children at different ages will respond in different ways, will have different needs and vulnerabilities, and will have different strengths and resilience. All of these developmental differences will play a role in how and why children respond to the sociocultural, familial, and political circumstances involved in becoming a refugee; and these developmental processes will all have cultural dimensions of their own (Webb and Davies 2003).

The Tiered or Pyramid Model

Critiques of a "mental health" perspective are important and many of them can be effectively addressed as part of a dialogue. In response to the broad critiques described above we might point out that there do seem to be experiences that are universal and there are ways of integrating different cultural models, even technological biomedical ones that seem so distinct from "traditional" cultures (terminology we would call into question if we had more time—these are, again, narratives about what constitutes culture itself). Furthermore, as narratives are shared, it is often discovered that we have much to learn from one another, but also much to teach. Stigma, an extensive incorporated narrative of exclusion, is a social reality that can be tempered with knowledge and compassion. Finally, it is widely recognized that in any population there may be some people who would indeed benefit from a "mental health" perspective that relies on biomedical paradigms and specialized psychological and psychiatric services.

The critiques and responses form a narrative as to what needs to be addressed, and it is one not without its own sociopolitical agenda; those who wish to address severe mental illness are cast as pathologizers who miss the larger picture while those who wish to address broader psychosocial needs risk neglecting the most vulnerable and those whose psychological needs are the greatest, and so on. But, we would argue, this is also an ethical problem; how do we manage these irreconcilable narratives and in so doing produce one that is responsive to the real lives of child refugees and resonates in the eyes of the public? Narrative approaches can develop complexity and richness, and so avoid caricature of opposing arguments, and can help develop the question at hand. If one is going to address the suffering that can be a consequence of political violence, and if one wants to bolster the innate resilience that can pull refugee children and families through difficult times what is it that we want to address and what is it that we want to bolster?

One narrative that is emerging out of this conflict is the tiered model (Hodes 2002; Wessells 2009). The broad foundation is to provide basic, general, and universal needs that can be addressed through broad public health interventions such as providing shelter and latrines in refugee camps, or language skills and work opportunities during the resettlement phase. The next level is to provide basic cultural needs, again reaching the majority of any population; the focus is more social than psychological, and includes safe places for children to play and access to education. The next level includes broad psychosocial interventions to address social fragmentation, and empowering individuals, families, and communities and include, for example, addressing reproductive health needs. Finally, one needs to address the frank psychopathology that requires specialist mental health interventions. For addressing specific mental health and psychosocial needs in emergency situations the Inter-Agency Standing Committee recommended a pyramid where the bottom layer includes basic services and security; the second layer, which may not be needed by everybody, covers services for family and community support, including family reunification and communal healing ceremonies; the third layer describes the supports necessary for a smaller number of people who additionally require more focused individual, family, or group interventions, such as psychological first aid and basic mental health; the tip of the pyramid includes the specialized psychiatric and psychological services that are required "for the small percentage of the population whose suffering, despite the supports already mentioned, is intolerable and who may have significant difficulties in basic daily functioning" (Inter-Agency Standing Committee 2007).

While inquiry into the cultural and practical value of psychiatric diagnoses is an important one, and the mutual critiques that stimulate discussion and editorials is academically healthy, few, to our knowledge, have disputed the pyramidal or tiered model as both an agenda and a praxis. The strengths of this narrative are that it seems fair and it matches clinical experience; even the epidemiological papers that seem to fit in the upper section of the pyramid by investigating psychopathology in the form of PTSD or depression tend to be accompanied by discussions acknowledging how the diagnoses and symptoms might be better explained in a model where most of those meeting criteria for psychopathology would benefit not from specialized services, but lower-tiered, broader services.

On the other hand, the model is not powerful enough; its widespread acceptance suggests that it would allow many people to continue doing what they are doing without adapting their strategies rather than improving what they do. The models also need to be tested; is the pyramidal or tiered approach effective in providing useful, culturally sound interventions to those who want help, and do they actually bolster and strengthen communities and families? Do they help us resolve the ethical problem of competing narratives or do they just segregate the narratives into different sections?

PSYCHOSOCIAL PERSPECTIVES

We want to turn now to three psychosocial approaches to show how different kinds of interventions can take place at different levels of the pyramid or tier, and how programs can responsibly locate themselves in relation to different domains in a child's life. Currently the evidence base for addressing the psychosocial needs of children and adolescents who have been displaced from their homes is slim (Henderson 2008; National Child Traumatic Stress Network 2005), but despite this lack of empirical support projects addressing the psychosocial needs of children and families have run the gamut from mental health programs identifying and seeking to prevent mental illness, through child-appropriate activities in refugee camps that seek to provide a safe place for children to be children, to educational and psychoeducational projects, and family reunification projects (e.g., Stepakoff et al. 2006; Mercy Corps 2005). While the costs of refugees' distress, suffering, and psychopathology are rarely addressed vast amounts of money, time, and expertise are spent annually on providing services to refugee communities (the UNHCR's operating budget for 2005 alone was $1.35 Billion [UNHCR 2006]).

Individual Approaches

Refugee children and adolescents who experience depression, post-traumatic stress disorder, or other psychiatric disorders whether caused by or exacerbated by their experiences deserve to have their psychological and psychiatric needs met. One way in which psychiatric services can be delivered is through individual encounters with a therapist. For example, Mohlen and colleagues (2004) studied a multimodal (family, individual, and group) intervention with ten Kosovar children and adolescents in Germany and reported decreased post-traumatic, anxiety and depressive symptoms. A common complaint is that this approach is too "egocentric" or "individually oriented" for children from "sociocentric" or "communal" societies; this much may be true, and it is worth bearing in mind. It is also worth bearing in mind that individual encounters can be constructive for the child, family, and communities, sensitive to the relative "egocentricity" or "sociocentricity" of the child, and that the same principles of autonomy, privacy, and confidentiality that benefit children from cultures that are more familiar with individual therapeutic modalities may also benefit children from less individualistic cultures.

As we alluded to earlier, one of the more powerful narratives has been "trauma," and a trauma-focused approach has produced some interesting studies. Layne and colleagues (2001) worked with 55 high-school-aged children from Bosnia and Herzegovina, using trauma and grief focused psychotherapy, and reported decreased psychosocial distress and improved psychosocial adaptation. One particular modality, trauma-focused cognitive behavioral therapy, is particularly promising for children who are symptomatic and impaired and should be further explored with refugee youth populations, with a close eye to the need for cultural adaptations and efficacy (Murray et al. 2008). The eminent questions for these approaches are how to identify children who would benefit from structured, individual psychotherapies; how to deliver these services in an effective and culturally acceptable way; and how to monitor these services to ensure that they are beneficial in the short and long term.

There are other personal, psychological, social, and cultural ways in which political violence impacts children beyond psychopathology. One increasingly well-established role for mental health professionals is listening to the stories that children, families, or communities tell, specifically to address and possibly mute the cynicism that meets people claiming persecution, a cynicism that may have been instrumental in their original persecution. Lustig and colleagues (2004) studied testimonial psychotherapy with three Somali adolescents in Boston finding that this was viewed as a safe and satisfying therapy. Conceiving psychotherapy as testimony and broadening the scope of mental health interventions to include legal and social concepts of truth-telling and forgiveness may counter prevailing doubts about the claims made by people subject to political violence (Weine et al. 1998; Lustig et al. 2004b). Narrative approaches recognize that patterns of distress may not be captured by psychiatric nosology and instead situate events, trauma, symptoms, and resilience in a person's own life story rather than on a checklist, and give the child the opportunity to identify his or her own sources of strength, need, and support (for a review please see Lustig and Tennakoon 2008).

As we think about this approach there are a number of questions worth asking. How do we adapt principles of belief and testimony to childhood? Do these projects tend to privilege the same type of narrative truths that are cast into doubt? That is, the stories tend to consolidate a "truthful" narrative, but as any story is partial and subjective, it can be critiqued for its veracity and its credibility. Children have different developmental relations to truth and fantasy, and are exposed to different expectations and norms regarding truth-telling; indeed, the same may be true of adults.

One of the more powerful and compelling narrative approaches of recent years has been part of this broader individual model: the novel and the memoir. One example that comes to mind is the writings of Alexander Hemon, who was born and raised in Bosnia-Herzegovina and came to Chicago as a young man just before the outbreak of war and subsequent genocide. Hemon's short stories and novels use the vantage points of exile and travel to describe the worlds of youth and adults impacted by war and refuge, giving us a view of the testimony narrative as a layered, nuanced, and complex part of the survivors' life, which is constantly being spoken, listened to, retold, reinterpreted, or not told at all (Hemon 2001; Hemon 2004). Another extraordinary example which directly looks at the world of child refugees is *What Is the What*, in which the novelist David Eggers imaginatively reconstructs the accounts told by Valentinto Achak Deng, a lost boy of Sudan (Eggers 2006).

Family Approaches

Political violence is commonly exacted against families whether indirectly through loss or murder, or directly through kidnapping, ransoming, and the shearing forces of political violence that forcibly separate families. As described above, preliminary research suggests that "family mental health" is an important concept, perhaps more important than "child mental health"; the social, medical, and psychological well-being of parents directly influences the well-being of children, and vice versa.

Directing psychosocial interventions towards helping families is a crucial step, but one that needs to be informed by a close understanding of cultural concepts of the family: Who is a member, and who is not? What are the obligations of family members, and what are the family roles? What sorts of pressures are brought to bear on the family and how does the family respond? Pertinent difficulties arise through generational tensions and conflicts, particularly apparent after migration, and through conflicting values about roles and family obligations in all stages of being a refugee including resettlement.

Dybdahl (2001) worked with 87 Bosnian-displaced mother-child dyads in Bosnia and Herzegovina, providing a five-month psychosocial intervention with an outcome suggesting improvement in mothers' mental health and psychosocial functioning. Weine and colleagues (2003) provided manualized family support and education groups for Bosnian refugees in Chicago and found that families who experienced more transitions, traumas, and adjustment difficulties were more likely to join a multiple family group, and that a multiple family group was able to increase access to additional mental health services through changing family communications. Adapting the group for 86 Kosovar refugees in Chicago, they found that the group improved mental health knowledge, services usage, and family hardiness, spanning different layers of the pyramid or tiered model. Weine and colleagues (2005) subsequently studied multiple family groups together with a family home visit for 30 families of people with mental illness in Kosova and reported improved use of services and decreased hospitalization rates. The multiple family group model has also been adapted and pre-piloted to address HIV prevention amongst adolescents in post-conflict Kosovo (Weine 2006), and educational disparities in U.S. refugee youth.

Before engaging in this type of intervention, one has to understand what a "family" is in any particular context; as already mentioned before, who is a member, and who is not? How is kinship determined, and who can speak to it? What gets people excluded from the family? One thing becomes quickly apparent in this work with families: families care deeply about each other and can provide support and guidance both within and across families. However, when families are overwhelmed with new problems in refuge, they often do not know how to effectively advocate for and help their children in the new context. One struggle that we often face is how to help parents reset their threshold of concern such that they not only care that their children can travel safely to school and are fed, but are also concerned enough about the quality of that educational experience that they get more involved with their children's teachers and schools.

School-Based Approaches

One of the roles of adults throughout the world is to educate children formally and informally. Through schools, home and religious instruction, and apprenticeships, children learn knowledge, skills, social rules, and social roles, and develop relationships, including peer relations. Evidence suggests that children with emotional difficulties can struggle with learning and schools are a place where we can have a positive impact (Barrett et al. 2000; Cortina et al. 2008; Rousseau et al. 2005). It is also an opportunity to address the world of the child, for the cultural shift that takes place with migration certainly includes the change in cultures of youth and adolescence: new peers, new peer relations, new exposures, new pop music, and so on.

School-based preventive programs can provide a structured, institutional framework for providing services, although there are several major obstacles: the problem of stigmatization for children and adolescents; the heterogeneity of children in schools (for example, refugee children from different countries, immigrant children from others, native-born children); and schools are substantially different in terms of their capacities (Rousseau and Guzder 2008). Rousseau and Guzder also summarize the promising aspects of school-based programs that can be sensitive to different needs in a tiered or pyramidal model: ecologic models that address the whole-school environment and encourage teacher sensitivity, parent-school interactions, and a broader educational mission about cultural diversity; classroom activities that support assimilation of past and present experiences as learning opportunities; the potential for preventive programs using specific treatment modalities that can be implemented in a school-room setting; and the opportunity to provide secondary prevention services to children who are identified with emotional and behavioral problems (Rousseau and Guzder 2008).

Given the importance of adults in the world of children, the input of teachers, principals, and school counselors provides an exciting opportunity to enrich the narratives about, and by, refugee children. Practically, the interventions can actively involve teachers who can be helpful in identifying children in need and facilitating service delivery (e.g., O'Shea et al. 2000; Ehntholt et al. 2005), or they can consult on the development of programs (Fazel et al. 2009).

ACCESSING NARRATIVES: DETENTION AND RADICALIZATION

All of the previous theoretical models and domains of intervention have questions that are not easily answered where one narrative comes into conflict with another; many of these debates occur within the field of psychosocial and mental health services. But as we discussed at the outset, there are broad complicated questions relating to legal and political status that may pose even greater problems as well as greater opportunities for psychosocial and mental health interventions. Narratives need to be spoken; they need to be heard. There must be a conversation, and every conversation requires access. Access can be understood in a number of different ways. For example, some of those who dispute "mental health perspectives" may say that such a biomedical universalist perspective closes down an ability to hear local, autochthonous ways of expressing and addressing suffering; on this reading, one narrative bars another when a dominant narrative prevents a quieter narrative from accessing its place in the discourse. These questions of access to discourse arise within communities as well; for example, in any particular community, are the stories told by boys the same as those told by girls, and would we be able to meet with the girls in such a way as to hear their stories? What happens when there are conflicting voices in the community?

In 2007 and 2008 over 20 Somali refugee youth from Minneapolis flew to Somalia to join jihadist training camps run by the Al Shabaab terrorist organization. Halima Abdi, a mother, said, "I had returned from work and asked my other children where my son Mohamed Yasin was but they said they hadn't seen him all day." After ten days she had almost given up when a young boy called from Somali: "Mum, it's your son Mohamed—I came to Mogadishu to fight against the enemies of Somalia." There is much to be said about what happened in Minneapolis, but we would like to point out the prominent, competing narratives and how these were shaped by the question of access. Parents felt like they did not have access to their children, that they had become American too fast; the children, however, had access to Somalia through storytelling and the Internet. One said, "When someone is killed, even in a village, we watch it on YouTube." They also had access to adults who were recruiting them for jihad; in some ways this was encouraged, if unwittingly; parents were pleased that their children attended the mosque but were not aware that the mosques may have been targeted by recruiters. The recruiters themselves may have come from the local community networked to jihadist organizations in Somalia, or they may have been outsiders. Stories and narratives are powerful; they can also be dangerous.

Access for those who want to develop psychosocial services can be stymied if it is thought that it will be too disruptive. Up to 80,000 unaccompanied children attempt to enter the United States each year (Knight 2004), and in 2001 it was estimated that on any given day some 500 unaccompanied alien children are in detention in the United States (Amnesty International 2001). In recent years, their numbers have increased dramatically from approximately 5,000 unaccompanied minors detained in 2002 to well over 8,000 in 2007 (Women's Refugee Commission 2009). Our current understanding of what is happening to these children comes from three main sources: advocacy groups, mental health research, and journalism. In a *New Yorker* article, Margaret Talbot (2008) reported on refugee families detained by the U.S. Department of Homeland Security (DHS) in the T. Don Hutto Residential Center, a former medium-security prison. Talbot drew attention to practices there such as prohibiting children from having stuffed animals, crayons, or pencils in their cells, restricting parents' access to their children at night, and conversely requiring parents to keep their children with them throughout the day—even, for example, as they disclosed their often traumatic stories to lawyers (Talbot 2008). In addition, studies have suggested a variety of adverse psychological consequences of detention for children (Mares and Jureidini 2004; Steel et al. 2004; Mares et al. 2002; McCallin 1992; Sourander 1998; Sultan and O'Sullivan 2001). It is particularly important to point out that these psychological symptoms may not be residual to previous trauma, risk factors, or experiences. A recent systematic review of the mental health impact of detention on adult and child asylum seekers in the UK, U.S., and Australia (Robjant et al. 2009) found evidence that detention itself is a cause of elevated psychopathology.

We suspect that children's experience of detention may vary widely according to a variety of factors including the country and specific facility they find themselves in, their experiences prior to detention, individual characteristics and personality variables, and whether they are with family members or unaccompanied (Michelson and Sclare 2009). For example, the presence of family members may or may not help protect the child against the stress of immigration custody; research suggests that the experience of parental distress, traumatization, and mental illness during detention may all increase children's vulnerability to emotional and behavioral disorders (Mares and Jureidini 2004). On the other hand unaccompanied minors may be particularly susceptible to mental health problems while in detention. Prior exposure to trauma may make people more susceptible to mental health problems while in detention (Robjant et al. 2009), and in a study in Holland, Bean and colleagues (2007) found that unaccompanied refugee minors had experienced twice as many stressful life events as refugee adolescents living with a family member or native Dutch adolescents, and were at significantly higher risk for psychopathology.

This raises a number of important questions about how we understand these youth; beyond the simple common denominator of uncertain immigration status there is little if anything which ties this "population"— marked as it is by considerable cultural, social, and linguistic heterogeneity—together as a group. And yet the biggest hurdle to face is one of access; those of us that want to hear their story a certain way are prevented from doing so by barriers erected by those who are curious about other aspects of their story (i.e., whether they can justify remaining in the United States, what they might say about the conditions of detention, and so on).

Narratives are complex and uncertain; they are constructed by individuals and communities, but often—as anybody who has listened to a parent and child describe the same argument only to hear two very different stories would know—can be markedly divergent and are sustained for reasons which are themselves narratives. A nation founded on a promise to immigrants, according to one story, may not want to hear another story about mistreating children who come over for the very same reasons as the Founding Fathers' ancestors, fleeing religious persecution.

CONCLUSION

Many in our field, including those trying to find innovative approaches, may be trying to solve problems that call for narrative approaches but are doing so without putting enough emphasis on narratives. The goal here has not been to idealize these narratives but instead to think about the many ways in which we can access, listen to, document, and understand what a refugee child in Minneapolis or Sydney or Jordan is going through. In the broadest sense, addressing the psychosocial needs of children and adolescents requires sensitivity to the cultural and historical forces that have shaped and been shaped by those children and to the familial and social environment in which the children have been raised, as well as to their own personal histories. Paying close attention to the local supports and structures is what will help programs and interventions become sustainable, and prevent them from undermining resilience and support that is in place, or replicating colonial or exploitative models (Wessells 2009; Betancourt 2008). The narrative approach sees conflicting narratives as neither an endpoint nor as something that must be solved, but rather as the beginning of a discussion, in which participants have something to share and where listening is conceived of as empowering. The narrative approach we are describing here is not unique to child refugees. Stewart and Rappaport (2005) have described a community narrative approach to HIV/AIDS which lends itself well to the trauma field as "an especially useful means to understanding, cultivating, and/or mobilizing shared experience and conceptualizations." Communities create narrative communities, whereby people are more than problem-ridden victims, where they can develop a way of explaining how and why they will commit to preventive activities.

We would never claim that narratives are all that we need in order to fulfill our obligations. We need resources and information, and especially scientific methods and empirical tools to provide us with reliable means of systematically understanding complex phenomena. But the science we need is not restricted to one methodological or theoretical framework. It is a mantra that there needs to be more research. In making sense of the psychosocial interdisciplinary work can be enormously productive and insightful as it includes a combination of research methodologies (e.g., Hundt et al. 2004). Ethnographic approaches that explore how refugee youth understand their situation, their needs, and their own strengths may not provide simple answers; indeed, there may be important tensions that arise. For example, in one study tensions between seeking support and valuing privacy and concealment were revealed (Whittaker et al. 2005). Moreover, just as there are pyramids and tiered models to describe the various needs of refugee populations so there need to be models of interdisciplinary collaboration, where different research methodologies can complement one another to tell a richer story, where different outcomes can be assessed, and, crucially, where we learn whether the work we do intending to help refugee children and families is actually helping them. In our opinion, the trauma field needs to evolve in a direction in which narratives will have more of a place, but with the recognition that we are not novelists. Working with narratives is a dominant organizing principle, but because we are committed to the real world in all its complexity and inconsistency, we must find the narrative approaches that best fit with the characteristics of that world.

Finally, to return to the issue we began with, we need a compelling narrative for psychosocial interventions that can successfully compete for public attention. The question is frequently asked; why address "psychosocial needs" when people are starving, herded together in refugee camps, or unemployed and marginalized in a host country that has little interest in them? A less frequent question turns this on its head; how can we expect to help people who are starving, who are unemployed, who are herded together in refugee camps, who are forgotten except for when their failure to assimilate becomes obvious, without attending to their needs as living human beings? It is a biological fact that a body needs food, water, and shelter; it is a triumph of public health that sanitation systems can channel human refuse away from homes, food stocks, and playgrounds; but people also need to be heard to live their lives—whether these are "inner" psychological lives or sociocultural lives.

In our experience, when asked, children, parents, professionals, and teachers will often say the same thing: they want help coping with the stresses of their life, they want help coping with how these stresses are tearing them apart, parents want help talking to their children, parents want help talking to teachers and other parents, and children want to be heard. Yes, they are bodies who need food, yes, they are bodies that need shelter, yes, they are citizens of a country that needs political stability, but they also need to be parents and children. These are substantial problems for "humanitarian" interventions where there is a frank prioritization of everyday living which is at once necessary but also part of the problem (Ticktin 2006; Fassin 2007). People become commodified as bodies that must be fed and clothed, and the "culture" as dynamic and responsive and individualized as it is enduring, stable, and generalized, can become similarly commodified. In the opening cartoon the comic journalist Roland Hedley sets up a dualism; the child has no food or school, but she has "hope." While this might seem to be a potential parody of mental health interventions, offering an inner psychic experience as compensation for lack of nutrition, it is in fact an astute indication of how the body and the psyche are split and played one against the other. Providing "food" and "shelter" without addressing or comprehending "meals" and "homes" risks the continued politicization of the refugees thus turning them into bodies, or "bare life" (Agamben 1999).

Psychosocial interventions do not just "rescue" people from the brink of death; psychosocial interventions are obliged to confront and repair the specific consequences of political violence, i.e., the disintegration of those emotional, psychological, and social bonds that make us human. As we noted at the outset the world of childhood is attacked specifically and intentionally. Psychosocial programs need to be aware of this and seek a remedy. The work needs to be holistic, rights oriented, and consistently evaluated not just for outcome efficacy but for how it addresses youth in an age-appropriate, culturally valid way (Jones 2008). Discussions around local healing, local structures, and local resilience are always tempered by the fact that these local strengths have not only been overwhelmed by circumstances, leading not to disintegration of social bonds but to some degree of social fragmentation. Without denigrating or dismissing local structures, it is important to see the fractures and blind spots that exist and existed. More disconcertingly, there needs to be a fuller discussion of how local healers, structures, and resilience were not just victims but contain their own reservoirs of violence and their own implication.

There are many questions left to be asked: Who is determining what services are needed, who is asking people in refugee communities what they need, and how do we understand their answers? What barriers are there to service delivery and service research? Is the fragmented research base a step in the right direction or part of the problem? But a final question worth considering is—what are the cultural, political, and social goals we hope to attain by providing psychosocial services? What do we expect of refugee children and families, and what is preventing us from seeing them as families, as when breast-feeding mothers are taken away from their infants for immigration violations or families are separated (Associated Press 2007; Gonzalez 2007)? These are difficult questions but ones worth considering and ones worth asking within the communities providing psychosocial services and about the communities who will be receiving these services.

REFERENCES

Agamben, G. *Homo Sacer: Sovereign Power and Bare Life.* Stanford: Meridian Books, 1999.

Amnesty International. *"Why Am I here?" Children in Immigration Detention.* Published 2001. Available at: http://www.amnestyusa.org/refugee/usa_children_summary.html. Accessed June 12, 2009.

Anagnostopoulos, D. C., Vlassopoulou, M., Rotsika, V., Pehlivanidou, H., Legaki, L., Rogakou, E., and Lazaratou, H. "Psychopathology and mental health service utilization by immigrants' children and their families." *Transcultural Psychiatry* 41 (2004): 465-486.

Associated Press. "US Immigration agency sets new policy after arrest of breastfeeding mother." November 9, 2007. Available at http://www.detentionwatchnetwork.org/node/475. Accessed June 12, 2009.

Bakhtin, M. *"Problems of Dostoevsky's Poetics."* Translated by Caryl Emerson. Minneapolis: University of Minnesota Press, 1984.

Barrett P.M., Moore A.F., and Sonderegger R. "The FRIENDS program for young former-Yugoslavian refugees in Australia: A pilot study." *Behaviour Change* 17(30) (2000): 124-133.

Bean, T., Derluyn, I., Eurelings-Bontekoe, E., Broekaert, E., and Spinhoven, P. "Comparing psychological distress, traumatic stress reations, and experiences of unaccompanied refugee minors with experiences of adolescents accompanied by parents." *Journal of Nervous and Mental Disease* 195(4) (2007): 288-297.

Betancourt, T.S. "Child soldiers: Reintegration, pathways to recovery, and reflections from the field." *Journal of Developmental and Behavioral Pediatrics* 29(2) (2008): 138-141.

Bhugra, D., and Minas, I.H. "Mental health and global movement of people." *Lancet* 370(9593) (2007): 1109-1111.

Cortina, M.A., Kahn, K., Fazel, M., Hlungwani, T., Tollman, S., Bhana, A., Prothrow-Stith, D., and Stein, A. "School-based interventions can play a critical role in enhancing children's development and health in the developing world." *Child: Care, Health and Development* 34(1) (2008): 1-3.

Dybdahl, R. "Children and mothers in war: An outcome study of a psychosocial intervention program." *Child Development* 72(4) (2001): 1214-1230.

Eggers, D. *What Is the What: The Autobiography of Valentino Achek Deng.* New York: McSweeney, 2006.

Ehntholt, K.A., Smith, P.A., and Yule, W. "School-based Cognitive-Behavioural Therapy Group Intervention for Refugee Children who have Experienced War-related Trauma." *Clinical Child Psychology and Psychiatry* 10 (2005): 235-250.

Emerson, C. *"The First Hundred Years of Mikhail Bakhtin."* Princeton, New Jersey: Princeton University Press, 1997.

Escobar, J.I. "Immigration and mental health: Why are immigrants better off?" *Archives of General Psychiatry* 55 (1998): 781-782.

Fairchild, A. *Science at the Borders.* Baltimore: Johns Hopkins University Press, 2003.

Fassin, D. "Humanitarianism as a Politics of Life." *Public Culture* 19 (2007): 499-520.

Fazel, M., Doll, H., and Stein, A. "A school-based mental health intervention for refugee children: An exploratory study." *Clinical Child Psychology and Psychiatry* 14 (2009):2 97-309.

Fazel, M., and Stein, A. "The mental health of refugee children." *Archives of Disease in Childhood* 87 (2002): 366-370.

Fazel M., and Stein A. "Mental health of refugee children: A comparative study." *British Medical Journal* 327(7407) (2003): 134.

Fazel, M,. Wheeler, J., and Danesh, J. "Prevalence of serious mental disorder in 7000 refugees resettled in western countries: A systematic review." *Lancet* 365(9467) (2005): 1309-14.

Gilligan, C. "'Highly Vulnerable'? Political Violence and the Social Construction of Childhood. *Journal of Peace Research* 46(2009): 119-134.

Gonzalez, C. "A family broken at the border." *Omaha World Herald.* December 17, 2007. Available at: http://www.detentionwatchnetwork.org/node/502. Accessed June 12, 2009.

Hemon, A. *The Question of Bruno.* New York: Vintage, 2001.

Hemon, A. *Nowhere Man.* New York: Vintage, 2004.

Henderson, S.W. "Preface." *Child and Adolescent Psychiatry Clinics of North America* 17(3) (2008): xv-xvi.

Hodes, M. "Three key issues for young refugees' mental health." *Transcultural Psychiatry* 39 (2002): 196 - 213.

Hundt, G.L., Chatty, D., Thabet, A.A., and Abuateya, H. "Advocating multi-disciplinarity in studying complex emergencies: The limitations of a psychological approach to understanding how young people cope with prolonged conflict in Gaza." *Journal of Biosocial Science* 36 (2004): 417-31.

Inter-Agency Standing Committee. "IASC guidelines on mental health and psychosocial support in emergency settings." Geneva: Inter-agency Standing Committee. 2007. Available at: http://www.who.int/mental_health/emergencies/guidelines_ iasc_mental_health_psychosocial_june_2007.pdf. Accessed June 12, 2009.

Jones, L. "Responding to the needs of children in crisis." *International Review of Psychiatry* 20(3) (2008): 291-303.

Knight, D. "Waiting in limbo, their childhood lost." U.S. News and World Report, March 7, 2004.

Kohrt, B.A., Jordans, M.J., Tol, W.A., Speckman, R.A,. Maharjan, S.M,. Worthman, C.M., and Komproe, I.H. "Comparison of mental health between former child soldiers and children never conscripted by armed groups in Nepal." *Journal of the American Medical Association* 300(6) (2008): 691-702.

Layne, C.M., Pynoos, R.S., Saltzman, W.R., Arslanagic, B., Black, M., Savjal, N., Popovic, T., Durakovic, E., Music, M., Campara, N., Djapo, N., and Houston, R. "Trauma/grief-focused group psychotherapy: School-based postwar intervention with traumatized bosnian adolescents." *Group Dynamics* 5(4) (2001): 277-290.

Lustig S.L., Kia-Keating M., Knight W.G., Geltman P., Ellis H., Kinzie J.D., Keane T., and Saxe, G.N. "Review of child and adolescent refugee mental health." *Journal of the American Academy of Child and Adolescent Psychiatry* 43(1) (2004a): 24-36.

Lustig S.T., and Tennakoon, L. "Testimonials, narratives, stories, and drawings: Child refugees as witnesses." *Child and Adolescent Psychiatry Clinics of North America.* 17(3) (2008): 569-584.

Lustig S.L., Weine S.M., Saxe G.N., and Beardslee, W.R. "Testimonial psychotherapy for adolescent refugees: A case series." *Transcultural Psychiatry* 41(1) (2004b): 31-45.

Mares S., and Jureidini, J. "Psychiatric assessment of children and families in immigration detention: Clinical, administrative and ethical issues." *Australian and New Zealand Journal of Public Health* 28(6) (2004).

Mares S., Newman L., Dudley M., and Gale, F. "Seeking refuge, losing hope: parents and children in immigration detention." *Australasian Psychiatry* 10 (2002): 91-96.

McCallin, M. "*Living in detention: A review of the psychological wellbeing of Vietnamese children in the Hong Kong detention centres.*" Geneva: International Catholic Child Bureau, 1992.

McKenzie, K., Fearon P., and Hutchinson, G. "Migration, ethnicity and psychosis." In *Society and Psychosis*, ed. C. Morgan, K. McKenzie, and P. Fearon. Cambridge: Cambridge University Press, 2008.

Mercy Corps. "Making a difference in Sudanese refugee camps." Available at: http://www.mercycorps.org/countries/sudan/10404. (June 7, 2005) Accessed June 12, 2009.

Michelson, D., and Sclare, I. "Psychological needs, service utilization and provision of care in a specialist mental health clinic for young refugees: A comparative study." *Journal of Clinical Child Psychology and Psychiatry* 14 (2009): 273-296

Möhlen H., Parzer P., Resch F., and Brunner R. "Psychosocial support for war-traumatized child and adolescent refugees: Evaluation of a short-term treatment program." *Australian and New Zealand Journal of Psychiatry* 39 (2005): 81-87.

Morson, G.S., and Emerson, C. *Mikhail Bakhtin: Creation of a Prosaics.* Palo Alto, CA: Stanford University Press, 1991.

Murray, L.K., Cohen, J.A., Ellis, B.H., and Mannarino, A. "Cognitive behavioral therapy for symptoms of trauma and traumatic grief in refugee youth." *Child and Adolescent Psychiatry Clinics of North America.* 17(3) (2008): 585-604.

National Child Traumatic Stress Network Refugee Trauma Task Force. "Mental Health Interventions for Refugee Children in Resettlement: White Paper II." 2005. Available at: http://www.nctsnet.org/nctsn_assets/pdfs/promising_practices/MH_Interventions_for_Refugee_Children.pdf. Accessed June 12, 2009.

Novins, D.K. "Participatory research brings knowledge and hope to American Indian communities." *Journal of American Academy of Child and Adolescent Psychiatry.* 48(2009): 585-586.

O'Shea, B., Hodes, M., Down, G., and Bramley, J. "A school-based mental health service for refugee children." *Clinical Child Psychology and Psychiatry* 5(2) (2000): 189-201.

Papageorgiou, V., Frangou-Garunovic, A., Iordanidou, R., Yule, W., Smith, P., Vostanis, P. "War trauma and psychopathology in Bosnian refugee children." *European Journal of Child and Adolescent Psychiatry* 9(2) (2000): 84-90.

Robjant, K., Hassan, R., and Katona, C. "Mental health implications of detaining asylum seekers: systematic review." *British Journal of Psychiatry* 194 (2009): 306-312.

Rousseau, C., Drapeau, A., Lacroix, L., Bagilishya, D., and Heusch, N. "Evaluation of a classroom program of creative expression workshops for refugee and immigrant children." *Journal of Child Psychology and Psychiatry* 46(2) (2005): 180-185.

Rousseau C., and Guzder, J. "School-based prevention programs for refugee youth." *Child and Adolescent Psychiatry Clinics of North America* 17(3) (2008): 533-550.

Shacknove, A.E. "Who is a refugee?" *Ethics* 95(2) (1985): 274-284.

Sourander, A. "Behavior problems and traumatic events of unaccompanied refugee minors." *Child Abuse and Neglect* 22(7) (2008): 719-727.

Steel, Z., Momartin, S., Bateman, C., Hafshejani, A., Silove, D.M., Everson, N., Roy, K., Dudley, M., Newman, L., Blick, B., and Mares, S. "Psychiatric status of asylum seeker families held for a protracted period in a remote detention centre in Australia." *Australian and New Zealand Journal of Public Health* 28(6) (2004): 527-536.

Stepakoff, S., Hubbard, J., Katoh, M., Falk, E., Mikulu, J.B., Nkhoma, P., and Omagwa, Y. "Trauma healing in refugee camps in Guinea : A psychosocial program for liberian and sierra leonean survivors of torture and war." *The American Psychologist* 61(8) (2006): 921-932.

Stewart, E., and Rappaport, J. "Narrative insurrections: HIV, circulating knowledges, and local resistances." In E.J. Trickett and W. Pequegnat (Eds). *Community Intervention and AIDS.* New York: Oxford University Press, 2005.

Sultan, A., and O'Sullivan, K. "Psychological disturbances in asylum seekers held in long term detention: a participant-observer account." *Medical Journal of Australia* 175 (2001): 593-96.

Summerfield, D. "The invention of post-traumatic stress disorder and the social usefulness of a psychiatric category." *British Medical Journal* 322 (2001): 95-98.

Summerfield, D. "How scientifically valid is the knowledge base of global mental health?" *British Medical Journal* 336 (2008): 992-994.

Talbot M. "The Lost Children." *The New Yorker.* 2008.

Thabet, A.A., Abu Tawahina, A., El Sarraj, E., and Vostanis, P. "Exposure to war trauma and PTSD among parents and children in the Gaza strip." *European Child and Adolescent Psychiatry* 17(4) (2008): 191-199.

Ticktin, M. "Where ethics and politics meet: The violence of humanitarianism in France." *American Ethnologist* 33(1) (2006): 33-49.

Tousignant, M., Habimana, E., Biron, C., Malo, C., Sidoli-LeBlanc, E., and Bendris, N. "The Quebec Adolescent Refugee Project: Psychopathology and family variables in a sample from 35 nations." *Journal of the American Academy of Child and Adolescent Psychiatry* 38(11) (1999): 1426-32.

Trudeau, G. *Doonesbury.* July 7, 2008. Available at: http://www.doonesbury.com/strip/dailydose/index.html?uc_full_date=20080709. Accessed July 31, 2008.

United Nations. "Rape and other grave sexual violence against children." Geneva: United Nations, Available at: http://www.un.org/children/conflict/english/sexual-violence.html. Accessed August 1, 2008.

United Nations. "Report of the Secretary-General: Children and Armed Conflict." United Nations: Geneva, 2009. Available at: http://daccessdds.un.org/doc/UNDOC/GEN/N09/282/44/PDF/N0928244.pdf Accessed June 12, 2009.

United Nations Children's Fund. "State of the World's Children 2006." Geneva: UNICEF, 2006. Available at: www.unicef.org/publications/index_30398.html. Accessed July 17, 2006.

United Nations High Commission for Refugees. "Convention and Protocol Relating to the Status of Refugees." Geneva: United Nations High Commission for Refugees, 1951.

United Nations High Commission for Refugees. "Note on Burden and Standard of Proof in Refugee Claims." Geneva: United Nations High Commission for Refugees, 1998. Available at: www.refugeelawreader.org/294/Note_on_Burden_and_Standard_of_Proof_in_Refugee_Claims.pdf. Accessed June 12, 2009.

United Nations High Commission for Refugees. "Extensive abuse of West African refugee children reported." Geneva: United Nations High Commission for Refugees, 2002. Available at: http://www.unhcr.org/cgi-bin/texis/vtx/news/opendoc. htm?tbl=NEWSandid=3c7bf8094. Accessed June 12, 2009.

United Nations High Commission for Refugees. "Basic Facts." Geneva: United Nations High Commission for Refugees, 2006. Available at: http://www.unhcr.org/cgi-bin/texis/vtx/basics/opendoc.htm?tbl=BASICSandid=3b028097c. Accessed July 17, 2006.

United Nations High Commission for Refugees. "The State of the World's Refugee: A Humanitarian Agenda." Geneva: United Nations High Commission for Refugees, 2007a. Available at: http://www.unhcr.org/publ/PUBL/3eb7ba414.pdf. Accessed June 12, 2009.

United Nations High Commission for Refugees. "The 1951 Refugee Convention: Questions and Answers." Geneva: United Nations High Commission for Refugees, 2007b. Pg 6. Available at: http://www.unhcr.org/basics/BASICS/3c0f495f4. pdf. Accessed June 12, 2009.

United Nations High Commission for Refugees. "Statistical Yearbook 2007." Geneva: United Nations High Commission for Refugees, 2007c. Available at: http://www.unhcr.org/statistics/STATISTICS/4981b19d2.html. Accessed June 12, 2009.

Vega, W.A., and Lopez, S.R. "Priority issues in Latino mental health services research." *Mental Health Services Research* 3(4) (2001): 189-200.

von Lersner, U., Elbert, T., and Neuner, F. "Mental health of refugees following state-sponsored repatriation from Germany." *BioMedCentral Psychiatry* 8(88) (2008).

Webb, E., and Davies, M. "Refugee children: Don't replace one form of severe adversity with another." *Archives of Disease in Childhood* 88(2003): 365-366

Weine, S.M. *"When History Is a Nightmare: Lives and Memories of Ethnic Cleansing in Bosnia-Herzegovina."* New Brunswick: Rutgers University Press, 1999.

Weine, S.M. *Testimony after Catastrophe: Narrating the Traumas of Political Violence.* Evanston, IL: Northwestern University Press, 2006.

Weine, S.M., Kulauzovic, Y., Besic, S., Lezic, A., Mujagic, A., Muzurovic, J., Spahovic, D., Feetham, S., Knafl, K., and Pavkovic, I. "A family beliefs framework for developing socially and culturally specific preventive interventions for refugee families and youth." *American Journal of Orthopsychiatry* 76(1) (2006): 1-9.

Weine, S. M., Kulenovic, T., Dzubur, A., Pavkovic, I, and Gibbons, R. "Testimony psychotherapy in Bosnian refugees: A Pilot Study." *American Journal of Psychiatry*, 155(1998): 1720-1726.

Weine, S.M., Raina, D., Zhubi, M., Delesi, M., Huseni, D., Feetham, S., Kulauzovic, Y., Mermelstein, R., Campbell, R.T., Rolland, J., and Pavkovic I. "The TAFES Multi-Family Group Intervention for Kosovar Refugees." *The Journal of Nervous and Mental Diseases* 191(2003): 100-107.

Weine, S.M., Ukshini, S., Griffith, J., Agani, F., Pulleyblank-Coffey, W., Ulaj, J., Becker, C., Ajeri, L., Elliott, M., Alidemaj-Sereq, V., Landau, J., Asllani, M., Mango, M., Pavkovic, I., Bunjaku, A., Rolland, J., Cala, G., Sargent, J., Saul, J., Makolli, S.,

Sluzki, C., Statovci, S., and Weingarten, K. "A family approach to severe mental illness in post-war Kosovo" *Psychiatry* 68(1) (2005): 17-27.

Wessels, M. "Supporting the mental health and psychosocial wellbeing of former child soldiers." *Journal of the American Academy of Child and Adolescent Psychiatry* 48(6) (2009): 587-590.

Whittaker, S., Hardy, G., Lewis, K., and Buchan, L. "An exploration of psychological well-being with young Somali refugee and asylum-seeker women." *Journal of Clinical Child Psychology and Psychiatry* 10 (2005): 177-196.

Women's Refugee Commission. "Halfway Home: Unaccompanied Children in Immigration Custody." Women's Refugee Commission, 2009. Available from: http://www.womensrefugeecommission.org/resources/reports. Accessed June 12, 2009.

World Vision. "Trapped! The Disappearing Hopes of Iraqi Children." World Vision, 2007. Available at: http://meero.worldvision.org/docs/57.pdf. Accessed June 12, 2009.

Zarowsky, C. "Writing trauma: Emotion, ethnography, and the politics of suffering among Somali returnees in Ethiopia" *Culture, Medicine and Psychiatry* 28(2) (2004):189.

II

INDIVIDUAL
DISORDERS/PROBLEMS

6

The Boundaries of Attention-Deficit/ Hyperactivity Disorder

*Guilherme Polanczyk, Rodrigo Chazan,
and Luis Augusto Rohde*

INTRODUCTION

Attention-deficit/hyperactivity disorder (ADHD) is a neurodevelopmental disorder characterized by pervasive and impairing symptoms of inattention, hyperactivity, and impulsivity. Approximately 5% of children and adolescents from the community around the world present with ADHD (Polanczyk et al. 2007) and this is the most frequent disorder in child and adolescent mental health services (Goldman et al. 1998; Pliszka 2007). ADHD is associated with a broad range of negative outcomes for affected individuals and with significant financial burdens to families and society (Pliszka 2007; Swanson et al. 1998).

Establishing a diagnosis of ADHD, as with any mental disorder during childhood and adolescence, is a complex task (Angold and Costello 2009). Specifically for ADHD, although the disorder is conceptualized as a distinct category its features (attentional ability, control over the motor activity and impulses) are continuously distributed within the population. Therefore, it is necessary to make the distinction between developmentally appropriate and inappropriate behaviors and abilities. Additionally, inattention, hyperactivity, and impulsivity may be the manifestation or may be complicated by other physical and mental disorders which should be promptly identified. Moreover, the clinical picture presented by a child or adolescent must be contextualized within the cultural background of the patient's family. Culture can influence the expression of behaviors, their identification as developmentally inappropriate, the access to medical care and appropriate diagnosis, and also acceptance of and adherence to treatment. These peculiarities, among others, make the evaluation and diagnostic process with a child who is referred for inattention or hyperactivity even more complex.

In situations characterized by blurred boundaries between the clinical picture presented by a patient and cultural issues, sub-threshold behaviors, and other conditions establishing the diagnosis of ADHD is a challenge. In this chapter the boundaries of ADHD diagnosis will be discussed specifically: (1) culture and ADHD; (2) ADHD as a dimensional or categorical entity; (3) the overlap between ADHD and conduct disorder; and (4) the overlap between ADHD and bipolar disorder.

CULTURE AND ADHD

Culture refers to shared language, values, beliefs, tradition, practices, and norms established in common social groupings, which may occur as a function of ethnic origins, economic income, religion, or professional activity (Greenfield et al. 2003). Cultural influences are always present in the clinical setting brought both by the patients (and their families) and the clinician (and the service system). These factors operate through biological and environmental/social mechanisms which are correlated and difficult to disentangle. The extent and implications of the impact of culture within the clinical setting must be promptly identified and adequately addressed to prevent the diagnostic and therapeutic processes being significantly affected.

Cultural aspects can influence the diagnostic and therapeutic processes of ADHD in a number of ways such as the way behavior is expressed, the way behavior is perceived, access to medical care and appropriate diagnosis, and the acceptance of diagnosis and adherence to treatment. Parental values and expectations towards their child may moderate the identification of symptoms or impairment. Also, the understanding and beliefs about the causes of their child's behavior are affected by cultural aspects such as the medicalization or not of behaviors, the avoidance of stigma or medical labels, the expectations that parents should solve all their child's problems, and narcissistic projections towards the child. The explanation parents give to their child's behavior and previous experiences with medical, psychological, educational, or other services for similar problems are likely to influence their attitudes toward the search for assistance (Kleinman 1987). The acceptance by parents of ADHD as a medical diagnosis and the necessity for and adherence to treatment are likely to be influenced by the extent to which the parents' first conceptualization of the behavior deviates from the scientific model, how rigid the parents are towards their beliefs, and the extent to which the provider can address these beliefs and correcting and informing the parents and patient where appropriate. On the other hand, the cultural background of clinicians can also moderate the likelihood of the diagnosis, the rapport established with the family, and the outcome (Mann et al. 1992).

Culture, Ethnicity, and Attitudes towards ADHD

A number of studies have been conducted to evaluate how different ethnic and cultural groups perceive the symptoms of ADHD and understand their origin and the differences in diagnosis and treatment (Margalit 1981; Holborow and Berry 1986; Mann et al. 1992; Reid et al. 1998; Rasmussen, Todd, et al. 2002; Pierce and Reid 2004; Norvilitis and Fang 2005; Gidwani, Opitz, and Perrin 2006; Mah and Johnston 2007; Norvilitis et al. 2008; Gomez and Vance 2008). However, this issue has not been examined in studies with representative samples of the population, and studies with limited sample size do not necessarily reflect the picture found in the general population. Also, the specificity and dynamic nature of culture, even within nations and groups that are believed to be homogeneous, make it difficult to delineate concrete pictures that can be widely generalized for each cultural background (Cooper and Denner 1998). Nevertheless, it was possible to identify a modest literature that compared the influence of ethnicity between African Americans and Caucasians with regard to explanatory models of ADHD, access to services, and clinical characteristics (Miller, Nigg, and Miller 2009). With regard to explanatory models of ADHD, Caucasian parents were more likely to refer to ADHD as a medical disorder, while African American parents were more likely to refer to ADHD as a behavior problem or as an inherent characteristic that implied that the child was "bad." African American parents were also more likely to anticipate a shorter duration of the problem behavior, in contrast to Caucasian parents who expected a prolonged course (Bussing, Gary, et al. 2003). African American parents were less informed about ADHD compared to Caucasian parents, and were more likely than Caucasian parents to attribute ADHD to causes not linked to the disorder (Bussing, Schoenberg, and Perwien 1998). Probably reflecting, in part, the different explanatory models for ADHD, African American children were less than half as likely to be assessed, diagnosed, and treated for ADHD as Caucasians (Bussing, Gary, et al. 2003; Zito et al. 1997). However, other barriers to treatment were also identified. Across race the most commonly endorsed barriers were system barriers (i.e., not knowing where to go for help), no perceived need (i.e., expecting the problem to improve without intervention), and negative expectations towards treatment, which was higher among African American parents (Bussing, Zima, et al. 2003). With regard to intensity and frequency of the disorder, studies identified a higher intensity of symptoms in African American children in comparison to Caucasians (Miller, Nigg, and Miller 2009). However, studies of ADHD diagnosis yielded lower prevalence rates for African American children (Miller, Nigg, and Miller 2009) which may reflect difficulties accessing services experienced by African Americans. Regarding the severity of cases, a small number of studies suggest that African American children manifest more severe cases, complicated by more comorbid conditions. The authors conclude that the limited literature on this issue is unable to address whether ADHD manifests in a unique way in African Americans or whether other factors besides lack of access to treatment account for differences in symptom severity or prevalence (Miller, Nigg, and Miller 2009). However, these findings indicate the necessity for interventions at the community level (e.g., schools, clubs, churches) that aim to educate parents and teachers about ADHD.

ADHD as a Cross-Cultural Diagnosis

Psychiatric nosology, as proposed both by the World Health Organization and the American Psychiatric Association, aims to generate cross-cultural diagnosis (Berganza 2003; Canino and Alegria 2008). A cross-cultural disorder is defined by a nosological construct that consistently reflects the same core phenomenon equally across cultural and ethnical groups (Westermeyer 1985). A number of studies have addressed the cross-cultural validity of ADHD from different perspectives. Studies have shown that the prevalence of the disorder is similar across different geographic locations when using equivalent methodological approaches (Polanczyk et al. 2007). The correlates (sex, age) and comorbid conditions associated with the disorder are comparable across different countries as well as the prognosis and response to treatment (Rohde et al. 1999; Rohde 2002; Bauermeister et al. 2003; Souza et al. 2004; Yang et al. 2004; Kooij et al. 2005; Rohde et al. 2005; Dopfner et al. 2006; Roessner et al. 2007; Bauermeister et al. 2007; Polanczyk et al. 2008; Nijmeijer et al. 2008; So, Leung, and Hung 2008). This consistent body of evidence is a strong indicator against the assumption that ADHD is a culture-bound diagnosis.

It is also possible to test the cross-cultural validity of ADHD by using factor analysis to assess whether the structure of the symptoms is equivalent in samples from different cultural and/or ethnic backgrounds. Factor analysis identifies the number of underlying dimensions contained in a set of symptoms. A number of studies have used this strategy in samples from different locations including the U.S. (Healey et al. 1993; Hudziak et al. 1998), Brazil (Brito, Pinto, and Lins 1995), Puerto Rico (Bauermeister 1992; Bauermeister et al. 1992), Finland (Lubke et al. 2007), South Africa (Meyer et al. 2004), Brazil (Rasmussen, Todd, et al. 2002; Rohde et al. 2001), and 11 European countries as well as Australia and Israel (Zhang et al. 2005). In general the studies are consistent with a two-model solution with inattentive and hyperactive-impulsive symptoms grouping in separate factors. The two-model solution was also frequently identified by studies that simultaneously assessed groups with different ethnic backgrounds (Reid et al. 1998; Beiser, Dion, and Gotowiec 2000; Wolraich et al. 2003; Gomez 2009).

It is also possible to test the cross-cultural validity of ADHD by using latent class analysis and assessing whether equivalent groups of individuals are identified based on the associations among a set of symptoms. Studies conducting latent class analysis, based on ADHD symptoms in samples of children and adolescents, were conducted in the U.S. (Acosta et al. 2008; Althoff et al. 2006; Hudziak et al. 1998; Neuman et al. 1999; Neuman et al. 2001; Neuman et al. 2005; Rasmussen, Todd, et al. 2002; Rasmussen et al. 2004; Todd et al. 2001; Todd et al. 2002; Volk, Neuman, and Todd 2005; Volk et al. 2009), Australia (Rasmussen, Neuman, et al. 2002; Rasmussen et al. 2004), Finland (Lubke et al. 2007), Brazil (Rohde et al. 2001; Rasmussen, Todd, et al. 2002), and the Netherlands (de Nijs, Ferdinand, and Verhulst 2007). These studies have identified six to eight classes that appear to account for the distribution of symptoms of ADHD using different methodologies in different samples and cultures. Two clinically relevant classes of severe symptoms that overlap with DSM-IV subtypes are frequently identified. Comorbidity does not seem to significantly impact the final solution, type of symptoms included, or level of endorsement in each class across different studies (Acosta et al. 2008; Neuman et al. 2001; Volk, Neuman, and Todd 2005; Volk et al. 2006), which is also true for different information sources (Althoff et al. 2006).

ADHD AS A DIMENSIONAL OR CATEGORICAL ENTITY

ADHD is defined as a discrete nosological entity which is delimited by the presence of at least six inattentive and/or hyperactive-impulsive symptoms (American Psychiatric Association 1994). This conceptualization is fundamental for purposes of research and communication between different professionals especially from different cultural backgrounds. However, it imposes limitations on clinicians who frequently see patients with subthreshold symptoms who clearly present with functional impairment and who are likely to benefit from interventions. In fact, the presence of functional impairment is frequently considered an external validation that indicates the necessity for treatment, even in situations where the symptom threshold is not reached (Rohde 2008). Therefore, the issue of when ADHD should be addressed as a categorical or dimensional entity has important limitations for future diagnostic definitions and for clinical practice (Rohde 2008).

Statistical Findings

Levy and colleagues (Levy et al. 1997) investigated the concordance of ADHD between twins and siblings in a large cohort of Australian children and demonstrated that its heritability was consistently high when defined either as a trait or a categorical entity. In the same vein Haslam (Haslam et al. 2006) used two taxometric procedures to examine the latent structure of ADHD and test whether it is best understood as categorical or dimensional. Results indicated the ADHD is best modeled as a continuum among both children and adolescents (Haslam et al. 2006).

Clinical Findings

Adults with sub-threshold inattentive or hyperactive symptoms presented significantly increased psychosocial impairment (Kooij et al. 2005). These individuals seem to be less severe in terms of comorbid profile than individuals with the diagnosis of ADHD (Faraone et al. 2006). However, sub-threshold ADHD is more common than the full syndrome in the community and, therefore, may have a greater impact in terms of public health (Lewinsohn et al. 2004). Also, individuals with sub-threshold symptoms are at greater risk of subsequently presenting with a full diagnosis of ADHD (Sanford et al. 1992; Scahill et al. 1999), and are more likely to present with other sub-threshold symptoms and other categorical diagnoses (Lewinsohn et al. 2004). In a random sample of approximately 2500 children from Korea 9% of the sample presented with three to five symptoms of ADHD, while 5.9% of the sample presented with the full diagnosis. Children with sub-threshold symptoms presented with an equivalent personality profile to those with the full disorder (i.e., high novelty seeking, low persistence, low self-directedness) as well as increased risk for externalizing disorders (Cho et al. 2009).

It is not clear, considering the scarcity of studies on this issue, how a dimensional approach can be incorporated in future classificatory systems for ADHD (Angold and Costello 2009). However, the evidence is consistent in indicating that inattention and hyperactivity are continuously distributed in the population and that individuals with sub-threshold symptoms are candidates for clinical attention. The question is whether these individuals will benefit from medical interventions and what kind of interventions are more cost-effective for this population. These issues should be addressed by future studies.

THE OVERLAP BETWEEN ADHD, CONDUCT DISORDER, AND ANTISOCIAL BEHAVIOR

Conduct disorder (CD) and ADHD overlaps in 30% to 50% of cases in both clinical and community samples (Biederman, Newcorn, and Sprich 1991).

Conduct disorder and antisocial behavior are frequently present in patients with ADHD with an early onset and persistent course and comorbid substance abuse or dependence (Biederman, Newcorn, and Sprich 1991; Pliszka 2007).

A study evaluating a clinical sample showed that ADHD was associated with higher than expected psychopathic traits and emotional dysfunctional scores, which are an important aspect of psychopathy (Fowler et al. 2009). The association between high psychopathy scores and ADHD symptom severity did not remain significant after statistically controlling for the presence of CD symptoms. The authors suggested that children with ADHD are at risk for elevated levels of psychopathy, although there is no evidence that those children will grow up as psychopaths (Fowler et al. 2009). In a sample of youths with ADHD, 42% of cases with CD followed a persistent course over time indicating that a poorer prognosis is present in a subsample of individuals with ADHD and comorbid CD (Biederman et al. 2001). It has been hypothesized that oppositional defiant disorder (ODD) would be a precursor of CD in children with ADHD. However, it seems that children with ADHD and comorbid ODD do not necessarily develop CD and two types of ODD, with different correlates, were identified (Biederman, Faraone, Milberger, Jetton, et al. 1996).

While some studies suggest a direct effect of ADHD on antisocial behavior in adulthood (Danckaerts et al. 2000) others demonstrate that ADHD is associated with adult antisocial behavior *only* when conduct disorder or substance use disorders are present in adolescence. This suggests a development pathway indicating that conduct disorder during adolescence mediates the relationship between childhood ADHD and adult antisocial behavior (Mannuzza, Klein, and Moulton 2008).

Clinical Aspects

The relationship between ADHD and CD was hypothesized to be mediated by deficits in self-regulation. Barkley (Barkley 2006) suggests a developmental-neuropsychological model of human self-control where executive functions are implicated in behavior inhibition control acting between an event and the person's response. One of the possible relationships between ADHD and antisocial behavior would lie in the executive deficits associated with ADHD, particularly in children with ADHD with impulsive behavior (Murphy, Barkley, and Bush 2002). Behavioral disinhibition would be a temperamental precursor to both disruptive behavior problems, which would explain the high rates of comorbidity (Hirshfeld-Becker et al. 2002).

Some clinical aspects of ADHD were found to predict later antisocial behavior. The ADHD subtypes bring different risks with the majority of studies showing a lesser risk for the inattentive type, although there are mixed results among studies (Burns and Walsh 2002; Murphy, Barkley, and

Bush 2002). Whether ADHD symptoms occur only at home or at both school and home is also related to later antisocial behavior, with the more pervasive type aggregating a higher risk for psychopathy (Thapar et al. 2006). Also, early onset of ADHD is supposed to carry an increased risk, as well as low IQ, impulsive behavior, and poor executive function (Thapar et al. 2006). Although few studies addressed these aspects the presence of comorbidity might also have some effect on later antisocial behavior as well as different patterns of temperament and personality characteristics (Thapar et al. 2006). There is evidence suggesting that even when ADHD diagnosis is not present, but there are ADHD symptoms, there is still a higher risk for antisocial behavior (Thapar et al. 2006).

Genetic Factors

An important etiological issue concerning the comorbidity between ADHD and CD is the extent to which genetic and environmental factors are implicated in the development of both disorders and the factors specific to each. Some research data support the idea that both genetic and environmental factors influence the development of antisocial behavior (Rhee and Waldman 2002) and that both conditions share the same genetic risk factors (Nadder et al. 2002; Silberg et al. 1996; Thapar, Harrington, and McGuffin 2001) with the hypothesis that the comorbidity between ADHD and CD represents a more severe form of ADHD in terms of genetic loading (Thapar, Harrington, and McGuffin 2001; Thapar et al. 2006).

Genes involved in the dopaminergic system are consistently related to vulnerability to ADHD (Smith, Mick, and Faraone 2009) but fewer studies have addressed the comorbidity between ADHD and antisocial behavior in terms of molecular genetics. Dopamine receptor D4 (DRD4) gene variants are implicated in ADHD diagnosis and some data also support the relation between this gene and antisocial behavior in ADHD patients (Holmes et al. 2002). Also, evidence from three independent samples indicates that the COMT valine/methionine polymorphism at codon 158 (COMT Val158Met) was associated with conduct disorder in individuals with ADHD. Individual valine/valine homozygotes presented more symptoms of conduct disorder, were more aggressive, and were more likely to be convicted of criminal offenses compared with methionine carriers (Caspi et al. 2008). This result was not replicated in a recent study with four different samples that aggregated more than 400 individuals with ADHD aged 6 to 55 years (Monuteaux et al. in press).

Environmental Factors

There is a considerable amount of data suggesting the influence of different types of environmental factors on the development of ADHD and antisocial behavior. Maternal smoking is one of the best studied prenatal factors associated with ADHD, remaining significant even after controlling for possible genetic bias (Thapar et al. 2003). Likewise, maternal smoking has been implicated in the development of antisocial behavior (Langley et al. 2007). However, establishing a direct causal relationship is difficult. Maternal smoking is related to different predictors and outcomes that are also associated with ADHD such as lower social class, low birth weight, and worse patterns of family functioning. Also, these factors are implicated in the development of other behaviors associated with ADHD like CD symptoms. In a clinical sample of children with ADHD where environmental risk factors were investigated, both maternal smoking and social class were associated with the severity of hyperactivity-impulsivity symptoms (no association was found with inattentive symptomatology). Maternal smoking and social class were also associated with CD diagnosis with an odds ratio of 3.14 for CD comorbidity in children with ADHD whose mothers smoked during pregnancy (Langley et al. 2007). There was an additive effect of low social class and maternal smoking during pregnancy with a more than five-fold increase in the risk for CD when both factors co-occurred (Langley et al. 2007). Another study detected an association between maternal smoking during pregnancy and psychopathy in adolescents independent of maternal ADHD, antisocial behavior, and the severity of ADHD and CD symptoms in adolescents (Fowler et al. 2009). Future studies should address the hypothesis of whether the association between maternal smoking during pregnancy and offspring ADHD and antisocial behavior might be mediated by psychopathic traits in the offspring.

Birth complications and later ADHD and CD have been the focus of research and positive results have been reported with a potential biologic mechanism implicating the prefrontal region and amygdala (Fowler et al. 2009). Although this same study could not find an association between family adversity and psychopathy investigators detected a significant association with CD symptoms within the ADHD group (Fowler et al. 2009). Other researchers have found an association between family adversity and ADHD as well as antisocial behavior. Also, there is data linking different patterns of family functioning especially lower cohesion and higher conflict with severity of ADHD symptoms (Biederman, Faraone, and Monuteaux 2002; Pressman et al. 2006). In a four-year follow-up study, increased family conflict and decreased cohesion were associated with the persistence of CD symptoms in a clinical sample of children and adolescents with ADHD (Biederman et al. 2001).

Likewise, other aspects of social adversity such as negative parenting and peer rejection are thought to be related to poorer outcomes in children with ADHD and conduct disorder. However, there is a lack of longitudinal studies to clarify the directional relationship between these factors; which is cause and which is effect? (Abikoff and Klein 1992; Biederman et al. 2001).

Gene-environmental interactions, i.e., the moderation effect of genetic variants on the development of mental disorders following exposure to adverse environmental factors, have been the focus of a great amount of research. Specifically for the development of CD in subjects with ADHD an interaction between birth weight and a variant in the COMT gene has been identified (Thapar et al. 2005). Further studies are necessary to replicate this finding especially considering the difficulty in establishing a causal relationship between the genetic and environmental risks and behavioral outcomes. Gene-environment correlation, that is, genetic vulnerability related to specific behaviors that in turn help to create a hostile environment that influences the outcome, is an important aspect to be studied regarding not only familial aspects but also extra-familial risks such as peer rejection (O'Connor et al. 1998).

Neuroimaging Findings

Although there is a considerable amount of research data on morphologic brain abnormalities in ADHD in pediatric samples most neuroimaging research on antisocial behavior comes from studies in adulthood. ADHD is found to be related with frontostriatal and frontocerebellar circuitries, while antisocial behavior has been linked with orbitofrontal and limbic system abnormalities (Huebner et al. 2008; Marsh, Gerber, and Peterson 2008). One study evaluated morphometric alterations in children with CD with and without comorbid ADHD compared to healthy controls. The CD and CD/ADHD group had a reduction of 6% in the total gray matter volume, particularly in the left orbitofrontal region and bilaterally in the temporal lobe, including the amygdala and the hippocampus on the left side (Huebner et al. 2008). The authors identified an association between hyperactivity-impulsivity symptoms and reduced gray matter volume of parts of the frontoparietal regions while CD symptoms were associated with reductions in the gray matter of the limbic structures. A recent study used the functional imaging paradigm to investigate differences and commonalities in neural networks mediating interference, inhibition, and attention allocation between children with pure ADHD and pure CD. The study showed shared dysfunction in both groups of patients in the right hemispheric temporal and parietal brain regions during interference inhibition and in the right dorsolateral prefrontal cortex during attention allocation. Ventrolateral prefrontal dysfunction, however, was specific to ADHD and not observed in patients with CD in the context of attention allocation (Rubia et al. 2009).

THE OVERLAP BETWEEN ADHD AND BIPOLAR DISORDER

Historically, ADHD has been characterized as a mental disorder of children and adolescents while bipolar disorder (BD) has been understood as a disorder of adults. In the past decades an increasing identification of ADHD in adulthood and BD in childhood and adolescence has turned scientific attention to a possible relationship between these two disorders (Galanter and Leibenluft 2008). Children and adolescents with ADHD and no mood disturbance, and children with classic euphoric episodic BD are easily recognized by trained clinicians. However, although unstable mood and irritability are not part of the diagnostic criteria for ADHD these features are frequently identified in individuals with the disorder (Skirrow et al. 2009). Therefore, when children with chronic inattention and hyperactive-impulsivity present with non-episodic irritability, questions emerge about how to differentiate ADHD from BD and what treatments should be indicated.

Epidemiology

There is high comorbidity between ADHD and BD in children and adolescents, with rates of BD in 10% to 22% of patients with ADHD, and rates of 57% to 98% in patients with BD (Kunwar, Dewan, and Faraone 2007). There are several hypothesis that might explain the high comorbidity rates: (1) a chance phenomenon; (2) an artifact of overlapping diagnostic criteria; (3) a common diathesis that leads to unspecific vulnerable states; and (4) the severe and chronic irritability commonly seen in ADHD is a developmental presentation of mania (Blacker and Tsuang 1992; Sachs et al. 2000; Galanter and Leibenluft 2008). The expression of ADHD in children, adolescents, and adults, although developmentally moderated, has similar clinical features as well as treatment response. However, since only a proportion of children and adolescents with ADHD maintain the full clinical picture during adulthood it has been suggested that the chronic and remitting ADHD might be a different subtype of the disorder, with different prognoses (Biederman, Faraone, Milberger, Curtis, et al. 1996). Some studies show a higher familial pattern in the non-remitting subtype when compared to the remitting form of the disorder (Skirrow et al. 2009). Until now, there have been no studies that evaluated the developmental aspects of mood instability in individuals with ADHD.

Data from three cross-sectional population-based studies analyzing rates of ADHD and BD suggest that people with BD are more likely than people without it to have ADHD (Galanter, Cohen, and Jensen 2003; Kessler et al. 2006; Lewinsohn, Klein, and Seeley 1995). The development of BD in ADHD clinical samples has yielded more conflicting results. Although two studies showed higher than expected rates of BD (Tillman and Geller 2006;

Biederman, Faraone, Mick, et al. 1996) others did not replicate this finding (Fischer et al. 2002; Rasmussen and Gillberg 2000; Mannuzza et al. 1993). In the sample from the Dunedin Multidisciplinary Health and Development Study this association was not detected (Kim-Cohen et al. 2003), while in the Children and Community study sample ADHD at mean age 13.7 years was a risk factor for BD during adolescence (mean age 16.3 years) but not in adulthood (Galanter, Cohen, and Jensen 2003). Based on the possibility that severe and chronic irritability seen in children with ADHD is an early manifestation of mania, two post-hoc analyses of the Children and Community sample and the Great Smoky Mountains Study were carried out to test its predictive validity in relation to later BD (Leibenluft et al. 2006; Brotman et al. 2006). Both analyses were negative and found that severe irritability predicted depressive disorders (Leibenluft et al. 2006; Brotman et al. 2006). Most studies show that early onset BD is associated with higher rates of ADHD (Perlis et al. 2004; Faraone et al. 1997). Some of the conflicting results in epidemiological studies may be the result of methodological and diagnostic disparities across studies such as the variation of sample ascertainment strategies. However, taken together, the findings suggest that ADHD imposes a risk for BD and BD is clearly a risk factor for ADHD.

Clinical Aspects

First of all, the phenomenology of ADHD and BD are to some extent overlapping. The core symptoms of ADHD can be part of BD: distractibility, hyperactivity, and impulsivity are found during hypomania and mania. Also, as previously noted, irritability is also found in children, adolescents, and adults with ADHD. The lack of a developmental perspective to the diagnostic criteria for ADHD (originally developed for children) and BD (originally developed for adults) complicates the possibility of accurately differentiating both disorders during childhood and adolescence (Kent and Craddock 2003). Nevertheless, there are points of non-convergence, which are useful for the differential diagnosis. Geller and colleagues (Geller et al. 2002) found that elation, grandiosity, flight of ideas/racing thoughts, decreased need for sleep, and hypersexuality were symptoms specific to BD, and that most accurately differentiated it from ADHD. Also, by definition BD is an episodic entity while ADHD symptoms are more persistent and stable over time, which, nevertheless, might worsen during a manic or depressive episode if BD is comorbid. The irritability commonly seen in children with ADHD might be explained by different comorbid disorders frequently observed in those patients such as depression, anxiety, ODD, and CD. Trying to characterize the stability of irritability over time (episodic or chronic) might be helpful to rule out the presence of a mood disorder. Using screening tools and different sources of information, as well as addressing these disorders in a developmental perspective, are interesting clinical strategies (Galanter and Leibenluft 2008).

Genetic Factors

The genetic aspects of ADHD and BD were the focus of several studies during the past decade. Relatives of children with ADHD present a fivefold increase in risk for the disorder when compared to controls (Kent and Craddock 2003). Twin studies show higher concordance rates for monozygotic (from 51% up to 82%) than dizygotic twins (0% to 40%) with an estimated heritability of approximately 80% (Kent and Craddock 2003). Similarly, BD is a highly familial disorder with a sevenfold to eightfold increase in risk for first-degree relatives (Craddock and Jones 1999). Monozygotic twins also have a higher concordance rate than dizygotic twins (eight times higher) with heritability remaining at around 80% (Kent and Craddock 2003). These results attest to an important genetic contribution to the pathogenesis of both disorders. Fewer studies addressed the relationship of both disorders in combination. Faraone and colleagues (Faraone et al. 1997) found that the comorbidity of ADHD and BD in youth predisposed to an increased risk for both disorders in first-degree relatives when compared to relatives of controls or ADHD-only patients. Geller and colleagues (Geller et al. 2006) found BD to be a risk factor for greater BD morbidity in first-degree relatives when compared to healthy or ADHD-only controls. Another study also found high rates of ADHD in first-degree relatives of BD youth, although it was not the most frequent diagnosis (Rende et al. 2007). A recent study (Birmaher et al. 2009) was conducted to examine the prevalence of psychiatric disorders in the offspring of parents with BD. The authors found a high risk for type I BD and BD-NOS, with an odds ratio of 13.4 when compared with the offspring of control parents, and an odds ratio of 9.1 when compared with offspring of parents with non-BD psychiatric disorders. The risk was also higher for other psychiatric conditions, including ADHD, with an odds ratio of 3.5 when compared with the offspring of control parents.

Taken together, this evidence indicates higher than expected rates of ADHD in family members of BD probands and weaker evidence to demonstrate elevated rates of BD in family members of children with ADHD (Galanter and Leibenluft 2008).

Neuropsychological Factors

From a neuropsychological point of view it has been suggested that the mood instability commonly observed in ADHD patients might be related to impairments in attention and other executive functions (Skirrow et al.

2009). The studies that evaluated the distinction between ADHD, BD, and comorbid conditions presented conflicting results. Patients with BD presented an impairment in executive functions independently of the comorbidity with ADHD, and the comorbid group presented the worst functioning (Pavuluri et al. 2006; Shear et al. 2002). Another study showed worse functioning when patients with ADHD with or without comorbid BD were compared with BD or healthy controls (Rucklidge 2006). A third study demonstrated different neuropsychological profiles between patients with ADHD and patients with BD with or without comorbid ADHD (Dickstein et al. 2005). Clearly, more research is needed in this field.

Neuroimaging Studies

There is robust evidence from structural and functional imaging studies implicating reduced size in frontal-striatal pathways, the corpus callosum, caudate nuclei, globus pallidum, and cerebellum in ADHD. Also, a dysfunction in the prefrontal, basal ganglia, and cingulate appears to be related to the disorder. In BD, evidence indicates differences in frontal, temporal, corpus callosum, and basal ganglia, although these associations have not been consistently reported. The main difference between these two disorders lies in the temporal area, which is not affected in ADHD. Apart from an overlap in some areas there is not enough evidence supporting a relationship between BD and ADHD (Kent and Craddock 2003). It is important to notice that most studies in ADHD were carried out in children while BD research is mainly assessed in adult populations (Kent and Craddock 2003). The lack of evidence for a common neuroanatomical substrate might be due to under-powered studies to detect differences.

Pharmacological Aspects

Treating ADHD with possibly comorbid BD can be a challenge. Usually it is recommended that BD symptoms should be addressed first and, if the ADHD symptomatology still poses impairment, treated subsequently. Two studies addressed the treatment of ADHD in youth who have BD. In one study, mixed amphetamine salts added to divalproex sodium were more effective than placebo in treating the symptoms of ADHD and no significant worsening of manic symptoms emerged (Scheffer et al. 2005). A chart review concluded that mood stabilization was a prerequisite for ADHD treatment (Biederman et al. 1999). In a post-hoc analysis of the Multimodal Treatment Study of Children with ADHD, the presence of manic symptoms without BD diagnosis was not associated with a poor stimulant treatment response (Biederman et al. 1999; Galanter et al. 2005). Carlson (Carlson et al. 2000) identified similar results and found no association between methylphenidate treatment and precipitation of BD in susceptible individuals. Two studies demonstrated that the comorbidity of ADHD and BD predicted a poorer response to typical antimanic medication in adolescents (State et al. 2004; Masi et al. 2004). On the other hand, another clinical trial did not support this evidence (Kafantaris et al. 1998). There is some evidence, mainly from case studies, that stimulants may precipitate manic symptoms or hasten the onset of BD (Cherland and Fitzpatrick 1999). These were retrospective and uncontrolled studies and this kind of evidence should be taken cautiously, especially due to the proven benefits that stimulants have on ADHD outcomes. Since methylphenidate acts mainly on dopaminergic systems and most antimanic medication action involves the same neurotransmitter systems the similar pharmacological profiles might be understood as evidence of a relationship between both disorders. However, the involvement of those systems are by no means specific to these disorders since the majority of psychiatric entities are thought to involve the same neurochemical systems (Kent and Craddock 2003).

FUTURE PERSPECTIVES

ADHD is a prevalent disorder that predicts several adverse events over the life of affected children, adolescents, and adults, and is associated with significant financial burden to societies. Future cross-national studies with large samples should aggregate the study of the impact of culture on different aspects of ADHD. These studies are likely to generate important data for future classificatory systems.

Also, prospective studies with representative samples of the population can better elucidate how sub-threshold symptoms should be addressed in the future. These studies will be able to answer some of the gaps in the literature about the comorbidity between ADHD, CD, and BD. Investigations should use standardized methodological approaches as much as possible, which can facilitate the interpretation and replication of results. Also, new methods integrating genetic, neuropsychological, and neuroimaging techniques can address the neurobiological characteristics specific to the disorders so that their relationship can be better understood.

Conflict of Interest

Dr. Polanczyk is on the speaker's bureau of Novartis. Dr. Rohde was on the speakers' bureau and/or acted as consultant for Eli-Lilly, Janssen-Cilag, and Novartis in the last three years. Currently, his only industry-related activity is taking part of the advisory board/speakers' bureau for Eli-Lilly and Novartis (less than US$10,000 per year and reflecting less than 5% of his gross income per year). The ADHD and Juvenile Bipolar Disorder Outpatient Programs chaired by him received unrestricted educational and research support from the following pharmaceutical companies in the last three years: Abbott, Bristol-Myers Squibb, Eli-Lilly, Janssen-Cilag, Novartis, and Shire.

REFERENCES

Abikoff, H., and R. G. Klein. 1992. Attention-deficit hyperactivity and conduct disorder: Comorbidity and implications for treatment. *J Consult Clin Psychol* 60 (6):881-92.

Acosta, M. T., F. X. Castellanos, K. L. Bolton, J. Z. Balog, P. Eagen, L. Nee, J. Jones, L. Palacio, C. Sarampote, H. F. Russell, K. Berg, M. Arcos-Burgos, and M. Muenke. 2008. Latent class subtyping of attention-deficit/hyperactivity disorder and comorbid conditions. *J Am Acad Child Adolesc Psychiatry* 47 (7):797-807.

Althoff, R. R., W. E. Copeland, C. Stanger, E. M. Derks, R. D. Todd, R. J. Neuman, T. C. Van Beijsterveldt, D. I. Boomsma, and J. J. Hudziak. 2006. The latent class structure of ADHD is stable across informants. *Twin Res Hum Genet* 9 (4):507-22.

American Psychiatric Association. 1994. *Diagnostic and Statistical Manual of Mental Disorders, Fourth Edition.* Washington, DC: American Psychiatric Association.

Angold, A., and E. J. Costello. 2009. Nosology and measurement in child and adolescent psychiatry. *J Child Psychol Psychiatry* 50 (1-2):9-15.

Barkley, R. A. 2006. *Attention-Deficit Hyperactivity Disorder.* New York: The Guilford Press.

Bauermeister, J. J. 1992. Factor analyses of teacher ratings of attention deficit-hyperactivity and oppositional defiant symptoms in children aged four through thirteen years. *J Clin Child Psychol* 21:27-34.

Bauermeister, J. J., M. Alegria, H. R. Bird, M. Rubio-Stipec, and G. Canino. 1992. Are attentional-hyperactivity deficits unidimensional or multidimensional syndromes? Empirical findings from a community survey. *J Am Acad Child Adolesc Psychiatry* 31 (3):423-31.

Bauermeister, J. J., G. Canino, M. Bravo, R. Ramirez, P. S. Jensen, L. Chavez, A. Martinez-Taboas, J. Ribera, M. Alegria, and P. Garcia. 2003. Stimulant and psychosocial treatment of ADHD in Latino/Hispanic children. *J Am Acad Child Adolesc Psychiatry* 42 (7):851-5.

Bauermeister, J. J., P. E. Shrout, R. Ramirez, M. Bravo, M. Alegria, A. Martinez-Taboas, L. Chavez, M. Rubio-Stipec, P. Garcia, J. C. Ribera, and G. Canino. 2007. ADHD correlates, comorbidity, and impairment in community and treated samples of children and adolescents. *J Abnorm Child Psychol* 35 (6):883-98.

Beiser, M., R. Dion, and A. Gotowiec. 2000. The structure of attention-deficit and hyperactivity symptoms among native and non-native elementary school children. *J Abnorm Child Psychol* 28 (5):425-37.

Berganza, C. E. 2003. Broadening the international base for the development of an integrated diagnostic system in psychiatry. *World Psychiatry* 2 (1):38-40.

Biederman, J., S. Faraone, E. Mick, J. Wozniak, L. Chen, C. Ouellette, A. Marrs, P. Moore, J. Garcia, D. Mennin, and E. Lelon. 1996. Attention-deficit hyperactivity disorder and juvenile mania: An overlooked comorbidity? *J Am Acad Child Adolesc Psychiatry* 35 (8):997-1008.

Biederman, J., S. Faraone, S. Milberger, S. Curtis, L. Chen, A. Marrs, C. Ouellette, P. Moore, and T. Spencer. 1996. Predictors of persistence and remission of ADHD into adolescence: Results from a four-year prospective follow-up study. *J Am Acad Child Adolesc Psychiatry* 35 (3):343-51.

Biederman, J., S. V. Faraone, S. Milberger, J. G. Jetton, L. Chen, E. Mick, R. W. Greene, and R. L. Russell. 1996. Is childhood oppositional defiant disorder a precursor to adolescent conduct disorder? Findings from a four-year follow-up study of children with ADHD. *J Am Acad Child Adolesc Psychiatry* 35 (9):1193-204.

Biederman, J., S. V. Faraone, and M. C. Monuteaux. 2002. Differential effect of environmental adversity by gender: Rutter's index of adversity in a group of boys and girls with and without ADHD. *Am J Psychiatry* 159 (9):1556-62.

Biederman, J., E. Mick, S. V. Faraone, and M. Burback. 2001. Patterns of remission and symptom decline in conduct disorder: A four-year prospective study of an ADHD sample. *J Am Acad Child Adolesc Psychiatry* 40 (3):290-8.

Biederman, J., E. Mick, J. Prince, J. Q. Bostic, T. E. Wilens, T. Spencer, J. Wozniak, and S. V. Faraone. 1999. Systematic chart review of the pharmacologic treatment of comorbid attention deficit hyperactivity disorder in youth with bipolar disorder. *J Child Adolesc Psychopharmacol* 9 (4):247-56.

Biederman, J., J. Newcorn, and S. Sprich. 1991. Comorbidity of attention deficit hyperactivity disorder with conduct, depressive, anxiety, and other disorders. *Am J Psychiatry* 148 (5):564-77.

Birmaher, B., D. Axelson, K. Monk, C. Kalas, B. Goldstein, M. B. Hickey, M. Obreja, M. Ehmann, S. Iyengar, W. Shamseddeen, D. Kupfer, and D. Brent. 2009. Lifetime psychiatric disorders in school-aged offspring of parents with bipolar disorder: The Pittsburgh Bipolar Offspring study. *Arch Gen Psychiatry* 66 (3):287-96.

Blacker, D., and M. T. Tsuang. 1992. Contested boundaries of bipolar disorder and the limits of categorical diagnosis in psychiatry. *Am J Psychiatry* 149 (11):1473-83.

Brito, G. N., R. C. Pinto, and M. F. Lins. 1995. A behavioral assessment scale for attention deficit disorder in Brazilian children based on DSM-IIIR criteria. *J Abnorm Child Psychol* 23 (4):509-20.

Brotman, M. A., M. Schmajuk, B. A. Rich, D. P. Dickstein, A. E. Guyer, E. J. Costello, H. L. Egger, A. Angold, D. S. Pine, and E. Leibenluft. 2006. Prevalence, clinical correlates, and longitudinal course of severe mood dysregulation in children. *Biol Psychiatry* 60 (9):991-7.

Burns, G. L., and J. A. Walsh. 2002. The influence of ADHD-hyperactivity/impulsivity symptoms on the development of oppositional defiant disorder symptoms in a 2-year longitudinal study. *J Abnorm Child Psychol* 30 (3):245-56.

Bussing, R., F. A. Gary, T. L. Mills, and C. W. Garvan. 2003. Parental explanatory models of ADHD: Gender and cultural variations. *Soc Psychiatry Psychiatr Epidemiol* 38 (10):563-75.

Bussing, R., N. E. Schoenberg, and A. R. Perwien. 1998. Knowledge and information about ADHD: Evidence of cultural differences among African-American and white parents. *Soc Sci Med* 46 (7):919-28.

Bussing, R., B. T. Zima, F. A. Gary, and C. W. Garvan. 2003. Barriers to detection, help-seeking, and service use for children with ADHD symptoms. *J Behav Health Serv Res* 30 (2):176-89.

Canino, G., and M. Alegria. 2008. Psychiatric diagnosis—is it universal or relative to culture? *J Child Psychol Psychiatry* 49 (3):237-50.

Carlson, G. A., J. Loney, H. Salisbury, J. R. Kramer, and C. Arthur. 2000. Stimulant treatment in young boys with symptoms suggesting childhood mania: A report from a longitudinal study. *J Child Adolesc Psychopharmacol* 10 (3):175-84.

Caspi, A., K. Langley, B. Milne, T. E. Moffitt, M. O'Donovan, M. J. Owen, M. Polo Tomas, R. Poulton, M. Rutter, A. Taylor, B. Williams, and A. Thapar. 2008. A replicated molecular genetic basis for subtyping antisocial behavior in children with attention-deficit/hyperactivity disorder. *Arch Gen Psychiatry* 65 (2):203-10.

Cherland, E., and R. Fitzpatrick. 1999. Psychotic side effects of psychostimulants: A 5-year review. *Can J Psychiatry* 44 (8):811-3.

Cho, S. C., B. N. Kim, J. W. Kim, L. A. Rohde, J. W. Hwang, D. S. Chungh, M. S. Shin, I. K. Lyoo, B. J. Go, S. E. Lee, and H. W. Kim. 2009. Full syndrome and subthreshold attention-deficit/hyperactivity disorder in a Korean community sample: Comorbidity and temperament findings. *Eur Child Adolesc Psychiatry* 18 (7):447-57.

Cooper, C. R., and J. Denner. 1998. Theories linking culture and psychology: Universal and community-specific processes. *Annu Rev Psychol* 49:559-84.

Craddock, N., and I. Jones. 1999. Genetics of bipolar disorder. *J Med Genet* 36 (8):585-94.

Danckaerts, M., E. Heptinstall, O. Chadwick, and E. Taylor. 2000. A natural history of hyperactivity and conduct problems: Self-reported outcome. *Eur Child Adolesc Psychiatry* 9 (1):26-38.

de Nijs, P. F., R. F. Ferdinand, and F. C. Verhulst. 2007. No hyperactive-impulsive subtype in teacher-rated attention-deficit/hyperactivity problems. *Eur Child Adolesc Psychiatry* 16 (1):25-32.

Dickstein, D. P., M. Garvey, A. G. Pradella, D. K. Greenstein, W. S. Sharp, F. X. Castellanos, D. S. Pine, and E. Leibenluft. 2005. Neurologic examination abnormalities in children with bipolar disorder or attention-deficit/hyperactivity disorder. *Biol Psychiatry* 58 (7):517-24.

Dopfner, M., H. C. Steinhausen, D. Coghill, S. Dalsgaard, L. Poole, S. J. Ralston, and A. Rothenberger. 2006. Cross-cultural reliability and validity of ADHD assessed by the ADHD Rating Scale in a pan-European study. *Eur Child Adolesc Psychiatry* 15 Suppl 1:I46-55.

Faraone, S. V., J. Biederman, A. Doyle, K. Murray, C. Petty, J. J. Adamson, and L. Seidman. 2006. Neuropsychological studies of late onset and subthreshold diagnoses of adult attention-deficit/hyperactivity disorder. *Biol Psychiatry* 60 (10):1081-7.

Faraone, S. V., J. Biederman, D. Mennin, J. Wozniak, and T. Spencer. 1997. Attention-deficit hyperactivity disorder with bipolar disorder: A familial subtype? *J Am Acad Child Adolesc Psychiatry* 36 (10):1378-87; discussion 1387-90.

Fischer, M., R. A. Barkley, L. Smallish, and K. Fletcher. 2002. Young adult follow-up of hyperactive children: Self-reported psychiatric disorders, comorbidity, and the role of childhood conduct problems and teen CD. *J Abnorm Child Psychol* 30 (5):463-75.

Fowler, T., K. Langley, F. Rice, N. Whittinger, K. Ross, S. van Goozen, M. J. Owen, M. C. O'Donovan, M. B. van den Bree, and A. Thapar. 2009. Psychopathy traits in adolescents with childhood attention-deficit hyperactivity disorder. *Br J Psychiatry* 194 (1):62-7.

Galanter, C. A., and E. Leibenluft. 2008. Frontiers between attention deficit hyperactivity disorder and bipolar disorder. *Child Adolesc Psychiatr Clin N Am* 17 (2):325-46, viii-ix.

Galanter, C. A., D. L. Pagar, M. Davies, W. Li, G. A. Carlson, H. B. Abikoff, L. E. Arnold, O. G. Bukstein, W. Pelham, G. R. Elliott, S. Hinshaw, J. N. Epstein, K. Wells, L. Hechtman, J. H. Newcorn, L. Greenhill, T. Wigal, J. M. Swanson, and P. S. Jensen. 2005. ADHD and manic symptoms: Diagnostic and treatment implications. *Clin Neurosci Res* 5:283-94.

Galanter, C.G., P. Cohen, and P. S. Jensen. 2003. ADHD does not predict adult bipolar disorder using longitudinal epidemiological data. Paper read at Annual Meeting of the American Academy of Child and Adolescent Psychiatry, at New York.

Geller, B., R. Tillman, K. Bolhofner, B. Zimerman, N. A. Strauss, and P. Kaufmann. 2006. Controlled, blindly rated, direct-interview family study of a prepubertal and early-adolescent bipolar I disorder phenotype: Morbid risk, age at onset, and comorbidity. *Arch Gen Psychiatry* 63 (10):1130-8.

Geller, B., B. Zimerman, M. Williams, M. P. Delbello, K. Bolhofner, J. L. Craney, J. Frazier, L. Beringer, and M. J. Nickelsburg. 2002. DSM-IV mania symptoms in a prepubertal and early adolescent bipolar disorder phenotype compared to attention-deficit hyperactive and normal controls. *J Child Adolesc Psychopharmacol* 12 (1):11-25.

Gidwani, P. P., G. M. Opitz, and J. M. Perrin. 2006. Mothers' views on hyperactivity: A cross-cultural perspective. *J Dev Behav Pediatr* 27 (2):121-6.

Goldman, L. S., M. Genel, R. J. Bezman, and P. J. Slanetz. 1998. Diagnosis and treatment of attention-deficit/hyperactivity disorder in children and adolescents. Council on Scientific Affairs, American Medical Association. *JAMA* 279 (14):1100-7.

Gomez, R. 2009. Invariance of parent ratings of the ADHD symptoms in Australian and Malaysian, and north European Australian and Malay Malaysia children: A mean and covariance structures analysis approach. *J Atten Disord* 12 (5):422-33.

Gomez, R., and A. Vance. 2008. Parent ratings of ADHD symptoms: Differential symptom functioning across Malaysian Malay and Chinese children. *J Abnorm Child Psychol* 36 (6):955-67.

Greenfield, P. M., H. Keller, A. Fuligni, and A. Maynard. 2003. Cultural pathways through universal development. *Annu Rev Psychol* 54:461-90.

Haslam, N., B. Williams, M. Prior, R. Haslam, B. Graetz, and M. Sawyer. 2006. The latent structure of attention-deficit/hyperactivity disorder: A taxometric analysis. *Aust N Z J Psychiatry* 40 (8):639-47.

Healey, J. M., J. H. Newcorn, J. M. Halperin, L. E. Wolf, D. M. Pascualvaca, J. Schmeidler, and J. D. O'Brien. 1993. The factor structure of ADHD items in DSM-III-R: Internal consistency and external validation. *J Abnorm Child Psychol* 21 (4):441-53.

Hirshfeld-Becker, D. R., J. Biederman, S. V. Faraone, H. Violette, J. Wrightsman, and J. F. Rosenbaum. 2002. Temperamental correlates of disruptive behavior disorders in young children: Preliminary findings. *Biol Psychiatry* 51 (7):563-74.

Holborow, P., and P. Berry. 1986. A multinational, cross-cultural perspective on hyperactivity. *Am J Orthopsychiatry* 56 (2):320-2.

Holmes, J., A. Payton, J. Barrett, R. Harrington, P. McGuffin, M. Owen, W. Ollier, J. Worthington, M. Gill, A. Kirley, Z. Hawi, M. Fitzgerald, P. Asherson, S. Curran, J. Mill, A. Gould, E. Taylor, L. Kent, N. Craddock, and A. Thapar. 2002. Association of DRD4 in children with ADHD and comorbid conduct problems. *Am J Med Genet* 114 (2):150-3.

Hudziak, J. J., A. C. Heath, P. F. Madden, W. Reich, K. K. Bucholz, W. Slutske, L. J. Bierut, R. J. Neuman, and R. D. Todd. 1998. Latent class and factor analysis of DSM-IV ADHD: A twin study of female adolescents. *J Am Acad Child Adolesc Psychiatry* 37 (8):848-57.

Huebner, T., T. D. Vloet, I. Marx, K. Konrad, G. R. Fink, S. C. Herpertz, and B. Herpertz-Dahlmann. 2008. Morphometric brain abnormalities in boys with conduct disorder. *J Am Acad Child Adolesc Psychiatry* 47 (5):540-7.

Kafantaris, V., D. J. Coletti, R. Dicker, G. Padula, and S. Pollack. 1998. Are childhood psychiatric histories of bipolar adolescents associated with family history, psychosis, and response to lithium treatment? *J Affect Disord* 51 (2):153-64.

Kent, L., and N. Craddock. 2003. Is there a relationship between attention deficit hyperactivity disorder and bipolar disorder? *J Affect Disord* 73 (3):211-21.

Kessler, R. C., L. Adler, R. Barkley, J. Biederman, C. K. Conners, O. Demler, S. V. Faraone, L. L. Greenhill, M. J. Howes, K. Secnik, T. Spencer, T. B. Ustun, E. E. Walters, and A. M. Zaslavsky. 2006. The prevalence and correlates of adult ADHD in the United States: Results from the National Comorbidity Survey Replication. *Am J Psychiatry* 163 (4):716-23.

Kim-Cohen, J., A. Caspi, T. E. Moffitt, H. Harrington, B. J. Milne, and R. Poulton. 2003. Prior juvenile diagnoses in adults with mental disorder: Developmental follow-back of a prospective-longitudinal cohort. *Arch Gen Psychiatry* 60 (7):709-17.

Kleinman, A. 1987. Anthropology and psychiatry. The role of culture in cross-cultural research on illness. *Br J Psychiatry* 151:447-54.

Kooij, J. J., J. K. Buitelaar, E. J. van den Oord, J. W. Furer, C. A. Rijnders, and P. P. Hodiamont. 2005. Internal and external validity of attention-deficit hyperactivity disorder in a population-based sample of adults. *Psychol Med* 35 (6):817-27.

Kunwar, A., M. Dewan, and S. V. Faraone. 2007. Treating common psychiatric disorders associated with attention-deficit/hyperactivity disorder. *Expert Opin Pharmacother* 8 (5):555-62.

Langley, K., P. A. Holmans, M. B. van den Bree, and A. Thapar. 2007. Effects of low birth weight, maternal smoking in pregnancy and social class on the phenotypic manifestation of attention deficit hyperactivity disorder and associated antisocial behaviour: Investigation in a clinical sample. *BMC Psychiatry* 7:26.

Leibenluft, E., P. Cohen, T. Gorrindo, J. S. Brook, and D. S. Pine. 2006. Chronic versus episodic irritability in youth: A community-based, longitudinal study of clinical and diagnostic associations. *J Child Adolesc Psychopharmacol* 16 (4):456-66.

Levy, F., D. A. Hay, M. McStephen, C. Wood, and I. Waldman. 1997. Attention-deficit hyperactivity disorder: A category or a continuum? Genetic analysis of a large-scale twin study. *J Am Acad Child Adolesc Psychiatry* 36 (6):737-44.

Lewinsohn, P. M., D. N. Klein, and J. R. Seeley. 1995. Bipolar disorders in a community sample of older adolescents: Prevalence, phenomenology, comorbidity, and course. *J Am Acad Child Adolesc Psychiatry* 34 (4):454-63.

Lewinsohn, P. M., S. A. Shankman, J. M. Gau, and D. N. Klein. 2004. The prevalence and co-morbidity of subthreshold psychiatric conditions. *Psychol Med* 34 (4):613-22.

Lubke, G. H., B. Muthen, I. K. Moilanen, J. J. McGough, S. K. Loo, J. M. Swanson, M. H. Yang, A. Taanila, T. Hurtig, M. R. Jarvelin, and S. L. Smalley. 2007. Subtypes versus severity differences in attention-deficit/hyperactivity disorder in the Northern Finnish Birth cohort. *J Am Acad Child Adolesc Psychiatry* 46 (12):1584-93.

Mah, J. W., and C. Johnston. 2007. Cultural variations in mothers' attributions: Influence of child attention-deficit/hyperactivity disorder. *Child Psychiatry Hum Dev* 38 (2):135-53.

Mann, E. M., Y. Ikeda, C. W. Mueller, A. Takahashi, K. T. Tao, E. Humris, B. L. Li, and D. Chin. 1992. Cross-cultural differences in rating hyperactive-disruptive behaviors in children. *Am J Psychiatry* 149 (11):1539-42.

Mannuzza, S., R. G. Klein, A. Bessler, P. Malloy, and M. LaPadula. 1993. Adult outcome of hyperactive boys. Educational achievement, occupational rank, and psychiatric status. *Arch Gen Psychiatry* 50 (7):565-76.

Mannuzza, S., R. G. Klein, and J. L. Moulton, III. 2008. Lifetime criminality among boys with attention deficit hyperactivity disorder: A prospective follow-up study into adulthood using official arrest records. *Psychiatry Res* 160 (3):237-46.

Margalit, M. 1981. Cultural differences in the hyperactive syndrome rated in the Conners abbreviated scale. *J Learn Disabil* 14 (6):330-1.

Marsh, R., A. J. Gerber, and B. S. Peterson. 2008. Neuroimaging studies of normal brain development and their relevance for understanding childhood neuropsychiatric disorders. *J Am Acad Child Adolesc Psychiatry* 47 (11):1233-51.

Masi, G., G. Perugi, C. Toni, S. Millepiedi, M. Mucci, N. Bertini, and H. S. Akiskal. 2004. Predictors of treatment nonresponse in bipolar children and adolescents with manic or mixed episodes. *J Child Adolesc Psychopharmacol* 14 (3):395-404.

Meyer, A., D. E. Eilertsen, J. M. Sundet, J. G. Tshifularo, and T. Sagvolden. 2004. Cross-cultural similarities in ADHD-like behaviour amongst South African primary school children. *S Afr J Psychol* 34:123-39.

Miller, T. W., J. T. Nigg, and R. L. Miller. 2009. Attention deficit hyperactivity disorder in African American children: What can be concluded from the past ten years? *Clin Psychol Rev* 29 (1):77-86.

Monuteaux, M., J. Biederman, A. Doyle, E. Mick, and S.V. Faraone. in press. Genetic risk for conduct disorder symptom subtypes in an ADHD sample: Specificity to aggressive symptoms. *J Am Acad Child Adolesc Psychiatry*.

Murphy, K. R., R. A. Barkley, and T. Bush. 2002. Young adults with attention deficit hyperactivity disorder: Subtype differences in comorbidity, educational, and clinical history. *J Nerv Ment Dis* 190 (3):147-57.

Nadder, T. S., M. Rutter, J. L. Silberg, H. H. Maes, and L. J. Eaves. 2002. Genetic effects on the variation and covariation of attention deficit-hyperactivity disorder (ADHD) and oppositional-defiant disorder/conduct disorder (ODD/CD) symptomatologies across informant and occasion of measurement. *Psychol Med* 32 (1):39-53.

Neuman, R. J., A. Heath, W. Reich, K. K. Bucholz, P. A. F. Madden, L. Sun, R. D. Todd, and J. J. Hudziak. 2001. Latent class analysis of ADHD and comorbid symptoms in a population sample of adolescent female twins. *J Child Psychol Psychiatry* 42 (7):933-42.

Neuman, R. J., N. Sitdhiraksa, W. Reich, T. H. Ji, C. A. Joyner, L. W. Sun, and R. D. Todd. 2005. Estimation of prevalence of DSM-IV and latent class-defined ADHD subtypes in a population-based sample of child and adolescent twins. *Twin Res Hum Genet* 8 (4):392-401.

Neuman, R. J., R. D. Todd, A. C. Heath, W. Reich, J. J. Hudziak, K. K. Bucholz, P. A. Madden, H. Begleiter, B. Porjesz, S. Kuperman, V. Hesselbrock, and T. Reich. 1999. Evaluation of ADHD typology in three contrasting samples: A latent class approach. *J Am Acad Child Adolesc Psychiatry* 38 (1):25-33.

Nijmeijer, J. S., R. B. Minderaa, J. K. Buitelaar, A. Mulligan, C. A. Hartman, and P. J. Hoekstra. 2008. Attention-deficit/hyperactivity disorder and social dysfunctioning. *Clin Psychol Rev* 28 (4):692-708.

Norvilitis, J. M., and P. Fang. 2005. Perceptions of ADHD in China and the United States: A preliminary study. *J Atten Disord* 9 (2):413-24.

Norvilitis, J. M., T. Ingersoll, J. Zhang, and S. Jia. 2008. Self-reported symptoms of ADHD among college students in China and the United States. *J Atten Disord* 11 (5):558-67.

O'Connor, T. G., K. Deater-Deckard, D. Fulker, M. Rutter, and R. Plomin. 1998. Genotype-environment correlations in late childhood and early adolescence: Antisocial behavioral problems and coercive parenting. *Dev Psychol* 34 (5):970-81.

Pavuluri, M. N., L. S. Schenkel, S. Aryal, E. M. Harral, S. K. Hill, E. S. Herbener, and J. A. Sweeney. 2006. Neurocognitive function in unmedicated manic and medicated euthymic pediatric bipolar patients. *Am J Psychiatry* 163 (2):286-93.

Perlis, R. H., S. Miyahara, L. B. Marangell, S. R. Wisniewski, M. Ostacher, M. P. DelBello, C. L. Bowden, G. S. Sachs, and A. A. Nierenberg. 2004. Long-term implications of early onset in bipolar disorder: Data from the first 1000 participants in the systematic treatment enhancement program for bipolar disorder (STEP-BD). *Biol Psychiatry* 55 (9):875-81.

Pierce, C. D., and R. Reid. 2004. Attention deficit hyperactivity disorder: Assessment and treatment of children from culturally different groups. *Semin Speech Lang* 25 (3):233-40.

Pliszka, S. 2007. Practice parameter for the assessment and treatment of children and adolescents with attention-deficit/hyperactivity disorder. *J Am Acad Child Adolesc Psychiatry* 46 (7):894-921.

Polanczyk, G., M. S. de Lima, B. L. Horta, J. Biederman, and L. A. Rohde. 2007. The worldwide prevalence of ADHD: A systematic review and metaregression analysis. *Am J Psychiatry* 164 (6):942-8.

Polanczyk, G., S. V. Faraone, C. H. Bau, M. M. Victor, K. Becker, R. Pelz, J. K. Buitelaar, B. Franke, S. Kooij, E. van der Meulen, K. A. Cheon, E. Mick, D. Purper-Ouakil, P. Gorwood, M. A. Stein, E. H. Cook, Jr., and L. A. Rohde. 2008. The impact of individual and methodological factors in the variability of response to methylphenidate in ADHD pharmacogenetic studies from four different continents. *Am J Med Genet B Neuropsychiatr Genet* 147B (8):1419-24.

Pressman, L. J., S. K. Loo, E. M. Carpenter, J. R. Asarnow, D. Lynn, J. T. McCracken, J. J. McGough, G. H. Lubke, M. H. Yang, and S. L. Smalley. 2006. Relationship of family environment and parental psychiatric diagnosis to impairment in ADHD. *J Am Acad Child Adolesc Psychiatry* 45 (3):346-54.

Rasmussen, E. R., R. J. Neuman, A. C. Heath, F. Levy, D. A. Hay, and R. D. Todd. 2002. Replication of the latent class structure of attention-deficit/hyperactivity disorder (ADHD) subtypes in a sample of Australian twins. *J Child Psychol Psychiatry* 43 (8):1018-28.

———. 2004. Familial clustering of latent class and DSM-IV defined attention-deficit/hyperactivity disorder (ADHD) subtypes. *J Child Psychol Psychiatry* 45 (3):589-98.

Rasmussen, E. R., R. D. Todd, R. J. Neuman, A. C. Heath, W. Reich, and L. A. Rohde. 2002. Comparison of male adolescent-report of attention-deficit/hyperactivity disorder (ADHD) symptoms across two cultures using latent class and principal components analysis. *J Child Psychol Psychiatry* 43 (6):797-805.

Rasmussen, P., and C. Gillberg. 2000. Natural outcome of ADHD with developmental coordination disorder at age 22 years: A controlled, longitudinal, community-based study. *J Am Acad Child Adolesc Psychiatry* 39 (11):1424-31.

Reid, R., G. J. DuPaul, T. J. Power, A. D. Anastopoulos, D. Rogers-Adkinson, M. B. Noll, and C. Riccio. 1998. Assessing culturally different students for attention deficit hyperactivity disorder using behavior rating scales. *J Abnorm Child Psychol* 26 (3):187-98.

Rende, R., B. Birmaher, D. Axelson, M. Strober, M. K. Gill, S. Valeri, L. Chiappetta, N. Ryan, H. Leonard, J. Hunt, S. Iyengar, and M. Keller. 2007. Childhood-onset bipolar disorder: Evidence for increased familial loading of psychiatric illness. *J Am Acad Child Adolesc Psychiatry* 46 (2):197-204.

Rhee, S. H., and I. D. Waldman. 2002. Genetic and environmental influences on antisocial behavior: A meta-analysis of twin and adoption studies. *Psychol Bull* 128 (3):490-529.

Roessner, V., A. Becker, A. Rothenberger, L. A. Rohde, and T. Banaschewski. 2007. A cross-cultural comparison between samples of Brazilian and German children with ADHD/HD using the Child Behavior Checklist. *Eur Arch Psychiatry Clin Neurosci* 257 (6):352-9.

Rohde, L. A. 2002. ADHD in Brazil: The DSM-IV criteria in a culturally different population. *J Am Acad Child Adolesc Psychiatry* 41 (9):1131-3.

———. 2008. Is there a need to reformulate attention deficit hyperactivity disorder criteria in future nosologic classifications? *Child Adolesc Psychiatr Clin N Am* 17 (2):405-20, x.

Rohde, L. A., G. Barbosa, G. Polanczyk, M. Eizirik, E. R. Rasmussen, R. J. Neuman, and R. D. Todd. 2001. Factor and latent class analysis of DSM-IV ADHD symptoms in A school sample of Brazilian adolescents. *J Am Acad Child Adolesc Psychiatry* 40 (6):711-8.

Rohde, L. A., J. Biederman, E. A. Busnello, H. Zimmermann, M. Schmitz, S. Martins, and S. Tramontina. 1999. ADHD in a school sample of Brazilian adolescents: A study of prevalence, comorbid conditions, and impairments. *J Am Acad Child Adolesc Psychiatry* 38 (6):716-22.

Rohde, L. A., C. Szobot, G. Polanczyk, M. Schmitz, S. Martins, and S. Tramontina. 2005. Attention-deficit/hyperactivity disorder in a diverse culture: Do research and clinical findings support the notion of a cultural construct for the disorder? *Biol Psychiatry* 57 (11):1436-41.

Rubia, K., R. Halari, A. B. Smith, M. Mohammad, S. Scott, and M. J. Brammer. 2009. Shared and disorder-specific prefrontal abnormalities in boys with pure attention-deficit/hyperactivity disorder compared to boys with pure CD during interference inhibition and attention allocation. *J Child Psychol Psychiatry.*

Rucklidge, J. J. 2006. Impact of ADHD on the neurocognitive functioning of adolescents with bipolar disorder. *Biol Psychiatry* 60 (9):921-8.

Sachs, G. S., C. F. Baldassano, C. J. Truman, and C. Guille. 2000. Comorbidity of attention deficit hyperactivity disorder with early- and late-onset bipolar disorder. *Am J Psychiatry* 157 (3):466-8.

Sanford, M. N., D. R. Offord, M. H. Boyle, A. Peace, and Y. A. Racine. 1992. Ontario child health study: Social and school impairments in children aged 6 to 16 years. *J Am Acad Child Adolesc Psychiatry* 31 (1):60-7.

Scahill, L., M. Schwab-Stone, K. R. Merikangas, J. F. Leckman, H. Zhang, and S. Kasl. 1999. Psychosocial and clinical correlates of ADHD in a community sample of school-age children. *J Am Acad Child Adolesc Psychiatry* 38 (8):976-84.

Scheffer, R. E., R. A. Kowatch, T. Carmody, and A. J. Rush. 2005. Randomized, placebo-controlled trial of mixed amphetamine salts for symptoms of comorbid ADHD in pediatric bipolar disorder after mood stabilization with divalproex sodium. *Am J Psychiatry* 162 (1):58-64.

Shear, P. K., M. P. DelBello, H. Lee Rosenberg, and S. M. Strakowski. 2002. Parental reports of executive dysfunction in adolescents with bipolar disorder. *Child Neuropsychol* 8 (4):285-95.

Silberg, J., M. Rutter, J. Meyer, H. Maes, J. Hewitt, E. Simonoff, A. Pickles, R. Loeber, and L. Eaves. 1996. Genetic and environmental influences on the covariation between hyperactivity and conduct disturbance in juvenile twins. *J Child Psychol Psychiatry* 37 (7):803-16.

Skirrow, C., G. McLoughlin, J. Kuntsi, and P. Asherson. 2009. Behavioral, neurocognitive and treatment overlap between attention-deficit/hyperactivity disorder and mood instability. *Expert Rev Neurother* 9 (4):489-503.

Smith, A. K., E. Mick, and S. V. Faraone. 2009. Advances in genetic studies of attention-deficit/hyperactivity disorder. *Curr Psychiatry Rep* 11 (2):143-8.

So, C. Y., P. W. Leung, and S. F. Hung. 2008. Treatment effectiveness of combined medication/behavioural treatment with Chinese ADHD children in routine practice. *Behav Res Ther* 46 (9):983-92.

Souza, I., M. A. Pinheiro, D. Denardin, P. Mattos, and L. A. Rohde. 2004. Attention-deficit/hyperactivity disorder and comorbidity in Brazil: Comparisons between two referred samples. *Eur Child Adolesc Psychiatry* 13 (4):243-8.

State, R. C., M. A. Frye, L. L. Altshuler, M. Strober, M. DeAntonio, S. Hwang, and J. Mintz. 2004. Chart review of the impact of attention-deficit/hyperactivity disorder comorbidity on response to lithium or divalproex sodium in adolescent mania. *J Clin Psychiatry* 65 (8):1057-63.

Swanson, J. M., J. A. Sergeant, E. Taylor, E. J. Sonuga-Barke, P. S. Jensen, and D. P. Cantwell. 1998. Attention-deficit hyperactivity disorder and hyperkinetic disorder. *Lancet* 351 (9100):429-33.

Thapar, A., T. Fowler, F. Rice, J. Scourfield, M. van den Bree, H. Thomas, G. Harold, and D. Hay. 2003. Maternal smoking during pregnancy and attention deficit hyperactivity disorder symptoms in offspring. *Am J Psychiatry* 160 (11):1985-9.

Thapar, A., R. Harrington, and P. McGuffin. 2001. Examining the comorbidity of ADHD-related behaviours and conduct problems using a twin study design. *Br J Psychiatry* 179:224-9.

Thapar, A., K. Langley, T. Fowler, F. Rice, D. Turic, N. Whittinger, J. Aggleton, M. Van den Bree, M. Owen, and M. O'Donovan. 2005. Catechol O-methyltransferase gene variant and birth weight predict early-onset antisocial behavior in children with attention-deficit/hyperactivity disorder. *Arch Gen Psychiatry* 62 (11):1275-8.

Thapar, A., M. van den Bree, T. Fowler, K. Langley, and N. Whittinger. 2006. Predictors of antisocial behaviour in children with attention deficit hyperactivity disorder. *Eur Child Adolesc Psychiatry* 15 (2):118-25.

Tillman, R., and B. Geller. 2006. Controlled study of switching from attention-deficit/ hyperactivity disorder to a prepubertal and early adolescent bipolar I disorder phenotype during 6-year prospective follow-up: Rate, risk, and predictors. *Dev Psychopathol* 18 (4):1037-53.

Todd, R. D., E. R. Rasmussen, R. J. Neuman, W. Reich, J. J. Hudziak, K. K. Bucholz, P. A. Madden, and A. Heath. 2001. Familiality and heritability of subtypes of attention deficit hyperactivity disorder in a population sample of adolescent female twins. *Am J Psychiatry* 158 (11):1891-8.

Todd, R. D., N. Sitdhiraksa, W. Reich, T. H. Ji, C. A. Joyner, A. C. Heath, and R. J. Neuman. 2002. Discrimination of DSM-IV and latent class attention-deficit/hyperactivity disorder subtypes by educational and cognitive performance in a population-based sample of child and adolescent twins. *J Am Acad Child Adolesc Psychiatry* 41 (7):820-8.

Volk, H. E., C. Henderson, R. J. Neuman, and R. D. Todd. 2006. Validation of population-based ADHD subtypes and identification of three clinically impaired subtypes. *Am J Med Genet B Neuropsychiatr Genet* 141B (3):312-8.

Volk, H. E., R. J. Neuman, and R. D. Todd. 2005. A systematic evaluation of ADHD and comorbid psychopathology in a population-based twin sample. *J Am Acad Child Adolesc Psychiatry* 44 (8):768-75.

Volk, H. E., A. A. Todorov, D. A. Hay, and R. D. Todd. 2009. Simple identification of complex ADHD subtypes using current symptom counts. *J Am Acad Child Adolesc Psychiatry* 48 (4):441-50.

Westermeyer, J. 1985. Psychiatric diagnosis across cultural boundaries. *Am J Psychiatry* 142 (7):798-805.

Wolraich, M. L., E. W. Lambert, A. Baumgaertel, S. Garcia-Tornel, I. D. Feurer, L. Bickman, and M. A. Doffing. 2003. Teachers' screening for attention deficit/hyperactivity disorder: Comparing multinational samples on teacher ratings of ADHD. *J Abnorm Child Psychol* 31 (4):445-55.

Yang, L., Y. F. Wang, Q. J. Qian, J. Biederman, and S. V. Faraone. 2004. DSM-IV subtypes of ADHD in a Chinese outpatient sample. *J Am Acad Child Adolesc Psychiatry* 43 (3):248-50.

Zhang, S., D. E. Faries, M. Vowles, and D. Michelson. 2005. ADHD Rating Scale IV: Psychometric properties from a multinational study as a clinician-administered instrument. *Int J Methods Psychiatr Res* 14 (4):186-201.

Zito, J. M., D. J. Safer, S. dosReis, L. S. Magder, and M. A. Riddle. 1997. Methylpheni-date patterns among Medicaid youths. *Psychopharmacol Bull* 33 (1):143-7.

7

Changes in Psychiatric Problems of Children and Adolescents in Japan

From Internalizing to Externalizing Symptoms

Sadaaki Shirataki and Kazu Kobayashi

INTRODUCTION

Child and adolescent psychopathology is perceived differently by professionals working inside and outside Japan. Self-injurious behavior, acute severe social withdrawal (known as Hikikomori), and school non-attendance have long been regarded as typical psychological problems of young people in Japan by those working outside the country. Japanese professionals, however, are currently addressing other types of symptoms such as hyperactivity, restlessness, inattentiveness, impulsivity, troublesome behavior and acting-out behaviors. Furthermore, these symptoms have been increasing dramatically recently, in line with their high frequency in other countries.

Rough estimates of the rates of symptoms observed in Japan in 6-16-year-olds in 2006 were as follows: 50/10,000 for suicide, 300/10,000 for school non-attendance, 630/10,000 for hyperactivity/inattentiveness, and 140/10,000 for antisocial behaviors (i.e., young people arrested by the police because of criminal offences) (White Paper on Child and Adolescent, Japanese Government, 2008).

A number of reports have described how social conditions in Japan including intra-familial conditions have changed over the past ten years. It has been postulated that these changes are likely to account for the observed variations in the psychopathology of children and adolescents. Differences in ways of thinking, attitudes, and behavior first manifested in children and adolescents and later in adults too. An early change was the loss of "reserve" in the attitudes and behaviors of young people; this in itself may in part constitute an

149

"externalizing" symptom as described by Achenbach (1966, 1983, 1991), in sharp contrast with the internalizing symptoms such as Hikikomori, school non-attendance, and self-injurious behavior which were based on Japanese thinking patterns that emphasize over-control and self-sacrifice.

Japanese child and adolescent psychiatrists work in a variety of ways and in collaboration with other professionals. This provides a real world view of how problematic behaviors, often involving externalizing symptoms, concern teachers in school. This chapter will begin by outlining the evidence on the nature of psychopathology among children and adolescents in present day Japan.

INTERNALIZING AND EXTERNALIZING SYMPTOMS

Achenbach (1966, 1983) developed a behavior checklist listing the psychiatric symptoms of children and adolescents. His assumption was that a group of symptoms forms a syndrome, and a group of syndromes comprises a disease entity. Through factor analyzing the symptoms he extracted two factors: internalizing/over-controlled and externalizing/under-controlled symptoms. We have adopted this classificatory system as fitting well the presentation of children and young people in Japan. Some ten years ago there was a predominance of internalizing symptoms while the present picture is an excess of externalizing symptoms. Nevertheless, there are limitations to his classification.

For example, similar symptoms could have different origins. Typically hyperactive/impulsivity may be caused both by psychological conflict and anxiety and by functional brain deficits (Baving et al., 2003). We could err on the side of ascribing hyperactivity/impulsivity ADHD as representing "externalizing" symptoms of psychological origin (Belsky et al., 2007; Burgess et al., 2003; McKee et al., 2008).

Another drawback is that internalizing and externalizing symptoms can occur sequentially and be observable at different time points. Furthermore, Achenbach's assumption that all symptoms can be assigned to either internalizing or externalizing symptom clusters is debatable. A recent report (Pesenti-Gritti et al., 2008) concluded that the two clusters can occur concurrently, something we ourselves have also observed. For example, impulsive and aggressive behavior towards a close friend in a school classroom may be a manifestation of ADHD, but the child may also shut himself away at home resulting in school non-attendance, thus presenting a mixture of externalizing and internalizing symptoms.

We have adopted Achenbach's dichotomous classification to describe the changes over time from internalizing to externalizing symptom clusters displayed by Japanese children. In the following paragraphs we will discuss our own experience from over 20 years providing consultations on difficult cases to the Governmental Board of Education in one Japanese city.

THE CHARACTERISTICS OF JAPANESE TRAITS IN THE PAST AND TODAY

The Characteristics of Japanese Traits in the Past

Japan is known by the words "Samurai," "Geisha," and "Fuyijama." The Japanese imperial system was transformed into a democratic one after Word War II. Consequently, there have been marked psychosocial and cultural changes which have influenced children and adolescents psychologically and spiritually. Macroscopically changes have involved social values, microscopically family situation and values.

Here we will focus on changes occurring since the 1980s. Around ten years earlier in 1967 Chie Nakane explained Japanese traits in *The Human Relationship in a Tate (Vertical) Society*, and in 1971 Takeo Doi published *The Anatomy of Dependence* (Amae) where he explained, in psychoanalytic terms, a trait akin to dependency that was found particularly in the Japanese; the origins of which could be rooted in the mother-child relationship. In 1974 *Identity and the Life Cycle* by E. H. Erikson (1959) was translated into Japanese (Keigo Okonogi, 1974). The concept of "identity" had a great influence in Japan, both on specialists and laypeople; it especially influenced thinking about the self-concept of adolescents who became involved in the serious school riots that took place at the time.

Looking back on adolescents living under the umbrella of militarism before World War II an identification with the group "for others," "for society," and "for their family" was very important to the self-concept. At that time in Japan this was particularly symbolized in "for the Emperor." A father took on the emperor's place in his family, and society therefore was centered on men. This is reflected in proverbs such as "a Man does not go into a kitchen," "a Man has seven enemies out of his house," and "a Man's words are like gold and metal." A woman was only somebody to complement a man. "Samurai" and "Geisha" were symbolic of this situation. Then after the war democracy was instituted and the equal rights of men and women were clearly stated. Nevertheless, it took nearly 30 years for this to become fully accepted by the nation and this was the basic motivation behind the national widespread school riots conducted by college students to which we previously alluded. Young people fought against authority and the nation, and fathers found themselves having to confront their "self-identity."

Prior to that, families were commonly large and extended; nuclear families were created with record-breaking speed in the fifteen years following the 1960s. In *The Chrysanthemum and the Sword* (R. Benedict, 1946) Japanese culture was described as a shame-sensitive society exemplifying how the group's logic took priority over individualism. The erythrophobia and anthropophobia peculiar to the Japanese symbolize the relationship between individuals and society (Kyoichi Kondoh, 1984). How to behave "for his/her nation," "for his/her family," "for his/her society," or "for his/her company" had long been regarded by adults as important issues. Hayao Kawai (1975) described this as "the ethics behind the scenes" and thought it based on the maternal principle. He contrasted it with Western countries' "ethics behind the individual" which he thought were based on the paternal principle, and which put great weight on satisfying one's desires and maximizing growth.

The Ajase complex was described by Heisaku Kosawa who presented it to Sigmund Freud in 1932. It was re-examined by Keigo Okonogi in 1979. In contrast to the Oedipus complex, which involves a guilt feeling connected with punishment, the Ajase complex involves a guilt feeling connected with sin and allowance/permission. It was also at that time that Masahisa Nisizono, another leader of Japanese psychoanalysis, became involved with anaclitic pharmacopsychotherapy in relation to psychoanalytic psychotherapy (1971).

As an historical overview the "Amae theory" by T. Doi, the "Ajase complex" by H. Kosawa, "ethics behind the scenes" by H. Kawai, and "anaclitic phamacotherapy" by M. Nisizono were all based on the relationships between the mother and child.

In conclusion, in the past, a commitment to the group as opposed to individual wishes was an important Japanese trait rooted on introjections and assimilation derived from maternal principles.

The Characteristics of Japanese Traits Today

About 25 years ago, deregulation—moving away from rules that had been used until then to maintain the public and group order—took place in schools. From 1984 expectations about issues such as hair length in boys changed over a short space of time. Eventually it came to look as if individual adolescents did not care about others very much. Behaviors such as loud shouting on trains, talking into mobile phones, or sitting on the compartment's floor were openly displayed with young people seemingly being oblivious to other people's feelings.

A Japanese sociologist, Yoji Morita (1991), based on his research on school non-attendance in Japan, coined the term "privatization" as the key for explaining the changes described above. In our view this accounts for some of the behavioral problems we are seeing at present. Some psychologists have highlighted the resulting changes in ego structure, including a narrowing of the ego structure and ability to contain or manage conflict (thus leading to conflict with others who regard the behavior as troublesome), and an inflexible ego structure which may be viewed by others as indicating a difficult person.

In summary, we are now seeing more troublesome behaviors and externalizing symptoms in children and adolescents as a result of changes in their value judgments or set of values. In the past it was thought natural to prioritize self-sacrifice over self-fulfilment, to maintain harmonious interpersonal relationships. Today, conversely, the priority is on satisfying individual needs and controlling behavior towards others. This can be accompanied by impulsivity, a low threshold for anger, and outbursts of acting-out behavior towards others. These constitute externalizing behavioral symptoms and they are causing much concern in present day Japan.

CHANGES IN SYMPTOM PATTERNS OBSERVED THROUGH SCHOOL MENTAL HEALTH CONSULTATIONS

Consultations by Child and Adolescent Psychiatrists to the Municipal Governmental Board of Education in a City in Japan

Over the past 20 years the authors have been providing school mental health consultations in collaboration with the municipal governmental board of education, in one city with a population of 475,000. This is a typical mid-sized urban city near the larger cities of Osaka and Kobe. It has 21 kindergartens, 42 primary schools, 20 junior high schools, and 3 high schools. All these schools have been involved in the mental health consultations, whereby a child and adolescent psychiatrist meets with all teachers including the principal and assistant principal. The purpose is to gain a better understanding of the psychopathology of individual children and adolescents and to help teachers in their management. Each school is able to request the municipal board for a number of consultations each year. Their frequency has ranged from 110 to 130 yearly, and 15 child and adolescent psychiatrists from surrounding areas have been recruited. During the consultation process the teacher responsible for the student reports on the presenting problem. Then, the consultant outlines the psychiatric aspects of the student's symptoms, and this is followed by a recommendation to the teacher on management strategies. We believe this kind of consultation is educative to teachers and helps them understand their students better through understanding their symptoms. We are also aware that most schoolteachers in neighboring areas are offered lectures by eminent academics; however, in our view these lectures cannot provide concrete, precise ways of handling the symptoms presented by pupils.

One of the authors, Shirataki, visits three kindergartens, seven elementary schools, four junior high schools, and one high school, two to four times a year, and has been doing so for the past five years, which has helped create a common ground and purpose with the teachers. Before the consultation the teacher writes a report summarizing the recent history and describing ways in which the student's behaviors are troublesome. This already helps teachers understand better the children's symptoms and observe relevant family dynamics. Whilst in the early stages teachers' reports tend to be lacking in necessary detail; after a few consultations the quality of reports improves considerably.

Trends of Symptoms Discussed in Consultations

As soon as the consultation has taken place schools send a brief report to the board that includes the relevant information discussed; for example, the key symptoms and a brief summary of what was learnt from the consultation. The reports are collated on a yearly basis and there is now statistical information available summarizing the work of more than 20 years. The data includes symptom and disorder frequency by gender. Here we have selected four symptoms (neurotic, school non-attendance, hyperkinetic/impulsive, and behavior problems) to document precise frequency trends between 1994 and 2008 (see Figure 7.1). Furthermore, we have grouped the first two symptoms into an internalizing symptom cluster and the latter two into an externalizing cluster and we have analyzed symptom cluster frequency over time (see Figure 7.2).

Figure 7.1 shows that school non-attendance and hyperkinetic/impulsive behavior have changed the most over the past 14 years. School non-attendance decreased dramatically from 2003, whilst hyperkinesis/impulsivity increased over the same time period. Behavioral problems have remained constant overall, in spite of sharp peaks every four to five years. We can see in Figure 7.2 the change in the pre-eminence of symptom clusters; before 2003 internalizing symptoms predominated and after 2003 externalizing symptoms did. We can also see that externalizing symptoms constitute some 35% of the student psychopathology reported by teachers as being a concern to them.

This data helps focus the management techniques required by teachers for dealing with pupils' symptoms. We can at the very least advise them not to wait until the difficult behavior causes damage to pupils, thus motivating them to want to change. Children with externalizing symptoms will not be helped by waiting, because some will need to be taught and supported in order to attend to educational problems caused by suboptimal cognitive and intellectual abilities.

Predominance of Internalizing over Externalizing
Symptoms and Area of Residence (Urban or Rural)

We have explained so far that children we see in kindergarten, elementary, and junior high schools tend to be referred for externalizing symptoms.

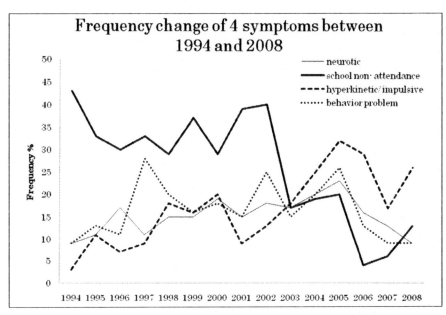

Figure 7.1. Frequency Change of Four Symptons between 1994 and 2008

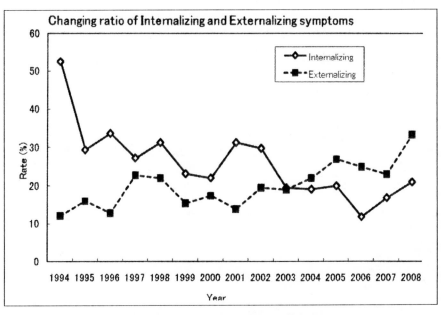

Figure 7.2. Changing Ratio of Internalizing and Externalizing Symptoms

However, this experience is based on children attending our local urban area. It is possible that the recent increase in internalizing symptoms—possibly resulting from changes in social attitudes and reduced closeness in family relationships—has only taken place in urban areas. As already mentioned, internalizing symptoms may be understood as a consequence of the very close intra-familial relationships prevalent in Japan until 20 years ago generating a conflicted and anxious inner world in young people.

One of the authors (S. Shirataki) has recently been asked to contribute to the medical treatment and attend to mental health in a local rural prefecture area approximately three hours by train from the urban center. The area has a modern public hospital with a sophisticated inner layout and atmosphere, but because of its remoteness psychiatric input is very limited. At the time of writing the author has worked in the local child psychiatric clinic for one month. Surprisingly, 80% of patients coming to the clinic had internalizing symptoms, school non-attendance being most prominent. It is entirely possible, therefore, that the relative predominance of internalizing over externalizing symptoms depends on geography even in a comparatively narrow country such as Japan. This experience also confirmed the fact that some adolescents present with a complex mixture of internalizing symptoms against a background of externalizing symptoms, particularly in young people who also have developmental disorders.

RELATIONSHIP BETWEEN EXTERNALIZING
SYMPTOMS AND DEVELOPMENTAL DISORDERS

Symptoms in Children with Developmental Disorders

In Japan there has been a great deal of recent interest in the developmental disorders. The Ministry of Education, Culture, Sports Science and Technology (MEXT, 2003) reported that 6.3% of children in mainstream elementary and junior high school have some kind of developmental disorder.

Japanese clinicians and researchers have traditionally concerned themselves with pervasive developmental disorders, and this accounts for the high number of presentations on this topic at IACAPAP congresses. It is, therefore, not difficult to find good research data on the incidence of PDD in Japan.

Honda and colleagues (2005) reported the incidence of childhood autism to be as high as 0.38% in boys, which in Japan is four to five times higher than some 30 years earlier. They also reported a remarkable increase in high functioning pervasive developmental disorders (PDD), which currently make up about a quarter of the all PDD diagnoses (see also chapter by Steiman et al. in this book).

Using checklist assessments with parents, Kanbayashi and colleagues (1994) reported a higher frequency of 5.3% for ADHD in schoolchildren aged six to ten years in a particular geographic area.

In our view the symptoms of the developmental disorders can be ordered within a hierarchical structure. Both our clinical observations and existing research indicates that symptoms in these children are not simply confined to key features. For example, PDD has three core symptoms: social aloofness and difficulty with smooth social relationships, problems communicating both verbally and nonverbally, and restricted/limited activities or interests. But affected children also display symptoms seen in other developmental disorders. Parents often complain that children with PDD forget events that happened only a few seconds earlier (an expression of dysfunctional working memory), and that these children also have anomalies in time perception. Some children with PDD and ADHD will have an unusual way of experiencing time spans or rhythmic time intervals. Furthermore, many children will show psychogenic reactions related to feelings of inferiority brought about by limited cognitive abilities. They will display symptoms such as school non-attendance, neurotic and psychosomatic complaints, and even self-injurious behaviors, all of which have long been recognized by Japanese child psychiatrists. The symptoms of developmental disorders may thus be understood as fitting within three separate levels. The basic level contains of course the symptoms characteristic of each type of disorder. The second level incorporates those common to all disorders, such as working memory and time perception dysfunction. Finally, the third level consists of symptoms of psychogenic origin within the internalizing/externalizing dimensions. This is depicted in Figure 7.3.

Problems with the Concept of ADHD

We have already discussed the fact that some externalizing symptoms in Japan may these days be erroneously attributed to developmental disorders such as ADHD, PDD, LD (learning disability), and MR (mental retardation). This may be due to ambiguities in the developmental disorder concept, especially with reference to ADHD. In line with other clinicians and researchers (Sonuga-Barke, 2005) we also wonder about the validity of ADHD as a separate disease entity. We summarize our arguments here:

1. The current DSM-IV-TR definition of ADHD only requires two symptom clusters: inattention and hyperkinesis/impulsivity, which is less strict than ICD-10's diagnostic criteria. Using the DSM definition may, therefore, be expected to identify more cases. Furthermore, DSM allows two types of ADHD, with predominant inattentiveness or alter-

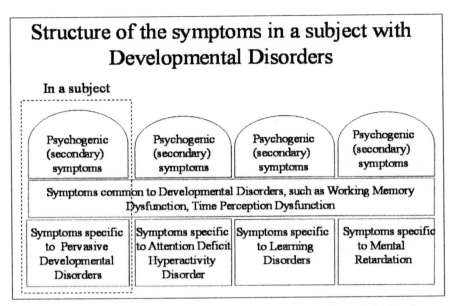

Figure 7.3.   Structure of the Symptoms in a Subject with Developmental Disorders

natively with hyperkinesis/impulsivity, which again increases the likelihood of reaching an ADHD diagnosis.

2. There are no objective tests to confirm the presence of the three core
   symptoms of ADHD nor are there clear criteria for defining appropriate or abnormal levels of activity, and the same applies to other childhood symptoms. Subjective decisions will therefore determine judg-
   ment on the presence or absence of ADHD.

3. Even if the symptoms of hyperkinesis were to be unequivocally identified, they might still have a psychogenic origin, for example, anxiety or
   deeply seated conflicts in the child's mind. At first glance, therefore, hyperkinesis of psychogenic origin could erroneously be ascribed to
   ADHD.

4. ADHD often accompanies other symptom clusters such as PDD, learning disability, and mental retardation. It might be best not regarded as a
   disease entity, but rather as a ubiquitous, or umbrella, concept in the
   same way as mental retardation (MR) was some 40 years ago when it
   was considered a disease entity related to disorders of the brain.

5. As an extension of this, ADHD could be construed as a common output
   of brain functional systems, or a "final common pathway" in the brain.
   This concept is familiar to neurologists and psychiatrists, though its
   precise nature and characteristics have been little studied so far.

6. Taking into account that some of the behaviors seen in ADHD are in line with behavioral styles that are culturally becoming common in children generally, the difficulty is in differentiating abnormal and excessive hyperkinesis and inattention from the normal, if highly active, behaviors of young people in the Japan of today.

CONCLUSIONS

This chapter has addressed an issue of concern to clinicians and researchers alike within child and adolescent psychiatry in Japan today, namely the remarkable increase in externalizing behaviors and in impulsive, restless behaviors which may be part of developmental disorders such as ADHD and pervasive developmental and conduct disorders. We conclude that changes in behavior are due on the one hand to broad changes in the Japanese character and ways of thinking. We believe we can successfully trace this back to the time when the Japanese modified their ways of relating to others. In the past parents and teachers inculcated in young people the importance of putting off self-fulfilment and the importance of perseverance. About 15 years ago, Japanese young people moved away towards a culture of self-preservation and self-fulfilment, and currently they seem not to recognize the concept of "public situations." Even on trains, high school students tend to sit directly on the floor of the carriage and group themselves into loud speaking circles, without any apparent consideration for fellow passengers. Psychiatrists observing this kind of behavior comment that over the past 20 years the young no longer seem to differentiate the private from the public space.

Researchers have attempted to explain the change in attitudes in the young as related to changes in the nurturing quality of the family. However, the fact that they are so widespread and pervasive makes them unlikely to be simply related to intra-familial changes, and suggests they are due to broader societal change. An additional factor complicates the situation further, namely, the recent increase in the number of young people with developmental disorders who present with symptoms comparable to those of children with externalizing behaviors. A remaining task for the future is explaining the increase in children and young people with developmental disorders (see also chapter by Steiman et al. in this book).

We wish to highlight our view that some researchers and clinicians put excessive emphasis on aggression as an expression of externalizing behavior in young children. Our clinical observations indicate that what may be interpreted as aggression may in fact be awkwardness but appearing to others as if carrying an aggressive intention. This becomes clear from the fact that those affected by these children's externalizing behaviors are often close or

Case Study of Externalizing Symptoms

An 11-year old, B, an elementary school fifth-grader, was the second child of a middle class family, consisting of parents and a 14-year-old brother. When B was born his elder brother was diagnosed with emotional disturbance and his parents had found this diagnosis hard to accept.

B attended a child psychiatric clinic with his parents because of difficult behavior in school. From the start of the fifth grade he had been consistently defiant to his teacher, and showed troublesome behaviors if thwarted; he had even been aggressive towards a teacher who was trying to restrain him. Teachers had become frightened of his aggression. It was not clear whether B was showing similar behaviors at home because his parents appeared unwilling to report difficulties, perhaps wanting to blame the problem on the teacher's management of the child.

The school decided to ask for a child psychiatric consultation and all teachers, including the schoolmaster and vice master, attended. The child psychiatrist advised the school to refer B for assessment, thinking about the possibility of an underlying developmental disorder such as high functioning pervasive developmental disorder. For six months the family failed to follow the school's advice, but finally they accepted the referral. Assessment at the clinic by a clinical psychologist and a child psychiatrist confirmed the suspected diagnosis of high functioning PDD and also of ADHD with marked impulsivity.

The assessment and diagnosis were followed by a collaborative relationship between B, the family, the school, and the clinic, and as a first step medication was tried for his ADHD. Several months of methylphenite followed, but neither B nor his parents reported any improvement and the treatment was discontinued. The consultant advised the school to request legal advice or intervention from the prefectural family-children's center. However, following a sudden attack by B on other students, one teacher was badly hurt whilst restraining B. The school approached the police because of the continuing antisocial violent behavior and B was referred to the family court for observation and therapeutic education.

This was an exceptionally difficult case in the sense that there was no single cause for such complex problems or a single management strategy. If the problem had presented ten years before, his parents probably would have been blamed as exercising poor discipline at home. We, as child and adolescent psychiatrists, however, know that impulsive/violent and antisocial behavior does not necessarily originate because of internal, conscious conflict in response to environmental stressors; we cannot, therefore, necessarily accept the notion of parents being blamed for mismanaging their child.

intimate friends; the child's difficult behavior may be an expression of ambivalent psychological attitudes.

REFERENCES

Achenbach, T.M. The classification of children's psychiatric symptoms: A factor-analytic study. *Psychological Monographs* 80(7) (1966): 1-37.

Achenbach, T.M., *Manual for the Child Behavior Checklist and Revised Child Behavior Profile.* Burlington: University of Vermont, 1983.

Achenbach, T.M. *Manual for the Child Behavior Checklist/ 4-18 and 1991 Profile.* Burlington: University of Vermont, 1991.

Baving, L., Laucht, M., & Schmidt, M.H. Frontal EEG correlates of externalizing spectrum behaviors. *European Child and Adolescent Psychiatry* 12 (2003): 36-42.

Belsky, J., Pasco Fearon, R.M., & Bell, B. Parenting, attention and externalizing problems: Testing mediation longitudinally, repeatedly and reciprocally. *Journal of Child Psychology and Psychiatry* 48(12) (2007): 1233-1242.

Benedict, R. *The Chrysanthemum and the Sword: Patterns of Japanese Culture.* New York: Houghton Mifflin, 1946.

Burgess, K.B., Marshall, P.J., Rubin, K.H., & Fox, N.A. Infant attachment and temperament as predictors of subsequent externalizing problems and cardiac physiology. *Journal of Child Psychology and Psychiatry* 44(6) (2003): 819-831.

Doi, T. *The Anatomy of Dependence.* Tokyo: Kobundo, 1971. (in Japanese)

Honda, H., Shimizu, Y., Imai, M., & Nitto, Y. Cumulative incidence of childhood autism: A total population study of better accuracy and precision. *Developmental Medicine & Child Neurology* 47 (2005): 10-18.

Kanbayashi, Y., Fujii, K., Kita, M., et al. (1994). *Study on the psychopathology of ADHD— from the DSM-III-R based checklist assessment by parents.* 1993 research report of the psychiatric and neurological disorders funded by Ministry of Health. (1994): 67-74.

Kawai, H. *Self, Shame, Fear—from the World of Anthrophobia.* Tokyo: Shiso, 1975. (in Japanese)

Kondoh, K. Characteristics in Japanese interpersonal-phobia. *Rinsho-SeishinIgaku* 11 (1984): 837-842.

McKee, L., Colletti, C., Rakow, A., Jones, D.J., & Forehand, R. Parenting and child externalizing behaviors: Are the associations specific or diffuse? *Aggression and Violent Behaviors* 13(3) (2008): 201-215.

Ministry of Education, Culture, Sports, Science and Technology. Final Report on the Special Needs Education, 2003.

Morita, Y. *Sociology of School Non-Attendance Phenomena.* Tokyo: Gakubunsha, 1991. (in Japanese).

Nakane, C. *The Human Relationship in the Tate (Vertical) Society.* Tokyo: Kodansha, 1967. (in Japanese)

Nishizono, M. The anaclitic drug-psychotherapy—A synthesis of psychoanalysis and high dose drug-therapy. *Folia Psychiatrica et Neurologica Japonica* 19(1) (1965): 9-15.

Okonogi, K. *Erikson's Ego-Identity*. Tokyo: Seishinshobo, 1974. (in Japanese)

Pesenti-Gritti, P., Spatola, C.A.M., Fagnani, C., Ogliari, A., Patricarca, V., Stazi, M.A., Battaglia, M. The co-occurrence between internalizing and externalizing behaviours. *European Child and Adolescent Psychiatry* 17(2) (2008): 82-92.

Sonuga-Barke, E.J.S. Causal models of ADHD: From common simple deficits to multiple developmental pathways. *Biological Psychiatry* 57(5) (2005): 1231-1238.

White Paper on Child and Adolescent. Japanese Government, 2009.

8

Trends in Autism Rates

Is There an Epidemic?

Mandy Steiman, Rebecca Simon,
Lisa Reisinger, and Eric Fombonne

INTRODUCTION

Autism is a neurodevelopmental disorder characterized by impairments in social and communication skills, with accompanied repetitive or restricted interests and behaviors. Autism involves both developmental delays and qualitative differences starting early in development. When the prevalence of autism was first studied in 1966, a rate of 4 per 10,000 was found. Today's best estimate of the prevalence of pervasive developmental disorders (PDD) is 60 to 70 per 10,000. The discrepancy between early rates and more current numbers has been the focus of much debate. Making sense of this increase poses a challenge for researchers who must provide explanations to an increasingly concerned public. The aim of this chapter is to provide an updated review of epidemiological surveys of pervasive developmental disorders, while commenting on the methodology of studies that document increased prevalence rates. Specific questions addressed include (a) What is the range of prevalence estimates for autism and other pervasive developmental disorder diagnoses? (b) What are the trends in prevalence rates over time? and (c) What methodological issues need to be considered in research on the prevalence of autism and other PDD diagnoses? In this chapter the terms "autism" and "autistic disorder" are used interchangeably, and the terms "PDD" and "autism spectrum disorder" (ASD) are considered as interchangeable.

Prevalence rates of autism are clearly higher than they were several decades ago. Based on increased autism rates, the existence of an "autism epidemic" has been questioned. The concern over a possible epidemic has led to an increased interest in studying environmental factors as possible causes. If there was indeed an increase in autism incidence over the course of several decades (i.e., a true increase in new cases over time), alterations in the gene pool alone could not be responsible for such a rapid change. If such a change were substantiated a major push to identify environmental and other causes would be expected to try and account for the increase. Without knowing whether there is a true increase in autism, embarking on the path of identifying environmental factors outside the context of possible genetic vulnerabilities is less compelling, especially in light of recent discoveries in genetics that may prove to be a more fruitful pursuit toward identifying underlying causes (e.g., Sebat et al. 2007). High prevalence rates provide the impetus to understand more about autism's causes, and existing data on prevalence and incidence could help to substantiate which paths to follow.

This chapter aims to address the question of an "autism epidemic" by summarizing current epidemiological research on autism. Studies were identified based on searches of major databases of scientific literature including MEDLINE, PsycINFO, and EMBASE, and from prior reviews (Fombonne 2003; Fombonne 2005; Fombonne et al. 2009; Williams et al. 2006). The studies considered are limited to those published in English and, to ensure that a more valid method of case ascertainment was used, excludes studies that relied on questionnaire-based approaches to define cases of autism. Included are 58 studies that were published between 1966 and 2009 that surveyed PDDs in clearly demarcated, non-overlapping samples. Of these, 48 provided information on rates of autistic disorder and 23 more recent studies provided estimates on all PDD diagnoses. Studies from 17 countries are included. The majority of studies have been conducted since 2001 and have widely varying sample sizes ranging from 826 (Kadesjö et al. 1999) to millions of individuals (e.g., CDC 2007a; CDC 2007b).

DIAGNOSIS OF AUTISM: CHANGES IN CASE DEFINITION

When trying to establish prevalence rates for particular disorders, methods of case definition and case ascertainment are essential to designing a study and greatly impact how results can be interpreted (Fombonne 2007). Although many core features of autism are understood similarly today as they have been in the past, finer distinctions in autism diagnosis began to be described about 30 years ago. Today, the umbrella term "autism spectrum disorder" (ASD) and its synonym "pervasive developmental disorder" are inclusive of a range of diagnoses. Definitions have broadened to include individuals with relatively mild symptoms, including individuals without cognitive delays, and with fewer and/or less severe symptoms. When trying to interpret prevalence rates, changes in nomenclature must be taken into account. Current epidemiological studies, using a broader definition of autism, are likely casting a much wider net.

The earliest description of autism was made by Kanner (1943), who identified 11 children with "autistic disturbances," including delayed and atypical communication skills, disturbances in social skills, and atypical responses to aspects of the environment. Since Kanner's relatively narrow definition of autism, definitions have changed over time to include broader criteria, as first proposed by Rutter (1970), and subsequently in the ninth edition of the International Classification of Diseases (ICD-9; World Health Organization 1977), the third edition of the Diagnostic and Statistical Manual of Mental Disorders (DSM-III; American Psychiatric Association 1980), and the revised third edition (DSM-III-R; American Psychiatric Association 1987). In these newer classification systems PDD presentations with fewer symptoms and less severe phenotypes began to be recognized. The two current worldwide diagnostic systems, DSM-IV (American Psychiatric Association 1994) and ICD-10 (World Health Organization 1992) are generally similar in their description of the PDD diagnoses and allow for broader criteria and milder presentations to be included. In contrast to the earliest conceptualizations of autism, PDDs now subsume diagnoses that occur without mental retardation. Specifically, use of the Pervasive Developmental Disorder—Not Otherwise Specified (PDD-NOS) category, introduced in the DSM-III-R and previously termed "atypical autism" in DSM-III, allows for a diagnosis to be made even if symptoms are few in number. Asperger's disorder, defined by Hans Asperger (1944), first appeared in classification systems in the 1990s (termed "Asperger syndrome" in ICD-10). This diagnosis also requires fewer symptoms than a classic autism diagnosis, although the validity of this diagnosis is debatable as a definable category separate from autism presentations without mental retardation (i.e., unofficially termed "high-functioning" autism) (Klin et al. 2005).

PDD diagnoses have high inter-rater reliability and expert clinicians can generally agree on diagnosis. As mentioned above, the ICD-10 and DSM-IV are mostly consistent in their descriptions of symptoms that are central to PDDs. However, the two major classification systems do have differences that add a layer of complexity when interpreting studies that have used case definitions based on one or other system. For example, presentations fitting the DSM-IV's broad PDD-NOS category (previously termed "atypical autism") are captured under several categories within ICD-10, including "atypical autism," "other PDD," and "PDD unspecified." As such, equivalence of the terms "PDD-NOS" and "atypical autism" across research studies cannot be assumed.

The broadening of classification systems to include milder forms of PDD is a likely contributing factor to the increased prevalence rates. Differences between available classification systems and changes within systems over time are factors that will continue to require careful consideration. As classification systems are updated, more changes are expected. For example, instead of understanding PDDs as being categorically different from normal development, and specific PDDs as categorically different from each other, there is an increasing emphasis on a dimensional understanding of the PDDs. This will potentially be formalized in future classification systems and will need to be considered in the forthcoming research on autism prevalence and incidence.

CASE ASCERTAINMENT: METHODS OF DEFINING PDD

In order to determine prevalence rates, valid and reliable methods of defining cases are required. In surveys on PDD numerous strategies including use of databases and registries, as well as multi-stage approaches, have been employed to ascertain cases within a population. Existing databases from service providers (Croen et al. 2002), special education databases (Gurney et al. 2003; Fombonne et al. 2006; Lazoff et al. 2009), and national registers (Madsen et al. 2002; Lin et al. 2009) have been relied upon for case ascertainment. Although these approaches can be convenient and provide an efficient method of case identification, they are not proactive in nature. Cases that are not yet identified within the databases and registries will be missed. Also, not all individuals will be in contact, and thus counted, by a given institution. The risk of underestimating the prevalence of cases exists within this methodology.

A multi-stage approach to identify cases includes various stages to help with case identification. At first, a large-scale screen is attempted in an effort to find all possible affected cases within a population. The second step includes a more intensive evaluation to verify the diagnostic status of potential cases. Methodological issues are often at issue at both these stages that impact the relative value and comparability of studies. At the screening stage, sampling techniques are not always adequate to ensure sampling of the entire target population, with some studies sampling in a more thorough manner than others. Comparison across countries is complicated by differences in service development and accessibility, reflecting differences in educational and health care systems across countries and over time.

Initial screeners range from diagnostic checklists written in colloquial language to more systematic screening tools that have known reliability and validity. Participation rates in this first stage of screening vary across studies although, on average, refusal rates tend to be low. Few studies provide an estimate of the reliability of the screening procedure, and the sensitivity of the screening method is difficult to establish. A typical approach to establish sensitivity involves random sampling of screened negative cases to estimate false negatives. Because PDD has a relatively low base rate in the population these kinds of estimations would be costly and are at risk of being imprecise. Due to these factors, prevalence estimates that use this kind of methodology may underestimate the true prevalence of PDD in the population, although the magnitude of the underestimation is not known.

At the second stage of multi-stage approaches, although participation rates tend to be high, similar methodological issues arise. To confirm a case at this stage different informants and data sources are used (e.g., medical records, health professionals). In some studies direct assessment of the individual with a PDD is completed. In the two surveys conducted by the American Centers for Disease Control and Prevention (CDC 2007a and 2007b) source files at multiple settings were screened (e.g., schools, state health facilities, hospitals, clinics, diagnosis centers, and other clinical providers for children with PDDs). For the more obvious cases a streamlined review was performed to confirm the status of the case. More intensive abstracted evaluations were performed for the less obvious cases. The process included clinician reviewers, the use of a scoring system based on diagnostic criteria to code the information, and reliability checks. For large samples this method seems adequate and is likely to be used again in future surveillance surveys.

In more recent surveys, direct assessment of a subset of cases is sometimes completed. When participants are directly examined, assessments may be conducted with standardized gold-standard measures to diagnose PDDs, such as the Autism Diagnostic Interview–Revised (ADI-R; LeCouteur et al. 1989) and/or the Autism Diagnostic Observation Schedule (ADOS; Lord et al. 2000). These tools gather detailed information on a child's developmental history and clinical presentation toward making a PDD diagnosis. At other times examination by a clinical expert without the use of standardized measures may be done.

PREVALENCE OF AUTISTIC DISORDER AND THE OTHER PDDS

Out of the 58 studies reviewed, some provide information on rates of autism or autistic disorder only, while others, generally the more recent studies, include information on prevalence of all the PDDs. Studies on autism only and studies on all the PDDs are represented separately in tables and figures.

Prevalence of Autistic Disorder

Prevalence estimates for 48 studies of autistic disorder are summarized in Table 8.1. These studies include 13 originating from the UK, 6 each from

Table 8.1 Prevalence of Autistic Disorder

Reference	Country	Age	Diagnostic Criteria	Number of Subjects with Autism / Size of Population	Prevalence Rate/10,000	95% CI*	Gender Ratio (M:F)	% without Cognitive Delay
Lotter (1966)	UK	8-10	Rating scale	32 / 78,000	4.1	2.7 - 5.5	2.6	15.6
Brask (1970)	Denmark	2-14	Clinical	20 / 46,500	4.3	2.4 - 6.2	1.4	-
Treffert (1970)	USA	3-12	Kanner	69 / 899,750	0.7	0.6 - 0.9	3.06	-
Wing et al. (1976)	UK	5-14	Rating scale of Lotter	17 / 25,000	4.8	2.1 - 7.5	16	30
Hoshino et al. (1982)	Japan	0-18	Kanner's criteria	142 / 609,848	2.33	1.9 - 2.7	9.9	-
Bohman et al. (1983)	Sweden	0-20	Rutter criteria	39 / 69,000	5.6	3.9 - 7.4	1.6	20.5
McCarthy et al. (1984)	Ireland	8-10	Kanner	28 / 65,000	4.3	2.7 - 5.9	1.33	-
Steinhausen et al. (1986)	Germany	0-14	Rutter	52 / 279,616	1.9	1.4 - 2.4	2.25	55.8
Burd et al. (1987)	USA	2-18	DSM-III	59 / 180,986	3.26	2.4 - 4.1	2.7	-
Matshuishi et al. (1987)	Japan	4-12	DSM-III	51 / 32,834	15.5	11.3 - 19.8	4.7	-
Bryson et al. (1988)	Canada	6-14	New RDC	21 / 20,800	10.1	5.8 - 14.4	2.5	23.8
Tanoue et al. (1988)	Japan	7	DSM-III	132 / 95,394	13.8	11.5 - 16.2	4.07	-
Cialdella & Mamelle (1989)	France	3-9	DSM-III (based on)	61 / 135,180	4.5	3.4 - 5.6	2.3	-
Ritvo et al. (1989)	USA	3-27	DSM-III	241 / 769,620	2.47	2.1 - 2.8	3.73	34
Sugiyama & Abe (1989)	Japan	3	DSM-III	16 / 12,263	13	6.7 - 19.4	-	-
Gillberg et al. (1991)	Sweden	4-13	DSM-III-R	74 / 78,106	9.5	7.3 - 11.6	2.7	18
Fombonne & du Mazaubrun (1992)	France	9 & 13	Clinical ICD (based on)	154 / 274, 816	4.9	4.1 - 5.7	2.1	13.3
Wignyosumarto et al. (1992)	Indonesia	4-7	CARS	6 / 5,120	11.7	2.3 - 21.1	2.0	0

Table 8.1 Prevalence of Autistic Disorder (contd.)

Study	Country	Age	Criteria	N	Rate	CI		
Honda et al. (1996)	Japan	5	ICD-10	18 / 8,537	21.08	11.4 - 30.8	2.6	50
Arvidsson et al. (1997)	Sweden	3-6	ICD-10	9 / 1,941	46.4	16.1 - 76.6	3.5	22.2
Fombonne et al. (1997)	France	8-16	Clinical; ICD-10 (based on)	174 / 325,347	5.35	4.6 - 6.1	1.81	12.1
Webb et al. (1997)	UK	3-15	DSM-III-R	53 / 73,301	7.2	5.3 - 9.3	6.57	-
Sponheim & Skjeldal (1998)	Norway	3-14	ICD-10	34 / 65,688	5.2	3.4 - 6.9	2.09	47.1
Kadesjö et al. (1999)	Sweden (Central)	6.7-7.7	DSM-III-R; ICD-10; Gillberg's criteria	6 / 826	72.6	14.7 - 130.6	5.0	50
Taylor et al. (1999)	UK	0-16	ICD-10	427 / 490,000	8.7	7.9 - 9.5	-	-
Baird et al. (2000)	UK	7	ICD-10	50 / 16,235	30.8	22.9 - 40.6	15.7	60
Kielinen et al. (2000)	Finland	5-7	DSM-IV	57 / 27,572	20.7	15.3 - 26.0	4.12	49.8
Powell et al. (2000)	UK	1.5	Clinical; ICD-10; DSM-IV	62 / 25,377	7.8	5.8 - 10.5	-	-
Bertrand et al. (2001)	USA	3-10	DSM-IV	36 / 8,896	40.5	28.0 - 56.0	2.2	36.7
Chakrabarti & Fombonne (2001)	UK	2.5-6.5	ICD-10; DSM-IV	26 / 15,500	16.8	10.3 - 23.2	3.3	29.2
Davidovitch et al. (2001)	Israel	7-11	DSM-III-R; DSM-IV	26 / 26,160	10	6.6 - 14.4	4.2	-
Fombonne et al. (2001)	UK	5-15	DSM-IV; ICD-10	27 / 10,438	26.1	16.2 - 36.0	8.0	55.5
Magnusson & Saemundsen (2001)	Iceland	5-14	Mostly ICD-10	57 / 43,153	13.2	9.8 - 16.6	4.2	15.8
Croen et al. (2002)	USA	5-12	CDER (full syndrome)	5,038 / 4,950,333	11	10.7 - 11.3	4.47	62.8

Table 8.1 Prevalence of Autistic Disorder (contd.)

Study	Country	Age	Criteria	Cases / Population	Prevalence	CI		
Madsen et al. (2002)	Denmark	8	ICD-10	46 / 63,859	7.2	5.0 - 10.0	-	-
Tebruegge et al. (2004)	UK	8-9	ICD-10	6 / 2,536	23.7	9.6 - 49.1	-	-
Barbaresi et al. (2005)	USA	0-21	DSM-IV	112 / 37,726	29.7	24.0 - 36.0	-	-
Chakrabarti & Fombonne (2005)	UK	4-7	ICD-10; DSM-IV	24 / 10,903	22	14.4 - 32.2	3.8	33.3
Honda et al. (2005)	Japan	5	ICD-10	123 / 32,791	37.5	31.0 - 45.0	2.5	25.3
Baird et al. (2006)	UK	9-10	ICD-10	81 / 56,946	38.9	29.9 - 47.8	8.3	47
Fombonne et al. (2006)	Canada	5-17	DSM-IV	60 / 27,749	21.6	16.5 - 27.8	5.7	-
Gillberg et al. (2006)	Sweden	7-12	Gillberg's criteria	115 / 32,568	35.3	29.2 - 42.2	3.6	-
Elleísen et al. (2007)	Denmark	8-17	ICD-10; Gillberg's criteria	12 / 7,689	16	7.0 - 25.0	3.0	-
Latif & Williams (2007)	UK	0-17	Kanner	50 / 39,220	12.7	9.0 - 17.0	-	-
Oliveira et al. (2007)	Portugal	6-9	DSM-IV	115 / 67,795	16.7	14.0 - 20.0	2.9	17
Williams et al. (2008)	UK	11	ICD-10	30 / 14,062	21.6	13.9 - 29.3	5.0	86.7
Lazoff et al. (2009)	Canada	5-17	DSM-IV	62 / 23,662	26.2	19.7 - 32.7	5.8	-
Lin J et al.(2009)	Taiwan	0-5 6-11 12-17	Not reported	1,019 / 1,299,004 3,161 / 1,826,201 1,999 / 1,928,991	7.8 17.3 10.4	7.4 - 8.3 16.7 - 17.9 9.9 - 10.8	6.6	-

the U.S. and Japan, 5 from Sweden, 3 each from Denmark, France, and Canada, and 2 or fewer studies each from Finland, Germany, Iceland, Indonesia, Ireland, Israel, Norway, Portugal, and Taiwan. The sample size ranged from 826 to 4.9 million subjects. The median sample size was 38,473 subjects. Studies differed in the age ranges that were considered, with some studies sampling a larger age range and others being limited to a more restricted age range (e.g., sampling only of children aged 11 years in Williams et al. 2008). Prevalence rates for autistic disorder ranged from 0.7 per 10,000 to 72.6 per 10,000, with a median value of 12.9 per 10,000. Prevalence rates of autistic disorder are represented in Figure 8.1.

The gender ratio for PDDs is generally reported to be around 4:1 males to females. In the 41 studies that reported on gender, males outnumbered females. The male to female ratio found in these studies ranged from 1.3 to 16.0, with a mean ratio of 4.4. IQ scores were reported for 26 studies; the percentage of individuals with autistic disorder who have an IQ outside the mentally retarded range ranges from 0 to 86.7%. This represents a large variation across studies in the level of cognitive functioning of individuals with autism, with some studies mostly sampling individuals who are

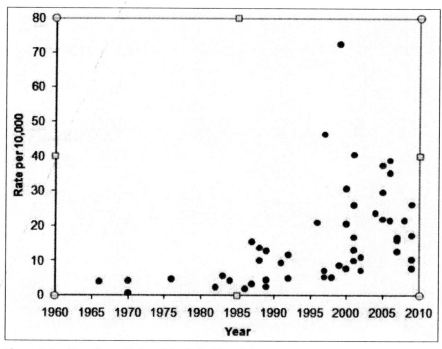

Figure 8.1. Prevalence Rates of Autistic Disorder

cognitively delayed, while others having a majority with relatively normal IQ. There was a trend toward a relationship between having a higher male to female ratio and more individuals without cognitive impairments. This result is consistent with previous research showing associations between gender and IQ, with females being more likely to have lower IQ scores.

Early studies, from pre-1989 (n = 15), before diagnostic criteria from DSM-III-R were available, reported a range of prevalence rates from 0.7 to 15.5 per 10,000, with a median value of 4.3 per 10,000. Studies from the 1990s (n = 10) reported a range of prevalence rates from 4.9 to 72.6 per 10,000 with a median prevalence rate of 9.1 per 10,000. Two studies within this group reported relatively high prevalence rates of 46.4 per 10,000 and 72.6 per 10,000 (Arvidsson et al. 1997; Kadesjö et al. 1999) respectively. Both these studies are from Sweden and included small populations from particular communities. Both studies included direct assessment of children suspected of having a PDD. These studies had the smallest sample sizes out of all the studies of autistic disorder that were reviewed, with the Arvidsson study finding 9/1,941 children with autistic disorder and the Kadesjö study finding 6/826 children with autistic disorder.

In the 23 most recent studies, from the year 2000 to 2009, prevalence rates ranged from 7.2 to 40.5 per 10,000 with a median value of 21.6 per 10,000. Sample sizes in the most recent studies were generally larger and in the majority of studies DSM-IV and ICD-10 criteria were used. Excluding the four studies with the smallest and the largest samples, the mean rate is similar to the median value at 22.9 per 10,000. There was a positive relationship between year of publication and prevalence rates (Spearman $r = 0.69$; $p = <.001$) suggesting that prevalence rates of autistic disorder have increased over time.

Prevalence of All the PDDs

Prevalence estimates for PDD (i.e., inclusive of autistic disorder and other PDD diagnoses) were available for a total of 23 studies and are summarized in Table 8.2. These studies are relatively recent, published between 2000 and 2009. Some of these studies overlap with those in Table 8.1, if they also report a separate figure for autistic disorder. All studies in this group used either DSM-IV or ICD-10 criteria to define cases as PDD. These studies included 9 from the United Kingdom, 6 from the United States, and 2 or fewer from Australia, Canada, China, Denmark, Japan, and Sweden. The sample size for these studies ranged from 2,536 to 4,247,206 (median = 32,568; mean = 270,026). Ages of individuals within the sampled populations ranged from 3 to 17 years. The median age of the samples ranged from 5 to 12.5 years with a modal and median age of 8 years. Prevalence rates for PDDs ranged from 30 to 181.1 per 10,000 with a median value of 61.9 per 10,000. Despite this range there is consistency between the median (61.9 per 10,000) and mean (66.0 per 10,000). The mean rate found across the 23 studies that are reviewed here is comparable to the 6.6 per 1,000 rate reported by the CDC (2007b) study that reported prevalence rates across 14 sites each in a different American state. There is no significant correlation between publication year and prevalence rates in these studies.

In the 21 studies that reported on gender males outnumbered females with the male to female ratio ranging from 2.7 to 15.7, with a mean ratio of 5.5. This range is comparable to the range in the studies on autistic disorder.

IQ scores were reported for 14 studies in this group. The percentage of individuals with PDDs who had an IQ not indicative of a significant cognitive impairment ranged from 30% to 85.3% (median = 54.4%; mean = 55.7%). Similar to the studies on autistic disorder, this represents a large variation across studies in the proportion of individuals who are cognitively impaired. However, when examining individuals with PDDs as a whole the percentage of those who are not cognitively impaired is higher compared to the autistic disorder group. This is not unexpected considering that the other common PDD diagnoses of Asperger's disorder and PDD-NOS are not as frequently associated with cognitive impairments; by definition, an individual with an Asperger disorder diagnosis cannot have a cognitive impairment, and individuals with PDD-NOS have milder impairments overall. Prevalence rates of PDD over time are represented in Figure 8.2, as is the proportion of children with IQ scores outside the mentally retarded range.

Asperger's Disorder and Childhood Disintegrative Disorder

Asperger's disorder (also termed "Asperger syndrome") is a PDD that is similar to autism in that individuals with this disorder present with impairments in social interaction as well as having circumscribed, repetitive, and stereotyped interests and behaviors. In both the DSM-IV and ICD-10 Asperger's disorder is distinguished from autistic disorder in that there are no associated impairments in relation to early language skills, cognitive development, or adaptive skills. Asperger's disorder has been specifically evaluated in 12 studies that were published between 1998 and 2009, and considered both Asperger's disorder and autistic disorder diagnoses. As Asperger's disorder was only recognized as a separate diagnostic category in versions ICD-10 and DSM-IV the reporting of separate rates is relatively recent. In the 12 studies there was a 160-fold variation in estimated rates of Asperger's disorder, ranging from 0.3 to 48.4 per 10,000 with a median value of 11 per 10,000. This variation suggests a lack of reliability for any given estimate. One issue is that individual clinicians may apply Asperger's disorder criteria differently and may be following different conventions

Table 8.2   Prevalence of Pervasive Developmental Disorders

Reference	Country	Age	Diagnostic Criteria	Number of Subjects with Autism / Size of Population	Prevalence Rate/10,000	95% CI*	Gender Ratio (M:F)	% without Cognitive Delay
Baird et al. (2000)	UK	7	ICD-10	94 / 16,235	57.9	46.8 – 70.9	15.7	60
Bertrand et al. (2001)	USA	3-10	DSM-IV	60 / 8,896	67.4	51.5 – 86.7	2.7	51
Chakrabarti and Fombonne (2001)	UK	4-7	ICD-10	96 / 15,500	61.9	50.2 – 75.6	3.8	74.2
Madsen et al. (2002)	Denmark	8	ICD-10	738 / unspecified	30.0	-	-	-
Scott et al. (2002)	UK	5-11	ICD-10	196 / 33,598	58.3	50 – 67	4.0	-
Yeargin-Allsopp et al. (2003)	USA	3-10	DSM-IV	987 / 289,456	34.0	32 – 36	4.0	31.8
Gurney et al. (2003)	USA	8 – 10	-		52.0 66.0	- -	-	-
Icasiano et al. (2004)	Australia	2-17	DSM-IV	177 / ≈ 54,000	39.2	-	8.3	53.4
Tebruegge et al. (2004)	UK	8-9	ICD-10	21 / 2,536	82.8	51.3 – 126.3	6.0	-
Chakrabarti and Fombonne (2005)	UK	4-6	ICD-10	64 / 10,903	58.7	45.2 – 74.9	6.1	70.2
Baird et al. (2006)	UK	9-10	ICD-10	158 / 56,946	116.1	90.4 – 141.8	3.3	45
Fombonne et al. (2006)	Canada	5-17	DSM-IV	180 / 27,749	64.9	55.8 – 75.0	4.8	-
Harrison et al. (2006)	UK	0-15	ICD-10, DSM-IV	596 / 134,661	44.2	39.5 – 48.9	7.0	-

Table 8.2 Prevalence of Pervasive Developmental Disorders (contd.)

Study	Country	Age	Criteria	Cases/Sample				
Gillberg et al. (2006)	Sweden	7-12	DSM-IV	262 / 32,568	80.4	71.3 – 90.3	3.6	-
CDC (2007a)	USA	8	DSM-IV-TR	1,252 / 187,761	67.0	-	2.8 to 5.5	38 to 60
CDC (2007b)	USA	8	DSM-IV-TR	2,685 / 407,578	66.0	63 – 68	3.4 to 6.5	55.4
Ellefsen et al. (2007)	Denmark	8-17	DSM-IV, Gillberg's criteria	41 / 7,689	53.3	36 – 70	5.8	68.3
Latif and Williams (2007)	UK	0-17	ICD-10, DSM-IV, Kanner's & Gillberg's criteria	240 / 39,220	61.2	54 – 69	6.8	-
Wong and Hui (2008)	China	0-14	DSM-IV	682 / 4,247,206	16.1 (1986-2005) 30.0 (2005)	- -	6.6	30
Nicholas et al. (2008)	USA	8	DSM-IV-TR	295 / 47,726	62.0	56 – 70	3.1	39.6
Kawamura et al. (2008)	Japan	5-8	DSM-IV	228 / 12,589	181.1	158.5 – 205.9	2.8	66.4
Williams et al. (2008)	UK	11	ICD-10	86 / 14,062	61.9	48.8 – 74.9	6.8	85.3
Lazoff et al. (2009)	Canada	5-17	DSM-IV	190 / 23,662	80.3	68.7 – 91.7	5.4	-

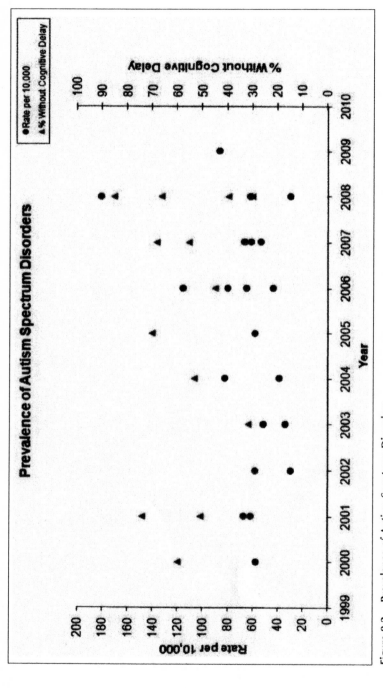

Figure 8.2. Prevalence of Autism Spectrum Disorders

when making diagnostic decisions (Lord et al. 2009). For instance, in one of the 12 studies, the prevalence of Asperger's disorder actually exceeded that of autism (Latif and Williams 2007), while in the other 11 studies rates of Asperger's disorder were lower than for autism. In the Latif and Williams study high-functioning autism was included in the Asperger's disorder definition. It is difficult to estimate how many of those diagnosed with Asperger's disorder would have instead met DSM-IV and/or ICD-10 diagnostic criteria for autistic disorder if strict hierarchical diagnostic rules were applied (i.e., not to diagnose Asperger's disorder if criteria for autistic disorder or another PDD are already met). This is an issue in two other studies, not included in the 12 above, which reported specifically on the prevalence of Asperger's disorder (Ehlers and Gillberg 1993; Kadesjö et al. 1999). Because there is not one universally applied method to differentiate Asperger's disorder from "high-functioning" autism, and due to the lack of clear boundaries around these diagnoses making meaningful comparisons across studies is difficult to accomplish.

Eleven studies provided data on childhood disintegrative disorder (CDD). CDD is a rare disorder within the PDDs which involves a marked regression and deterioration in skills that follows a period of at least 2 years of normal development. Following the regression, autism-like symptoms emerge. For this rare condition, prevalence estimates ranged from 0 to 9.2 per 100,000. The pooled estimate based on 11 identified cases and a surveyed population of about 604,000 children was 1.8 per 100,000 with a male to female ratio of 9:1.

Regression and PDD

Early regression of skills is thought to occur in a subset of children diagnosed with PDD. Nine of the reviewed studies reported the frequency of regression in their respective samples (Baird et al. 2008; Bertrand et al. 2001; CDC 2007a, CDC 2007b; Fombonne and Chakrabarti 2001; Icasiano et al. 2004; Lotter 1966; Sugiyama and Abe 1989; Taylor et al. 2002). Regression was not defined in a similar way across studies. The earliest study reporting rates of regression found that a "setback" had occurred in about a third of children with autism. In this study a setback was defined as either a loss of ability or as a failure to progress after a "satisfactory beginning" where the child met early milestones in the first 17 months of life (Lotter 1966). Perhaps due to this broad definition of regression some children meeting these criteria were as old as 4.5 years while in other later studies the age at regression was usually between 18 and 24 months. An early age of regression differentiates autism/PDD from regression associated with a childhood disintigrative disorder diagnosis where the loss in skills occurs later, after a child's second birthday. In the 8 later studies regression focused on a loss of language and/or skills in other domains such as social, play, and motor skills. The percentage of cases where regression occurred ranged from 12.5% (Sugiyama and Abe 1989) to 38.6% (Baird et al. 2008) with a median rate of 24%.

Summary of Studies on Prevalence Rates

Based on the 58 studies reviewed, estimates of PDD converge to around 60 to 70 per 10,000. There is a notable amount of variability in rates across and within some studies, depending on the methods and definitions used, and some studies report figures that are two to three times higher than this estimate (Baird et al. 2006; Kawamura et al. 2008). The mean figure of PDDs at 66 per 10,000 translates into 1 child out of 150 suffering from a PDD. Compared to several decades ago there is a trend toward increasing rates, but there is no evidence that prevalence has continued to rise in the more recent past—the last decade.

TRENDS IN RATES OF PDD

There has been an increase in prevalence rates of autistic disorder when comparing current rates to those found between the 1960s and 1980s. However, there are challenges inherent to interpreting this increase because an increase in prevalence rate does not necessarily translate into a true increase in the manifestation of a particular condition. There is a risk of misinterpreting increases in prevalence data as meaning there is an increase in new cases (i.e., incidence). Prevalence refers to the proportion of individuals in a population who suffer from a defined disorder at any one point in time. To truly understand whether there is an autism "epidemic," incidence rates are required. Incidence refers to the number of new cases occurring in a population over time. Both prevalence and incidence rates can be inflated when case definitions are broadened to include a wider variety of symptom presentation, and when better methods of case ascertainment become available. Only when definitions and methods of case ascertainment remain stable, along with other potentially confounding factors, can studies be compared in a reasonable manner. The methods used in particular studies need to be carefully considered before conclusions about the epidemic hypothesis can be made.

Understanding the Variation in Rates across
Studies: Methodological Differences

There is notable variation in prevalence rates of PDD across studies and even within studies. This complicates interpretation of time trends in rates of autism and PDD and raises the distinct possibility that the significant correlation between publication year and prevalence of autistic disorder merely reflects differences in methodologies and practices, including factors such as better case identification and changes in diagnostic conventions (Webb et al. 1997; Kielinen et al. 2000; Magnusson et al. 2001; Shattuck 2006; Bishop et al. 2008).

Evidence that methodological factors could account for most of the variability in published prevalence estimates comes from a direct comparison of eight recent surveys on the prevalence of PDD conducted in the United Kingdom and the United States (Fombonne 2005). In each country, four surveys were conducted around the same year and with similar age groups. As there is no reason to expect large between-area differences in rates, prevalence estimates should be comparable within each country. However, there was a sixfold variation in rates among the United Kingdom studies, and a fourteenfold variation in rates among the United States studies. In each set of studies, high rates were found when intensive population-based screening techniques were used and lower rates were found when studies relied on passive administrative methods to find cases of PDD. Since these studies were conducted around the same time differences in case identification methods across studies likely contributed to the variation.

Similarly, in the large CDC (2007b) study from the United States, an average prevalence for PDD of 66 per 10,000 was reported for 14 states. However, there was a threefold variation in state rates, ranging from 33 per 10,000 for Alabama to 106 per 10,000 in New Jersey. The same methods were used in each state and surveys were conducted within the same time period. If so much variation in rates occurs in a study like this it is difficult to have confidence in any simple comparison of prevalence rates for PDDs over time because studies from different time periods are likely to have even more variation in the methods used. As surveillance efforts continue it is likely that awareness and services will develop in states that were previously lagging behind, which leads to an expectation that there will be an overall increase in the average rate of PDDs in the United States in the future.

Prevalence estimates from studies from all countries need to be understood within the context of imperfect methods of case ascertainment that can result in downward biases in prevalence proportions (Harrison et al. 2006). Some of the lowest rates in Table 8.2 (i.e., those below 40 per 10,000) probably underestimate true population rates. For example, studies using national registries, such as the Danish Madsen and colleagues (2002) study, are using a less sensitive methodology for case ascertainment. Less systematic ascertainment techniques may also have been an issue in the Hong Kong (Wong and Hui 2008) and Australian (Icasiano et al. 2004) studies.

When very young children are included in studies this may also lower the overall rate because they may be too young to have been identified with PDD. Also, if older children are not included in the study rates can be underestimated. Some children with PDD are only diagnosed when they are of school age, or later in adolescence, and many 3- and 4-year-olds with PDD do not receive early diagnoses even if symptoms have already begun to manifest. For example, in the Atlanta study by Yeargin-Allsopp and colleagues (2003), the overall prevalence of PDD was 3.4 per 1,000 overall, which is relatively low. However, age-specific rates showed that the prevalence of PDD was 1.9 per 1,000 in 3-year-olds, but 4.7 per 1,000 in 8-year-olds.

Increased confidence in results is possible when case finding techniques are completed as part of a multi-stage process and include multiple and repeated population screenings, multiple informants, and surveillance of the same cohorts at different ages; direct assessment using standardized PDD assessment tools also increases confidence. When these more thorough methods are used the sensitivity of case identification is maximized (e.g., Chakrabarti and Fombonne 2005; Baird et al. 2006). As new studies on the prevalence and incidence of PDDs emerge methods of case identification must be evaluated as interpretations of rates are made.

Repeated surveys, using the same methodology and conducted in the same geographical area at different points in time, can potentially yield useful information on time trends, provided that methods are kept relatively constant. Studies from Göteborg, Sweden, provided three prevalence estimates of PDD which increased over a short period of time from 40 (1980) to 66 (1984) to 95 per 10,000 (1988) (Gillberg 1984; Gillberg et al. 1991). However, methodological issues obscure results because comparing the rates is complicated by improved detection, changes in local services, broadening definitions of autism, and increased migration over the surveyed period. Similarly, studies conducted in Japan at different points in time in Toyota (Kawamura et al. 2008) and Yokohama (Honda et al. 1996 and 2005) showed rises in prevalence rates that their authors interpreted as reflecting improved population screening of preschoolers and a broadening of diagnostic concepts and criteria.

Two separate surveys of children born between 1992-1995 and between 1996-1998 in Staffordshire in the United Kingdom (Chakrabarti and Fombonne 2001 and 2005) were performed with rigorously identical methods of case definition and case identification. The prevalence for combined PDDs was comparable and not statistically different in the two surveys (Chakrabarti and Fombonne 2005) suggesting no upward trend in overall rates of PDDs during the time interval between studies. In the two recent CDC surveys (2007a and 2007b) the prevalence rates in the 2000 and 2002 surveys remained constant in four sites, and increased in two sites (Georgia and West Virginia) most likely due to improved quality of survey methods at these sites. As long as confounding factors are minimized, continued efforts to conduct repeated surveillance in specific areas will continue to be informative about trends in PDDs over time.

In large surveys encompassing a wide age range, increasing prevalence rates among more recent birth cohorts could be interpreted as indicating a secular increase in the incidence of the disorder, provided that alternative explanations can confidently be eliminated. This analysis was used in two large French surveys (Fombonne and du Mazaubrun 1992 and Fombonne et al. 1997). The surveys included birth cohorts from 1972 to 1985 (735,000 children, 389 of whom had autism) and when pooling the data of both surveys age-specific rates showed no upward trend (Fombonne et al. 1997).

An analysis of special education disability data from Minnesota showed a sixteenfold increase in the number of children identified with a PDD from 1991-1992 to 2001-2002 (Gurney et al. 2003). The increase was not specific to autism since, during the same period, an increase of 50% was observed for all disability categories (except severe mental handicap), especially for the category including attention-deficit/hyperactivity disorder (ADHD). The large sample size allowed the authors to assess age, period, and cohort effects. Prevalence increased regularly in successive birth cohorts. For example, among 7-year-olds the prevalence rose from 18 per 10,000 in those born in 1989, to 29 per 10,000 in those born in 1991, and to 55 per 10,000 in those born in 1993 suggestive of birth cohort effects. Within the same birth cohorts age effects were also apparent because for children born in 1989 the prevalence rose with age from 13 per 10,000 at age 6, to 21 per 10,000 at age 9 to 33 per 10,000 at age 11. Their analysis identified the early 1990s as the period where rates started to increase in all ages and birth cohorts. Gurney and colleagues (2003) noted that this phenomenon coincided closely with the inclusion of PDDs in the Federal Individual with Disabilities Educational Act's (IDEA) funding and reporting mechanism in the U.S. Similar interpretations of upward trend had been put forth for analyses of the California Department of Disability Services (DDS) data (Croen et al. 2002), and in a well-executed analysis of trends of the Department of Education data (Shattuck 2006).

Interpreting Increasing Referral Rates

In order to establish whether there is an autism epidemic some investigators have turned to evidence of increased referrals of children to specialized services for PDDs. In numerous countries upward trends of rates of PDD were documented in national registries and medical and educational databases in the late 1980s and early 1990s (Taylor et al. 1999; Gurney et al. 2003; Madsen et al. 2002; Shattuck 2006). However, it would be erroneous to assume that even large numbers of newly referred cases are equivalent to an actual increase in incidence. An increase in referrals is confounded by factors including, but not limited to, public awareness of a disorder, referral patterns by professionals, decreasing age of diagnosis, and availability of services to assess and treat particular conditions (see chapter in this volume by K. Sayal and T. Ford).

Confounding factors are not always possible to control and even when controlled they may be overlooked leading to a misinterpretation of results (Fombonne 2001). This issue is highlighted by the case of the California Developmental Database Services (DDS) reports (California DDS 1999 and 2003) which indicated increased referrals to services in California and have been cited as evidence of an autism epidemic. These reports indicated an increasing percentage of persons with autism relative to the total client population served. Although this kind of evidence does suggest that more individuals with PDD are entering a system and requesting services a true increase in PDD cannot be assumed. To correctly calculate changes in prevalence it would be important to compare the number of referrals in a given year to the number of individuals in the population, which was not done in these reports. Populations can increase over time and it would follow that referral rates would thus increase.

To illustrate this point, in December 2007 the total number of individuals aged 3 to 21 years with a PDD was found to be 31,332, according to the 2007 California DDS report (December 2007). This number must be understood as relative to a total population of 9,976,768 individuals aged 3 to 21 years as reported for July 1, 2007 (United States Census Bureau 2009). The California DDS did not include the number of the population in their report. If the referral numbers are compared to the population figure, it appears that the reported number by the California DDS is below what would be expected based on recent epidemiological estimates of the prevalence of PDD. Applying an expected rate of 66 per 10,000 individuals with PDD, as described earlier, the expected number of individuals in California in 2007 with a PDD in this age group would be much greater and would total 65,846 individuals. Although the sheer number of referrals is essential to note when developing services for individuals with PDD care must be taken to refrain from using these figures as evidence for an increase in incidence.

Additional confounds in the California DDS data include that trends in diagnostic concepts were not taken into account. Over the years considered in the reports (1987 to 2002) major changes in classification systems were made and broader diagnostic conventions began to be used. Furthermore, the preponderance of younger children with PDD was presented as evidence of increasing rates in successive birth cohorts (Fombonne 2001). Disentangling age from period and cohort effects in such observational data is known to be problematic, as understood in epidemiological literature, and requires careful statistical handling. Decreasing age at diagnosis is in itself a confounding factor and could result in increased numbers of referrals to services (Wazana et al. 2007) as parents and professionals become more aware that a diagnosis is possible at a young age. However, as the cohort becomes older this effect would be expected to attenuate. A more refined analysis of the effect of a younger age at diagnosis, using cumulative incidence data by age 5, showed that 12% of the increase in incidence from the 1990 to the 1996 birth cohort could be explained by this factor and up to 24% with an extrapolation to the 2002 cohort (Hertz-Picciotto and Delwiche 2009).

Another study of this dataset was completed and the results were interpreted as supporting an "epidemic" of PDD (MIND Institute 2002). In this study the authors attempted to assess whether changes in diagnostic practices and immigration rates into California could be ruled out as reasons for increased referral rates. Immigration was ruled out as a cause for increased numbers. However, due to low response rates the data was not clear about whether diagnostic practices account for the increase. Similar to the problems in the earlier California DDS reports, rates were based on the number of individuals accessing services. Increased numbers may merely reflect an increased proportion of individuals who are aware of existing services and are registering to obtain them. In order to use this information correctly it would be important to track over time both referred and non-referred subjects (i.e., including those who are perhaps referred for other services). Without this information inferences about true increases in rates are unfortunately impossible to make (Fombonne 2003).

Changing Definitions of PDD and Diagnostic Substitution

The earliest studies on the prevalence of autism showed awareness that some children were presenting with similar or related disorders but falling short of the diagnostic criteria that were in use at the time. These studies from the 1960s and 1970s used different labels to capture these "sub-threshold" groups (see Fombonne 2003 and 2005). For example, Lotter (1966) referred to three groups: one with classic autism symptoms; a second with symptoms of autism but who had fewer, less severe, and more heterogeneous presentations; and a third "non-autistic" handicapped group who were reported to share some behaviors with the autism group. Other groups have used different labels to capture children whom they felt presented with sub-threshold symptoms. These labels have included the "triad" of impairments in reciprocal social interaction, communication, and imagination (Wing and Gould 1979), autistic mental retardation (Hoshino et al. 1982), borderline childhood psychoses (Brask 1970), and "autistic-like" syndromes (Burd et al. 1987).

In today's conceptualization these individuals could potentially be captured under the newer PDD-NOS or atypical autism labels. Higher rates for these milder atypical forms have been found, compared to the rates of autistic disorder which is more narrowly defined. For example, the rate reported by Lotter would increase from 4.1 to 7.3 per 10,000 if all three groups of children with some form of autism symptoms were included as cases. Similarly, in Wing and colleagues' study (1976) the prevalence was 4.9 per 10,000 for autistic disorder, but, adding the figure of 16.3 per 10,000 (Wing and Gould, 1979) corresponding to the triad of impairments the prevalence of PDD for the whole PDD would arguably become 21.2 per 10,000.

In addition to changes in diagnostic criteria in DSM-III-R, DSM-IV, and ICD-10, several additional factors have led to the broadening of the diagnostic concept of autism since the 1960s (see Rutter 2005). These factors have included the growing understanding that autism represents a qualitative impairment in social and communication skills that can co-occur with mental retardation and should not be discounted when the deficits in social and communication are abnormal, relative to the level of intellectual ability. Today, it is common to diagnose a child with autism and co-occurring mental retardation, whereas in the past the child may have only received the mental retardation diagnosis. Similarly, cases of autism with co-occurring medical and genetic conditions began to be recognized rather than being dismissed as medical disorders with secondary autistic symptoms. For example, a child with Trisomy 21, tuberous sclerosis, or neurofibromatosis may also receive a comorbid autism diagnosis. Twin and family studies have also highlighted how milder presentations were relatively frequent in relatives of individuals with autism, which has led to more awareness of milder forms of PDD. Finally, the recognition of Asperger's disorder helped solidify the broadening of diagnostic criteria to include individuals with normal cognitive functioning and language development.

As another factor contributing to the difficulty of interpreting PDD rates, health professionals may have become increasingly likely to use a PDD diagnosis instead of labelling children with other diagnoses. Diagnostic substitution refers to the phenomenon whereby an individual presenting with identical symptoms may receive one diagnosis at one point in time and another diagnosis at a later point in time. This may occur when new diagnostic categories are introduced and become increasingly recognized and employed by health professionals. Also, this may occur when a new diagnostic category ensures better access to health and educational services. If this pattern were in effect it would be expected that there would be an accompanying corresponding decrease in the use of another classification label.

Indeed, there is evidence from an analysis of United States Department of Education data from 50 states indicating that as the PDD diagnosis gained popularity there were corresponding declines in the odds of being classified under both mental retardation and learning disability categories

(Shattuck 2006). The declining prevalence of mental retardation and learning disabilities from 1994 to 2003 immediately followed the introduction of the new autism reporting category in 1993 and 1994. The pre-existing trajectories of mental retardation and learning disabilities were deflected downward as the autism category began to be used. Although this pattern was evident in most of the United States it was thought that California was one of the few American states that were exceptions (Croen et al. 2002; Eagle 2004). However, a new study using individual level data has re-examined this issue in the California DDS dataset described above and has shown that 24% of the increase in caseload could be attributed to diagnostic substitution (King and Bearman, in press).

In addition to decreased use of mental retardation and learning disabilities other forms of diagnostic substitution that are not as well studied may also be occurring. The milder forms of PDD and Asperger's disorder could potentially be replacing other psychiatric diagnoses such as childhood schizoid personality disorder (Wolff and Barlow 1979), ADHD, and obsessive-compulsive disorder. In one study in the United Kingdom, the incidence of specific developmental disorders, including language disorders, for boys born between 1990-1997 decreased by about the same amount as the increase in the incidence of autism (Jick et al. 2003). Another United Kingdom study has found that up to two-thirds of adults previously diagnosed with developmental language disorders (e.g., specific language impairments and pragmatic language impairments) have behaviors that would meet diagnostic criteria for a broad definition of PDD (Bishop et al. 2008).

The Possibility of Environmental Contributions to PDD

It would be essential to look at environmental factors as possible causes of PDDs if there were an increase in incidence. Since evidence for an increase in the incidence of PDDs is lacking the study of environmental causes becomes less compelling, especially in light of strong evidence for genetic contributions to PDDs which continues to accumulate. Even though no such increase has been established some environmental factors have been proposed as explanations for why more children are now being given a PDD label, including pesticides, metals, pollutants, exposure to viruses, and medical procedures or pharmaceuticals (Hertz-Picciotto et al. 2006). In addition, an alleged link between the measles mumps rubella (MMR) vaccine and autism has been proposed and has received much media attention. A related hypothesis alleging links between thimerosal, a vaccine preservative containing ethyl mercury, has also sparked public debate. Causal hypotheses implicating vaccines seem to offer much explanatory power and have the appeal of an "easy answer" to why autism happens.

However, the evidence to date argues strongly against vaccines and vaccine preservatives contributing to the cause of autism (IOM 2004; Fombonne et al. 2006; Offit 2008). There is no association between autism rates and stopping or starting the MMR vaccine, or exposure to thimerosal and if there are true environmental risk factors for autism the medical community is in agreement that vaccines are unlikely candidates (Rutter 2005). Other proposed factors include exposure to valproic acid and thalidomide (e.g., Miller et al. 2005; Snow et al. 2008), folate deficiency (e.g., Moretti et al. 2008), the use of pesticides (e.g., Roberts et al. 2007), and increased use of in-vitro fertilization. So far, evidence is extremely scant for any of these playing a role in an alleged increase in PDD incidence. However, the contribution of environmental factors to PDDs cannot be ruled out and worthy contenders should continue to be studied.

CONCLUSION

Epidemiological surveys of autism and PDDs have now been conducted within many countries, but methodological differences in case definition and case finding procedures make between-survey comparisons difficult to perform. A best estimate of 60 to 70 per 10,000 (about 1 in 150) can be confidently derived for the prevalence of PDDs. Current evidence does not strongly support the hypothesis of a secular increase in the incidence of autism but the ability to detect time trends is seriously limited in existing studies. The possibility that a true increase in the incidence of PDDs has also partially contributed to the upward trend in prevalence rates cannot, and should not, be eliminated based on available data. Too many confounding factors and varying methodologies obscure interpretation and the contribution of factors such as changing diagnostic criteria, diagnostic substitution, and different kinds of ascertainment methods. Also, social changes cannot be discounted and these moving targets include increased awareness, changing policies and classification labels, increased funding for services for children with PDD, and possible willingness to seek services to address symptoms of PDD. It is also noteworthy that the rise in number of children diagnosed occurred at the same time in many countries when radical shifts occurred in the diagnostic approaches to identifying and treating children with PDDs. Alternatively, this might of course reflect the effect of environmental influences operating simultaneously in different parts of the world. However, there has been no proposed and legitimate risk mechanism to account for this kind of worldwide effect.

To date, there is not enough evidence to support the contention of an autism epidemic. Upward trends in prevalence cannot be directly attributed to increases in incidence or true new cases. However, continued efforts need to be made to monitor the prevalence and incidence of autism and other PDDs. To assess whether or not the incidence has increased factors that account for variability in rates must be tightly controlled. New survey methods have been developed for use in multinational comparisons and ongoing surveillance programs are expected to be more informative.

What is clear is that autism and the other PDDs are much more common than many other childhood disorders, including Type I diabetes, childhood cancer, and cystic fibrosis. These numbers support the imperative to address the needs of children and families affected by autism. Timely diagnosis and intensive treatments for autism are in high demand. The needs of children with autism and their families require ongoing attention and action within the spheres of public health and educational institutions.

REFERENCES

American Psychiatric Association. *Diagnostic and Statistical Manual of Mental Disorders, 3rd Edition*. Washington, DC: APA, 1980.

American Psychiatric Association. *Diagnostic and Statistical Manual of Mental Disorders, 3rd Edition, Revised*. Washington, DC: APA, 1987.

American Psychiatric Association. *Diagnostic and Statistical Manual of Mental Disorders, 4th Edition*. Washington, DC: APA, 1994.

American Psychiatric Association. *Diagnostic and Statistical Manual of Mental Disorders, 4th Edition, Text Revision*. Washington, DC: APA, 2000.

Arvidsson, T., B. Danielsson, P. Forsberg, C. Gillberg, M. Johansson, and G. Kjellgren. Autism in 3-6-year-old children in a suburb of Göteborg, Sweden. *Autism* 1 (1997): 163-173.

Asperger, H. Die "autistichen psychopathen" im kindersalter. *Archive für Psychiatrie und Nervenkrankheiten* 117 (1944): 76-136.

Baird, G., T. Charman, S. Baron-Cohen, et al. A screening instrument for autism at 18 months of age: A 6-year follow-up study. *Journal of the American Academy of Child and Adolescent Psychiatry* 39 (2000): 694-702.

Baird, G., T. Charman, A. Pickles, et al. Regression, developmental trajectory and associated problems in disorders in the autism spectrum: The SNAP study. *Journal of Autism and Developmental Disorders* 38 (2008): 1827-1836.

Baird, G., E. Simonoff, A. Pickles, et al. Prevalence of disorders of the autism spectrum in a population cohort of children in South Thames: The special needs and autism project (SNAP). *Lancet* 368 (2006): 210-215.

Barbaresi, W. J., S. K. Katusic, R. C. Colligan, A. L. Weaver, and S. J. Jacobsen. The incidence of autism in Olmsted County, Minnesota, 1976-1997: Results from a population-based study. *Archives of Pediatrics and Adolescent Medicine* 159 (2005): 37-44.

Bertrand, J., A. Mars, C. Boyle, F. Bove, M. Yeargin-Allsopp, and P. Decoufle. Prevalence of autism in a United States population: The Brick Township, New Jersey, investigation. *Pediatrics* 108 (2001): 1155-1161.

Bishop, D. V., A. J. Whitehouse, H. J. Watt, and E. A. Line. Autism and diagnostic substitution: Evidence from a study of adults with a history of developmental language disorder. *Developmental Medicine and Child Neurology* 50 (2008): 341-345.

Bohman, M., I. Bohman, P. Bjorck, and E. Sjoholm. Childhood psychosis in a northern Swedish county: Some preliminary findings from an epidemiological survey. In *Epidemiological Approaches in Child Psychiatry*, eds. M. Shmidt and H. Remschmidt, 164-173. Stuttgart, Germany: Georg Thieme Verlag, 1983.

Brask, B. A prevalence investigation of childhood psychoses. Paper presented at the Nordic Symposium on the Care of Psychotic Children, Oslo, 1970.

Bryson, S. E., B. S. Clark, and I. M. Smith. First report of a Canadian epidemiological study of autistic syndromes. *Journal of Child Psychology and Psychiatry and Allied Disciplines*, 29 (1988): 433-445.

Burd, L., W. Fisher, and J. Kerbeshan. A prevalence study of pervasive developmental disorders in North Dakota. *Journal of the American Academy of Child and Adolescent Psychiatry* 26 (1987): 700-703.

California Department of Developmental Services (DDS). *Changes in the Population of Persons with Autism and Pervasive Developmental Disorders in California's Developmental Services System: 1987 through 1998*, March 1999.

California Department of Developmental Services (DDS). *Autism Spectrum Disorders: Changes in the California Caseload. An Update: 1999 through 2002*, April 2003.

California Department of Developmental Services (DDS). http://www.dds.ca.gov/FactsStats/docs/Dec07_QRTTBLS.pdf, December 2007 (accessed January 29, 2009).

Centers for Disease Control and Prevention. Prevalence of autism spectrum disorders—autism and developmental disabilities monitoring network, six sites, United States, 2000. *Morbidity and Mortality Weekly Report: Surveillance Summaries* 56 (2007a): 1-11.

Centers for Disease Control and Prevention. Prevalence of autism spectrum disorders—autism and developmental disabilities monitoring network, 14 sites, United States, 2002. *Morbidity and Mortality Weekly Report: Surveillance Summaries* 56 (2007b): 12-28.

Chakrabarti, S., and E. Fombonne. Pervasive developmental disorders in preschool children. *Journal of the American Medical Association* 285 (2001): 3093-3099.

Chakrabarti, S., and E. Fombonne. Pervasive developmental disorders in preschool children: Confirmation of high prevalence. *American Journal of Psychiatry* 162 (2005.): 1133-1141.

Cialdella, P., and N. Mamelle. An epidemiological study of infantile autism in a French department (Rhone): A research note. *Journal of Child Psychology and Psychiatry and Allied Disciplines* 30 (1989): 165-175.

Croen, L. A., J. K. Grether, J. Hoogstrate, and S. Selvin. The changing prevalence of autism in California. *Journal of Autism and Developmental Disorders* 323 (2002): 207-215.

Davidovitch, M., G. Holtzman, and E. Tirosh. Autism in the Haifa area—an epidemiological perspective. *Israeli Medical Association Journal* 3 (2001): 188-189.

Eagle, R. S. Commentary: Further commentary on the debate regarding increase in autism in California. *Journal of Autism and Developmental Disorders* 34 (2004): 87-88.

Ehlers, S., and C. Gillberg. The epidemiology of Asperger syndrome: A total population study. *Journal of Child Psychology and Psychiatry & Allied Disciplines* 34 (1993): 1327-1350.

Ellefsen, A., H. Kampmann, E. Billstedt, I. C. Gillberg, and C. Gillberg. Autism in the Faroe Islands: An epidemiological study. *Journal of Autism and Developmental Disorders* 37 (2007): 437-444.

Fombonne, E. Is there an epidemic of autism? *Pediatrics* 107 (2001): 411-413.

Fombonne, E. Epidemiological surveys of autism and other pervasive developmental disorders: An update. *Journal of Autism and Developmental Disorders* 33 (2003): 365-382.

Fombonne, E. Epidemiology of autistic disorder and other pervasive developmental disorders. *Journal of Clinical Psychiatry* 66 (2005): 3-8.

Fombonne, E. Epidemiology. In *Child and Adolescent Psychiatry: A Comprehensive Textbook, 4th Edition*, eds. A. Martin & F. Volkmar, 150-171. Philadelphia: Lippincott, Williams and Wilkins Publishing, 2007.

Fombonne, E., and S. Chakrabarti. No evidence for a new variant of measles-mumps-rubella-induced autism. *Pediatrics* 108 (2001): e58.

Fombonne, E., and C. du Mazaubrun. Prevalence of infantile autism in four French regions. *Social Psychiatry & Psychiatric Epidemiology* 27 (1992): 203-210.

Fombonne, E., C. du Mazaubrun, C. Cans, and H. Grandjean. Autism and associated medical disorders in a French epidemiological survey. *Journal of the American Academy of Child & Adolescent Psychiatry* 36 (1997): 1561-1569.

Fombonne, E., S. Quirke, and A. Hagen. Epidemiology of pervasive developmental disorders. In *Autism Spectrum Disorders*, eds. D. G. Amaral, G. Dawson, and D. H. Geschwind DH. Oxford: Oxford University Press, (2009).

Fombonne, E., H. Simmons, T. Ford, H. Meltzer, and R. Goodman. Prevalence of pervasive developmental disorders in the British nationwide survey of child mental health. *Journal of the American Academy of Child & Adolescent Psychiatry* 40 (2001): 820-827.

Fombonne, E., R. Zakarian, A. Bennett, L. Meng, and D. McLean-Heywood. Pervasive developmental disorders in Montreal, Quebec, Canada: Prevalence and links with immunizations. *Pediatrics* 118 (2006): 139-150.

Gillberg, C. Infantile autism and other childhood psychoses in a Swedish urban region. Epidemiological aspects. *Journal of Child Psychology and Psychiatry* 25 (1984): 35-43.

Gillberg, C., M. Cederlund, K. Lamberg, and L. Zeijlon. Brief report: "The autism epidemic". The registered prevalence of autism in a Swedish urban area. *Journal of Autism and Developmental Disorders* 36 (2006): 429-435.

Gillberg, C., S. Steffenburg, and H. Schaumann. Is autism more common now than ten years ago? *British Journal of Psychiatry* 158 (1991): 403-409.

Gurney, J. G., M. S. Fritz, K. K. Ness, P. Sievers, C. J. Newschaffer, and E. G. Shapiro. Analysis of prevalence trends of autism spectrum disorder in Minnesota [comment]. *Archives of Pediatrics and Adolescent Medicine* 157 (2003): 622-627.

Harrison, M. J., A. E. O'Hare, H. Campbell, A. Adamson, and J. McNeillage. Prevalence of autistic spectrum disorders in Lothian, Scotland: An estimate using the "capture-recapture" technique. *Archives of Disease in Childhood* 91 (2006): 16-19.

Hertz-Picciotto, I., L. A. Croen, R. Hansen, C. R. Jones, J. van de Water, and I. N. Pessah. The CHARGE study: An epidemiologic investigation of genetic and environmental factors contributing to autism. *Environmental Health Perspectives* 114 (2006): 1119-1125.

Hertz-Picciotto, I., and L. Delwiche. The rise in autism and the role of age at diagnosis. *Epidemiology* 20 (2009): 84-90.

Honda, H., Y. Shimizu, K. Misumi, M. Niimi, and Y. Ohashi. Cumulative incidence and prevalence of childhood autism in children in Japan. *British Journal of Psychiatry* 169 (1996): 228-235.

Honda, H., Y. Shimizu, and M. Rutter. No effect of MMR withdrawal on the incidence of autism: A total population study. *Journal of Child Psychology and Psychiatry* 46 (2005): 572-579.

Hoshino, Y., H. Kumashiro, Y. Yashima, R. Tachibana, and M. Watanabe. The epidemiological study of autism in Fukushima-Ken. *Folia Psychiatrica et Neurologica Japonica* 36 (1982): 115-124.

Icasiano, F., P. Hewson, P. Machet, C. Cooper, and A. Marshall. Childhood autism spectrum disorder in the Barwon region: A community based study. *Journal of Paediatrics and Child Health* 40 (2004): 696-701.

Institute of Medicine (IOM). *Immunization Safety Review: Vaccines and Autism.* Washington, DC: National Academies Press, 2004.

Jick, H., J. A. Kaye, and C. Black. Epidemiology and possible causes of autism: Changes in risk of autism in the UK for birth cohorts 1990-1998. *Pharmacotherapy* 23 (2003): 1524-1530.

Kadesjö, B., C. Gillberg, and B. Hagberg. Brief report: Autism and Asperger syndrome in seven-year-old children: A total population study. *Journal of Autism and Developmental Disorders* 29 (1999): 327-331.

Kanner, L. Autistic disturbances of affective contact. *Nervous Child* 2 (1943): 217-250.

Kawamura, Y., O. Takahashi, and T. Ishii. Re-evaluating the incidence of pervasive developmental disorders: Impact of elevated rates of detection through implementation of an integrated system of screening in Toyota, Japan. *Psychiatry and Clinical Neurosciences* 62 (2008): 152-159.

Kielinen, M., S.-L. Linna, and I. Moilanen. Autism in northern Finland. *European Child and Adolescent Psychiatry* 9 (2000): 162-167.

King, M., and P. Bearman. Diagnostic change and the increase in prevalence of autism. *International Journal of Epidemiology* (in press).

Klin, A., J. McPartland, and F. Volkmar. Asperger syndrome. In *Handbook of Autism and Pervasive Developmental Disorders (3rd Edition): Diagnosis, Development, Neurobiology, and Behaviour*, eds. F. Volkmar, R. Paul, A. Klin, and D. Cohen. Hoboken, NJ: Wiley, 2005.

Latif, A. H., and W. R. Williams. Diagnostic trends in autistic spectrum disorders in the South Wales valleys. *Autism,* 11 (2007): 479-487.

Lazoff, T., T. Piperni, E. Clarke, L. Lewis, and E. Fombonne. *Prevalence rates of PDD among children at the English Montreal School Board.* Poster presented at the 8th annual International Meeting for Autism Research (IMFAR), Chicago, 2009.

Le Couteur, A., M. Rutter, C. Lord, et al. Autism diagnostic interview: A standardized investigator-based instrument. *Journal of Autism and Developmental Disorders* 19 (1989): 363-387.

Lin, J. D., L. P. Lin, and J. L. Wu. Administrative prevalence of autism spectrum disorders based on national disability registers in Taiwan. *Research in Autism Spectrum Disorders* 3 (2009): 269-274.

Lord, C., L. Harvey, S. Petkova, et al. *Representing behavioural phenotype heterogeneity within autism spectrum disorders (ASD): Questions and answers from the Simons Simplex Collection.* Poster presented at the 8th annual International Meeting for Autism Research (IMFAR), Chicago, 2009.

Lord, C., S. Risi, L. Lambrecht, et al. The autism diagnostic observation schedule-generic: A standard measure of social and communication deficits associated with the spectrum of autism. *Journal of Autism and Developmental Disorders* 30 (2000): 205-223.

Lotter, V. Epidemiology of autistic conditions in young children: I. Prevalence. *Social Psychiatry* 1 (1966): 124-137.

Madsen, K. M., A. Hviid, M. Vestergaard, et al. A population-based study of measles, mumps, and rubella vaccination and autism. *The New England Journal of Medicine* 347 (2002): 1477-1482.

Magnusson, P., and E. Saemundsen. Prevalence of autism in Iceland. *Journal of Autism and Developmental Disorders* 31 (2001): 153-163.

Matsuishi, T., M. Shiotsuki, K. Yoshimura, H. Shoji, F. Imuta, and F. Yamashita. High prevalence of infantile autism in Kurume City, Japan. *Journal of Child Neurology* 2 (1987): 268-271.

McCarthy, P., M. Fitzgerald, and M. Smith. Prevalence of childhood autism in Ireland. *Irish Medical Journal* 77 (1984): 129-130.

Miller, T. M., K. Strömland, L. Ventura, M. Johansson, J. M. Bandim, and C. Gillberg. Autism associated with conditions characterized by developmental errors in early embryogenesis: A mini review. *International Journal of Developmental Neuroscience* 23 (2005): 201-219.

MIND Institute. *MIND Institute Report to the Legislature on the Principal Findings from the Epidemiology of Autism in California: A Comprehensive Pilot Study.* University of California, Davis, October 17, 2002.

Moretti, P., S. U. Peters, D. del Gaudio, et al. Brief report: Autistic symptoms, developmental regression, mental retardation, epilepsy, and dyskinesias in CNS folate deficiency. *Journal of Autism and Developmental Disorders* 38 (2008): 1170-1177.

Nicholas, J. S., J. M. Charles, L. A. Carpenter, L. B. King, W. Jenner, and E. G. Spratt. Prevalence and characteristics of children with autism-spectrum disorders. *Annals of Epidemiology* 18 (2008): 130-136.

Offit, P. A. *Autism's False Prophets: Bad Science, Risky Medicine, and the Search for a Cure.* New York: Columbia University Press, 2008.

Oliveira, G., A. Ataíde, and C. Marques. Epidemiology of autism spectrum disorder in Portugal: Prevalence, clinical characterization, and medical conditions. *Developmental Medicine and Child Neurology* 49 (2007): 726-733.

Powell, J., A. Edwards, M. Edwards, B. Pandit, S. Sungum-Paliwal, and W. Whitehouse. Changes in the incidence of childhood autism and other autistic spectrum disorders in preschool children from two areas of the West Midlands, UK. *Developmental Medicine and Child Neurology* 42 (2000): 624-628.

Ritvo, E., B. Freeman, C. Pingree, et al. The UCLA-University of Utah epidemiologic survey of autism: Prevalence. *American Journal of Psychiatry* 146 (1989): 194-199.

Roberts, E. M., P. B. English, J. K. Grether, G. C. Windham, L. Somberg, and C. Wolff. Maternal residence near agricultural pesticide applications and autism spectrum disorders among children in the California Central Valley. *Environmental Health Perspectives* 115 (2007): 1482-1489.

Rutter, M. Autistic children: Infancy to adulthood. *Seminars in Psychiatry* 2 (1970): 435-450.

Rutter, M. Incidence of autism spectrum disorders: Changes over time and their meaning. *Acta Paediatrica* 94 (2005): 2-15.

Scott, F. J., S. Baron-Cohen, P. Bolton, and C. Brayne. Brief report: Prevalence of autism spectrum conditions in children aged 5-11 years in Cambridgeshire, UK. *Autism*, 6 (2002): 231-237.

Sebat, J., B. Lakshmi, D. Malhotra, et al. Strong association of de novo copy number mutations with autism. *Science* 20 (2007): 445-449.

Shattuck, P. T. The contribution of diagnostic substitution to the growing administrative prevalence of autism in US special education. *Pediatrics* 117 (2006): 1028-1037.

Snow, W. M., K. Hartle, and T. L. Ivanco. Altered morphology of motor cortex neurons in the VPA rat model of autism. *Developmental Psychobiology* 50 (2008): 633-639.

Sponheim, E., and O. Skjeldal. Autism and related disorders: Epidemiological findings in a Norwegian study using ICD-10 diagnostic criteria. *Journal of Autism and Developmental Disorders* 28 (1998): 217-227.

Steinhausen, H. C., D. Gobel, M. Breinlinger, and B. Wohlloben. A community survey of infantile autism. *Journal of the American Academy of Child Psychiatry* 25 (1986): 186-189.

Sugiyama, T., and T. Abe. The prevalence of autism in Nagoya, Japan: A total population study. *Journal of Autism and Developmental Disorders* 19 (1989): 87-96.

Tanoue, Y., S. Oda, F. Asano, and K. Kawashima. Epidemiology of infantile autism in southern Ibaraki, Japan: Differences in prevalence in birth cohorts. *Journal of Autism and Developmental Disorders* 18 (1988): 155-166.

Taylor, B., E. Miller, C. Farrington, et al. Autism and measles, mumps, and rubella vaccine: No epidemiological evidence for a causal association. *The Lancet* 353 (1999): 2026-2029.

Taylor, B., E. Miller, R. Lingam, N. Andrews, A. Simmons, and J. Stowe. Measles, mumps, and rubella vaccination and bowel problems or developmental regression in children with autism: Population study. *British Medical Journal* 324 (2002): 393-396.

Tebruegge, M., V. Nandini, and J. Ritchie. Does routine child health surveillance contribute to the early detection of children with pervasive developmental disorders? An epidemiological study in Kent, UK. *BMC Pediatrics* 4 (2004): 4.

Treffert, D. A. Epidemiology of infantile autism. *Archives of General Psychiatry* 22 (1970): 431-438.

U.S. Census Bureau. http://www.census.gov/popest/states/asrh/SC-EST2007-01.html, 2009 (accessed January 28, 2009).

Wazana, A., M. Bresnahan, and J. Kline. The autism epidemic: Fact or artifact? *Journal of the American Academy of Child and Adolescent Psychiatry* 46 (2007): 721-730.

Webb, E., S. Lobo, A. Hervas, J. Scourfield, and W. Fraser. The changing prevalence of autistic disorder in a Welsh health district. *Developmental Medicine and Child Neurology* 39 (1997): 150-152.

Williams, E., K. Thomas, H. Sidebotham, and A. Emond. Prevalence and characteristics of autistic spectrum disorders in the ALSPAC cohort. *Developmental Medicine and Child Neurology* 50 (2008): 672-677.

Williams, J. G., J. P. Higgins, and C. E. Brayne. Systematic review of prevalence studies of autism spectrum disorders. *Archives of Disease in Childhood* 91 (2006): 8-15.

Wing, L., and J. Gould. Severe impairments of social interaction and associated abnormalities in children: Epidemiology and classification. *Journal of Autism and Developmental Disorders* 9 (1979): 11-29.

Wing, L., S. Yeates, L. Brierly, and J. Gould. The prevalence of early childhood autism: Comparison of administrative and epidemiological studies. *Psychological Medicine* 6 (1976): 89-100.

Wignyosumarto, S., M. Mukhlas, and S. Shirataki. Epidemiological and clinical study of autistic children in Yogyakarta, Indonesia. *Kobe Journal of Medical Sciences* 38 (1992): 1-19.

Wolff, S., and A. Barlow. Schizoid personality in childhood: A comparative study of schizoid, autistic, and normal children. *Journal of Child Psychology and Psychiatry* 20 (1979): 29-46.

Wong, V. C., and S. L. Hui. Epidemiological study of autism spectrum disorder in China. *Journal of Child Neurology* 23 (2008): 67-72.

World Health Organization. *The International Statistical Classification of Diseases and Related Health Problems, Ninth Revision (ICD-9)*. Geneva: WHO, 1977.

World Health Organization. *The ICD-10 Classification of Mental and Behavioural Disorders: Clinical Descriptions and Diagnostic Guidelines*. Geneva, WHO, 1992.

Yeargin-Allsopp, M., C. Rice, T. Karapurkar, N. Doernberg, C. Boyle, and C. Murphy. Prevalence of autism in a US metropolitan area [comment]. *The Journal of the American Medical Association* 289 (2003): 49-55.

9

PTSD in Mothers Coping with Trauma in Their Children

Charlotte Allenou, Bertrand Olliac, Franck Hazane,
Philippe Birmes, and Jean-Philippe Raynaud

INTRODUCTION

Psychotraumatology in children and adolescents has been the subject of a greater amount of research over the last few years, in particular owing to the frequency and impact of different types of traumatic events in patients undergoing development. At the forefront of these potentially highly traumatic events are road traffic accidents and being confronted with a disease.

In France in 2007, the Observatoire National Interministériel de la Sécurité Routière (O.N.I.S.R.) [National Interministerial Observatory on Road Safety] (Chapelon et al. 2007) carried out a census of a million individuals covering all age groups, which showed that there were 690 victims of road traffic accidents aged 0-14 years, and 3,713 victims aged 15-17 years. The accidents represent the major cause of mortality amongst children from the age of one upwards and almost half of all accidental deaths are caused by road traffic accidents (Chapelon et al. 2007). Road traffic accidents in industrialized countries are the most common cause of post-traumatic stress disorder (PTSD) (Norris 1992). In the United States, road traffic accidents are likewise one of the most common events experienced by children; more than 300,000 children are injured each year in such accidents (National Highway Traffic Safety Administration 1999).

Facing up to an illness is also a particularly stressful event for children and adolescents. In France, cancer and leukemia strike roughly 1,500 children each year (Desandes et al. 2004). Although the rate of cure has been improving over the last 30 years these illnesses are the second most common cause of death amongst children aged 1-15 years (20% of deaths) after accidents (40%) (High Committee of Public Health 1997). The treatment of cancer takes a long time (between 4 and 18 months) and causes significant side effects. Sooner or later a relapse is quite common, which involves medical supervision over several years.

In this context, the majority of studies are centered on traumatological mortality and morbidity. However, PTSD, as an anxiety and adaptation disorder, is the main secondary psychiatric disorder following a traumatizing event. The prevalence of PTSD amongst the general population varies from 2% to 7% according to samples (Alonso et al. 2004; Brunet, Akerib, and Birmes 2007; Kessler et al. 2005). In western Europe, the traumatic events most frequently linked with the onset of PTSD include rape, private events that have not been revealed, serious illnesses affecting children, being beaten by the spouse, being ill, and being beaten by the person looking after you, and so on (Darves-Bornoz et al. 2008).

In its definition of PTSD, the *Diagnostic and Statistical Manual of Mental Disorders*, fourth edition (DSM-IV) defines the exposure criteria. According to criterion A1, a person is exposed to a traumatic event, during the course of which he/she has been confronted with one or more events, which involved death, the threat of death, serious injury, or the threat to the person's own or other people's physical integrity; or as a result of being a witness to an event that could result in death, injury, or a physical threat to another person; or as a result of learning about a violent or unexpected death, serious aggression, or the threat of death or injury by a family member or somebody close (American Psychiatric Association 1994). In its fourth version the DSM introduced criterion A2, as a diagnostic criterion for PTSD: "The reaction of the person involved is a feeling of intense fear, a feeling of powerlessness or horror, and disorganised or agitated behaviour in the child" (American Psychiatric Association 1994). This concept also takes account of the severity of the initial traumatic effects. From a medical point of view, from the Greek *traumatos* (injury), trauma is the "injury or wound produced by an outside agent on a specific part of the organism as a result of a mechanical action inflicted on the latter, leading to different problems according to the force involved." Traumatism represents "all the psychic, physical or secondary phenomena that have been triggered in the organism as a result of a trauma."

Psychic or psychological traumatism is "a violent psychological shock which exceeds the patient's ability to adapt and the major emotional repercussions of which can lead to long-lasting pathological effects on the patient's psyche or personality." Hence the current traumatic event is defined in DSM-IV as the addition of an objective exposure to an event entailing a threat to life or physical integrity and an immediate subjective response in the form of intense fear and/or powerlessness and/or horror.

In some aspects, the psychotraumatic effects in children may be similar to those described in adults: repetitive, invasive nightmares and flashbacks;

the feeling of distress when reminded of these events or when exposed to elements serving to remind of such events; more or less conscious efforts to avoid thinking or talking about them; avoiding situations associated with the traumatism; reduced interest in certain activities; and sleeping disorders, problems concentrating, etc. But other aspects show that the effects in children vary considerably from those observed in adults, depending on their onset and developing psychism, with different levels and ability of emotional control, depending on the age and level of maturity of the child. Hence, we observe frequent behavioral manifestations, either in the form of inhibition and withdrawal or in the form of more external manifestations, i.e., altering games and drawings, agitation, aggression, regression (secondary bed-wetting, sucking the thumb), fear of separation, etc. Added to this symptomatology, which may differ from that of adults, are the consequences on brain development and neurobiological functioning (Nader 2008). The developing central nervous system can be particularly vulnerable when subject to intense stress which can lead to long-lasting, if not definitive change, to the modulation and organization of neuronal systems and can also upset the hormonal systems, such as growth hormone secretion control or the corticotropic axis.

Terr (1991) specifically defined two types of psychotraumatism in the child. Type I traumatism is where the event is unique and sudden and has a massive impact, whilst the consequences of type II are due to exposure to repeated or long-lasting events which can therefore be anticipated (Terr 1991). Some symptoms are common to both types of traumatism: repetitive behavior, i.e., repetitive games or actions re-creating some aspects of the traumatic situation; repetitive dreams which are rare in the child are mostly merely scary dreams lacking in recognizable content; intrusive and repetitive memories (visual but also tactile, olfactory, or proprioceptive); specific fear associated with the traumatism, which is the most easy to identify, or fear that can extend to other objects or situations not associated with the traumatism; and loss of confidence and pessimism regarding the future, as well as a change in attitude towards others. Following type I traumas all or only some of these manifestations may be observed.

The victims of such traumas may be affected in that they avoid situations reminding them of the trauma, are unable to perceive reality in the initial stages and for a time following the trauma (such as false recognition, visual hallucinations, illusions, and time distortions), and are permanently looking for an explanation with regard to the event.

For type II trauma other symptoms can be added to this table. Defense reactions when faced with repeated events may be the cause of such symptoms. Hence, most frequently one notes an important denial, emotional dulling of the senses, greater avoidance, loss of memory of entire episodes of childhood, depersonalization and dissociation reactions, expressions of anger, and self or heteroaggression. However, it must be pointed out that the distinction between type I and II is not always very clear or well defined. Account should also be taken of the fact that some everyday life events may have long-lasting consequences for the child (e.g., death of a parent, disability, or their consequences).

Whatever the context, comorbidities may occur. It is not unusual to witness the development of anxiety disorders (obsessive ideas, phobic manifestations, free anxiety, or anxiety of separation); depressive or dysthymic disorders; behavioral problems; and somatic problems or regressive type behavior (in particular bed-wetting). With respect to type II traumas this could also give rise to the question of the early onset of personality disorders (borderline, narcissist, antisocial, etc.).

The observed consequences of traumatic exposure are the three classical manifestations of re-experiencing, avoidance, and hyper-vigilance. The victims may initially present with re-experiencing in the form of images, intrusive memories, nightmares, and the impression of reliving the event, as well as symptoms of avoidance and dulling of their senses, coupled with, for example, emotional detachment and a feeling of a bleak future, etc. Finally symptoms of hyper-vigilance coupled with sleeping disorders, hyper-vigilance and permanent states of being alert, and reactions of being startled may complete the clinical picture.

For a number of years the literature reported on the impact of the mother's psychic disorders on the child, particularly in the context of psychotraumatology. Hence, a child is more likely to develop PTSD when his/her parents themselves show high levels of anxiety, distress, or PTSD symptoms (Green et al. 1991). The parental reactions would be the crucial predictors of the manner in which children will respond to traumatism (Pelcovitz et al. 1998). Where a child is suffering from cancer it has been shown that the mother plays a crucial role in mediating between the child and PTSD symptomatology (Stuber et al. 1994). The transgenerational link seems to have been demonstrated for transmitting the mother's disorder to the child. Nonetheless, it would be interesting to also assess the impact on the mother of traumatism in the child, e.g., how to regulate, organize, and transform their emotions, memories, and anxious anticipations for the immediate or more long-term future? A traumatic event could affect the nearest and dearest, who had witnessed or suddenly learned that one of their family members had, for example, been involved in an accident. The DSM-IV (American Psychiatric Association 1994) acknowledged with respect to criterion A1, that the fact of learning about a threat of death or an injury suffered by a member of the family is an extreme stress factor and can lead to intense fear and subsequent PTSD symptoms in the same way as for direct victims. However, little work has been undertaken concerning the "indirectly" exposed victims. From one of our observations a mother learning about her child's accident over the telephone only has a little information about the seriousness of this accident; she therefore imagines the worst for her child and feels completely at a loss. Consequently, even if, on arrival at the scene of the accident she is reassured about her child's condition she is aware from that day onwards that she could have lost her child. This feeling may persist well after the accident and possibly be accompanied by a feeling of guilt for not having been able to avoid her child's accident.

EPIDEMIOLOGY OF PTSD IN MOTHERS COPING WITH THEIR CHILD'S TRAUMATISM

The epidemiology of PTSD essentially concerns the victims and witnesses of a particularly stressful event. Studies concerning the parents, mothers in particular, of children having suffered a trauma are still rare to the present day.

General Population

According to the Breslau and colleagues' study (1998), the incidence of discovering a traumatic event during the course of their lives, affected 63.1% of men and 61.8% of women (Breslau et al. 1998). However, the prevalence of PTSD in response to the fact of discovering the event was 1.4% for men and 3.2% for women (Breslau et al. 1999). In Table 9.1 data from the Detroit Area Survey of Trauma is presented showing the rates of exposure to indirect trauma and the resulting prevalence of PTSD due to exposure to indirect trauma.

Table 9.1: PTSD Following the Announcement of a Traumatic Event

Type of trauma	% Exposed (SD)	% PTSD (SD)
Learning about the traumatization of another person	62.4 (1.2)	2.2 (0.7)
Learning that a close person (family/friend) had been raped or sexually abused	32.6 (1.2)	3.6 (1.7)
Learning that a close person (family/friend) had been seriously physically attacked	16.1 (0.9)	4.6 (2.9)
Learning that a close person (family/friend) had been seriously injured in a road traffic accident	39.4 (1.2)	0.9 (0.5)
Learning that a close person (family/friend) had been seriously injured in another type of accident	12.2 (0.8)	0.4 (0.4)
Learning of the unexpected death of a friend or close relation	60.0 (1.2)	14.3 (2.6)

Although this data on the prevalence of indirect victims is less than that normally found in the literature these figures should be analyzed with interest. In the months following the traumatic exposure, the rate of PTSD amongst the direct victims fluctuated from 9.2% (Breslau et al. 1998) to 32%. (Jehel et al. 2003). These "indirect" victims may develop post-traumatic symptoms following this type of exposure. We shall now make distinctions between the mothers of child victims according to different types of traumatism. This data is not exhaustive but relates to those types of traumatic events that are most widespread in the literature.

Mothers of Children Who Have Been the Victim of Road Traffic Accidents

In 2004 (Bryant et al. 2004) conducted a yearlong study amongst a group of 86 children, aged 5 to 16 years, who were admitted to the accident and emergency unit following a road traffic accident;15% of the children suffered from acute stress, 25% had PTSD symptoms after three months, and 18% still had these symptoms after six months. Three-quarters of the mothers described feeling moderate to severe fear and half of these feared that their child had been seriously injured or were even dead. Eighty-four percent of all the mothers reported symptoms of reliving the incident and 81% had hyper-vigilant symptoms. At three and six months, 50% of the mothers showed signs of reliving the incident and hyper-vigilant symptoms. On the other hand, only two mothers (4%) suffered from the characteristic PTSD.

The other group studies on parents with children involved in road traffic accidents showed comparable rates. The study conducted by Landolt and colleagues (2005) showed that 20% of mothers had symptoms that were clinically significant of acute PTSD four and six weeks after the accident; 6% of mothers still had significant symptoms, and 13.2% showed partial symptoms one year following the accident involving their child. The prevalence of PTSD symptoms in a group of children and adolescents who were victims of a road traffic accident rose to 15% in the study conducted by De Vries and colleagues (1999) for the parents who developed clinically significant symptoms of PTSD 7 and 12 months following the road traffic accident involving their child. Of the sample, 35% of children developed significant PTSD symptoms. Fifteen percent of parents whose children were involved in a road traffic accident also reported that they suffered from clinically significant PTSD symptoms 3 to 13 months following their exposure to the trauma, according to a study by Winston and colleagues (2003). In 1998, Winje and Ulvik analyzed the psychological sequelae for children and their parents one and three years following a bus accident which had occurred in 1988. Twelve children and four parents died in the accident. One year later the symptoms suffered by the child and mother were similar. Nonetheless, beyond one year the children made far greater and more rapid improvements than the parents. The children seemed to need more special attention from the professionals who surrounded them only during the following year. As for the parents, professional assistance could last for several years following the trauma. The development of symptoms amongst parents of children who had been victims of a road traffic accident is frequent but, up to now, has not been fully examined.

Mothers of Children Who Suffered Burns

Child burns are amongst the most stressful trauma events for the parents (Byrne et al. 1986; Cella et al. 1988; Mason and Hillier 1993a, 1993b; Rizzone et al. 1994). Several stress factors for the parents can be analyzed: the burn itself, the fact of having to witness the pain suffered by one's child, being far from home, and the impact of the wound on the future development of the child. Although studies suggested that the parents of children suffering from burns could develop symptoms including guilt, depression, anxiety, and hostility (Byrne et al. 1986; Cella et al. 1988; Kent, King, and Cochrane 2000), only a few studies examined the post-traumatic responses from amongst this population. From a study of severely burnt children (the average extent of the burn being 37.9%), 52% of mothers suffered PTSD symptoms (Rizzone et al. 1994) as opposed to only 25% of the children. Thirty-one percent of mothers still showed these symptoms roughly seven years following admission of their severely burnt child to a hospital. In 1998, Fukunishi (1998) examined the symptoms of PTSD and depression amongst those mothers of children who suffered accidental burns at bath time; 12.5% of mothers suffered from PTSD symptoms and 18.8% suffered from depression. With respect to the intense distress when exposed to a similar event restricting outcomes to the affect and hyper-vigilance symptoms, the rates were greater amongst the mothers than the children (Fukunishi 1998). Four years later, 13% of parents suffered increased irritability and sleeping problems. Hall and colleagues (2006) conducted a trial on 62 parents of children having suffered burns; 47% of parents indicated that they experienced one PTSD criterion (reliving the event or avoidance/dulling of the senses or hyper-vigilance) three months after the burn, 28% experienced two criteria, and 9% experienced all three criteria.

Other Events

After the sinking of the vessel *Jupiter* in 1988, which was carrying children, 35% of mothers suffered PTSD symptoms three months following the catastrophe and 8% six months later (Mirzamani 2005). Sexual aggression involving the child as a victim also occurred, as did traumatic exposure for the parents (Kelley 1990).

Mothers of Children Suffering from a General Illness

The noxious effects of cancer and its necessary treatment extend beyond the physical consequences. Cancer in the child involves long and restrictive treatment which obliges the family to organize itself around the child's illness. The psychosocial impact of cancer on the child and parents cannot be denied. Cancer, by its very nature, involves multiple and chronic stress agents such as announcing the diagnosis, the severity of the illness, the prognosis, invasive treatments, and their side effects. Research has shown that these children and their parents are at high risk of intense psychological distress (Greenberg et al. 1994; Kangas, Henry, and Bryant 2002; Kornblith et al. 1992) particularly with regard to PTSD symptoms (Brown, Madan-Swain, and Lambert 2003; Hobbie et al. 2000; Pelcovitz et al. 1998).

According to studies, the incidence of PTSD can be observed in 6.2% (Manne et al. 1998) to 25% (Pelcovitz et al. 1996) of mothers whose children suffered from cancer. With regard to PTSD symptoms, the rates varied between 10.2% (Kazak et al. 1997) and 44% (Fuemmeler, Mullins, and Marx 2001). The studies of mothers with children suffering from cancer show, as classically described in psychotraumatology, that the symptoms of PTSD may be temporary or persist over several years (Kazak 1997; Manne et al. 1998; Pelcovitz et al. 1996). These results highlight the psychotraumatological impact on the family circle and particularly on the mothers (Bruce 2006). For the mothers, the experience of a child suffering from cancer is more traumatic than the fact of themselves having survived cancer (Kangas et al. 2002; Smith et al. 1999).

Diabetes may likewise induce stress for the patient's family circle. This stress may be associated with long-term treatment and the repercussions this entails with the hypoglycemic and hyperglycemic phases and the shock of diagnosis. This latter situation could correspond to acute stress whilst the treatment would correspond to chronic stress. According to Landolt and colleagues (2002) these two forms of stress could be etiological factors for PTSD. These authors show that 24% of mothers of children recently diagnosed as suffering from type 1 diabetes experienced PTSD symptoms. These figures were similar to those found in studies involving mothers of children suffering from an illness or chronic wound, such as burns (Pelcovitz et al. 1996; Rizzone et al. 1994).

Some studies leaned towards the post-traumatic consequences for mothers with children suffering from epilepsy. The unforeseeable development, the terrifying aspect of the fit, and the uncertain damage caused by each fit make it very difficult for family members to deal with epilepsy. Iseri, Ozten, and Aker (2006) assessed the prevalence of PTSD symptoms and depression amongst the parents of epileptic children (77 mothers and 3 fathers). The results showed that 88% of parents experienced symptoms of re-experiencing and 80% of hyper-vigilance symptoms. The prevalence of PTSD was 31.5%. The rate of prevalence of PTSD in this study was similar to that found in parents of children suffering from another illness potentially endangering life (Andrykowski and Cordova 1998; Breslau 2002).

These studies confirm that learning that one's child has experienced a traumatic event could be an extreme stress factor associated with the development of PTSD. In order to offer such mothers the best support the literature should provide information about the factors likely to contribute to PTSD as soon as their children receive medical care.

PREDICTIVE FACTORS LEADING TO THE DEVELOPMENT OF PTSD IN MOTHERS

Studies were carried out to highlight to predictive link between certain pre-, peri-, and post-traumatic variables and the onset of subsequent PTSD in the close family circle of the victim.

Pretraumatic Variables

Socio-Demographic Characteristics

In the study conducted by De Vries and colleagues (1999), distress following a road traffic accident was greater in mothers whilst their child was young. The mother's emotional commitment and her feelings of responsibility for the trauma experienced by her child were more important whilst the child was young (De Vries et al. 1999). The female gender of the child (Winston et al. 2003), the young age of the child (Winston et al. 2003; De Vries et al. 1999), and the moderate social-economic level (Landolt et al. 2003) constitute, for some studies, predictive PTSD variables for the mother. However, other studies show no relationship with respect to gender (Landolt et al. 2005; Landolt et al. 2002), the child's age (Landolt et al. 2005; Bryant et al. 2004; Landolt et al. 2002), social-economic status (Goldenberg Libov et al. 2002), and the onset of PTSD symptoms in the mother.

Life Events

As concerns (Landolt et al. 2005), only the quantitative assessment of life events in the 12 months preceding the accident (moving house, divorce, etc.) was related to PTSD symptoms in the mother one year after the event. These results were likewise described for mothers with children suffering from cancer. There is a relationship between stressful life events and the onset of PTSD symptoms in mothers of children suffering from cancer (Baraka et al. 1997; Manne et al. 1998).

It should also be pointed out that mothers themselves, having survived cancer during their childhood, are more likely to suffer from PTSD symptoms if their child also suffers from cancer (Fuemmeler et al. 2000; Kazak et al. 1997; Landolt et al. 2003: Stuber et al. 1996).

Peritraumatic Variables

Peritraumatic Dissociation and Distress

Exposure to a traumatic event may, at the time of the event or within hours following it, lead to peritraumatic reactions, such as distress and dissociation. Peritraumatic distress refers to the negative emotions (e.g., feelings of helplessness, sadness and grief, frustration, or anger), and to the perceived threat of life and bodily arousal (feeling afraid for one's safety, feeling worried about the safety of others, experiencing physical reactions like sweating, shaking, pounding heart, etc.) that are experienced during and immediately after the trauma (Brunet et al. 2001; Birmes et al. 2005). Peritraumatic dissociation is defined as a way of processing information during and immediately after the trauma which involves an altered perception of time, place, and self: moments of losing track of time or blanking out; finding oneself acting on "automatic pilot"; a sense of time changing during the event; the event seeming unreal; a feeling as if floating above the scene; a feeling of body distortion; confusion as to what was happening to the self and others; and not being aware of things that happened during the event, and disorientation (Lensvelt Mulders et al. 2008; Birmes et al. 2005). These two concepts hold a significant place in the current literature on PTSD. Numerous studies showed that the victims who experienced these peritraumatic reactions were a "high risk" group likely to develop subsequent PTSD (Birmes et al. 2005; Brunet et al. 2001).

Numerous studies have been conducted with the close family members of victims and especially mothers. In their study on mothers of children who have sustained burns, Hall and colleagues (2006) suggested that parental, peritraumatic dissociation predicted PTSD symptoms in the mother (Hall et al. 2006). As regards peritraumatic distress, only the predictor role of the feeling of powerlessness in the mother leading to the subsequent development of PTSD symptoms has already been demonstrated at the time of accidents involving her children (Iseri, Ozten, and Aker 2006; Winston et al. 2003).

Involvement of the Mother in the Incident

Some studies failed to illustrate that the mother's level of involvement in the accident is likely to influence the subsequent development of PTSD symptoms (Bryant et al. 2004; Landolt et al. 2005; Winston et al. 2003). Not all studies confirmed this result.

Posttraumatic Variables

Severity of the Trauma

Rizzone and colleagues showed for mothers of children having suffered burns that the most powerful predictor for the development of PTSD was the extent of the burns on the child (Rizzone et al. 1994). Hall and colleagues (2006) highlighted that the risk factors (peritraumatic dissociation, PTSD symptoms in the child) leading to the development of PTSD were mediated by the extent of the burns on the child (Hall et al. 2006). With regard to road traffic accidents, the majority of studies did not show that the severity of the child's wound (Landolt et al. 2005; De Vries et al. 1999; Bryant et al. 2004) was instrumental as a high risk factor leading to the development of PTSD in the mother. For diabetic or epileptic children, neither the hospital stay nor the characteristics of the epileptic fit were associated with PTSD symptoms in the mother (Williams et al. 2003; Baki et al. 2004).

Symptoms of the Child

Mirzamani and colleagues (2005) established that the mothers of children who were victims in the *Jupiter* shipwreck showed increased symptoms when their child suffered PTSD symptoms. Other studies developed the analysis of the relationship between PTSD symptoms in the child and those of the mother (Barakat et al. 1997; Kazak et al. 1997; Stuber et al. 1996). The study conducted by Laor, Wolmer, and Cohen (2001) provided more details. Out of 81 Israeli children aged 8-10 years and their mothers, whose houses were damaged by missile attacks during the first Gulf War, the relationship between the PTSD symptoms in the mother and those of her child were greater the younger the child. Other authors confirmed the relationship between the mother's symptoms and those presented by the child (Pelcovitz et al. 1998). However, some authors undermine the relationship between PTSD symptoms in the child and those suffered by the mother (Kazak et al. 2004; Landolt et al. 2003; Bruce 2006). There is not as yet any consensus on the predictor role of symptoms in the child to the development of PTSD symptoms in the mother.

DISCUSSION

The current studies confirm that the parents, especially the mothers of traumatized children, may permanently suffer quite widespread psychotraumatological scars. A small percentage of mothers may develop characteristic PTSD but most show PTSD symptoms. In some studies the mothers of the child victims would even, in some cases, be more exposed to the development of PTSD symptoms than their child. Following the consequences of the accident involving their child, or any other trauma, the mother may recall her arrival at the place of the accident and the first images of her child and then subsequently avoid the area or any situation reminding her of this accident. This can then go hand in hand with symptoms of hyper-vigilance where the mother becomes much more vigilant as soon as her child goes out alone or even when she is in the car.

Moreover, a serious wound or threat to the child's life is extremely stressful for the parents (Kazak 1997; Stuber et al. 1996; Stuber et al. 1998; Winston et al. 2002). The parents of a sick or injured child must fight when faced with the possibility of their child dying or with the consequences of the child's condition. The parents also suffer stress when admitting their child to hospital, learning of the treatment, witnessing the pain, waiting for examination results, and so on. These experiences can exhaust the most resilient of parents.

On the other hand, the symptoms which are most widely reported by the mothers in different studies essentially relate to symptoms of hyper-vigilance (insomnia, irritability, lack of concentration, state of being alert, being startled). These symptoms may have consequences for the children. Faced with their mother's anxiety in situations reminiscent of the event the children may feel overprotected and deprived of their own independence and confidence in themselves. Moreover, some parents find themselves in a conflicting situation between the fear that the event would have negative repercussions for members of their family and the desire to start afresh and put such a painful event behind them.

It is also important to note that 46% of parents with children suffering from PTSD symptoms request help for their child, whilst only 20% request help for themselves when they suffer PTSD symptoms (De Vries et al. 1999). These results confirm the under-utilization of the mental health services for children and their families in distress and point to the need to track down those families at high risk of developing PTSD symptoms on arrival at the accident and emergency department.

PTSD has many consequences for the family: reduced and limited privacy, poor communication and the inability to resolve conflicts, and unsatisfactory relationships. Assisting families in this situation seems vital. Consideration of the repercussions on the mother should provide a global view of the family. It is necessary, even with the sole aim of helping the child, to take charge of the different members of the family when faced with trauma. Because of her unique relationship with the child it is the mother who is an essential support in the treatment of her child. A reaction of distress in the mother may, for example, exacerbate the trauma suffered by the child. During emergency treatment it is the current acknowledgment that all family members are suffering that could have direct, practical consequences. Treatment procedures are often difficult for the parents. They may suffer on account of a lack of information or understanding of the problems affecting their child. Better information on traumatism and its consequences could have a beneficial effect on the satisfaction and distress of the parents (Birmes, Raynaud, Daubisse, Brunet et al. 2009). Research over the past few years on the post-traumatic consequences of mothers confronted with the traumatic exposure of their child is still quite sparse. Nonetheless, the introduction in DSM-IV of the announced disorder in the child has contributed to broader research in this field and particularly concerning the announcement of a cancer in the child. This expansion in research is extending, little by little, to the other types of trauma. However, these results still remain to be verified and details must be provided about the still controversial risk factors, especially by analyzing the peritraumatic variables in play at the time of the trauma such as peritraumatic distress and dissociation. The perception of a vital threat and peritraumatic dissociation amongst the direct victims seem to be better predictors of PTSD than objective measures such as the severity of the wound in the adult (Ehlers, Mayou, and Bryant 1998; Birmes et al. 2005). At present, the emphasis on the secondary prevention of PTSD is placed on the peritraumatic variables associated with the subsequent development of PTSD. As these indices are widely acknowledged amongst the populations of direct victims they remain to be explored amongst the closest family members of victims in order to provide the appropriate assistance to the parties involved as early as possible.

CONCLUSION

When a traumatic event strikes family life, all members of the family are shaken. Each person will live through this event in his or her own way and with his or her own resources. Following a traumatizing event mothers can subsequently show PTSD symptoms. The difficulty for such mothers is to project themselves into the future and their feeling of guilt sometimes means that they take a long time to find solutions and obtain assistance. What is more, the mother's role in looking after her child is all the more fundamental today, owing to the development and transfer of technologies, given that the pattern of patient treatment is being shifted more and more from the hospital to the patient's home. Analyzing the screening indices for early PTSD symptoms and taking on overall care will provide better assistance to the children and their mothers following a traumatic event.

REFERENCES

American Psychiatric Association. 1994. *Diagnostic and Statistical Manual of Mental Disorders (4th ed.)*. Washington, DC: Author.

Alonso, J., Angermeyer, M. C., Bernert, S., Bruffaerts, R., Brugha, T. S.,Bryson, H., et al. 2004. Prevalence of mental disorders in Europe: Results from the European Study of the Epidemiology of Mental Disorders (ESEMeD) project. *Acta Psychiatr Scand* Suppl (420): 21-27.

Andrykowski, M. A., and M. J. Cordova. 1998. Factors associated with PTSD symptoms following treatment for breast cancer: Test of the Andersen model. *J Trauma Stress* 11 (2):189-203.

Baki, O., A. Erdogan, O. Kantarci, G. Akisik, L. Kayaalp, and C. Yalcinkaya. 2004. Anxiety and depression in children with epilepsy and their mothers. *Epilepsy Behav* 5 (6):958-64.

Barakat, L. P., A. E. Kazak, A. T. Meadows, R. Casey, K. Meeske, and M. L. Stuber. 1997. Families surviving childhood cancer: A comparison of posttraumatic stress symptoms with families of healthy children. *J Pediatr Psychol* 22 (6):843-59.

Birmes, P, A. Brunet, M. Benoit, S. Defer, L. Hatton, H. Sztulman, and L. Schmitt. 2005. Validation of the Peritraumatic Dissociative Experiences Questionnaire self-report version in two samples of French-speaking individuals exposed to trauma. *European Psychiatry* 20 (2):145-51.

Birmes, P., Raynaud, J.-P., Daubisse, L., Brunet, A., Arbus, C., Klein, R., Cailhol, L., Allenou, C., Hazane, F., Grandjean, H., Schmitt, L. 2009. Children's enduring PTSD symptoms are related to their family's adaptability and cohesion. *Journal of Community Mental Health* 45 (4):290-99.

Breslau, N. 2002. Epidemiologic studies of trauma, posttraumatic stress disorder, and other psychiatric disorders. *Can J Psychiatry* 47 (10):923-9.

Breslau, N., H. D. Chilcoat, R. C. Kessler, E. L. Peterson, and V. C. Lucia. 1999. Vulnerability to assaultive violence: Further specification of the sex difference in post-traumatic stress disorder. *Psychol Med* 29 (4):813-21.

Breslau, N., R. C. Kessler, H. D. Chilcoat, L. R. Schultz, G. C. Davis, and P. Andreski. 1998. Trauma and posttraumatic stress disorder in the community: The 1996 Detroit Area Survey of Trauma. *Archives of General Psychiatry* 55 (7):626-32.

Brown, R. T., A. Madan-Swain, and R. Lambert. 2003. Posttraumatic stress symptoms in adolescent survivors of childhood cancer and their mothers. *J Trauma Stress* 16 (4):309-18.

Bruce, M. 2006. A systematic and conceptual review of posttraumatic stress in childhood cancer survivors and their parents. *Clin Psychol Rev* 26 (3):233-56.

Brunet, A., Akerib, V., & Birmes, P. 2007. Don't throw out the baby with the bathwater (PTSD is not overdiagnosed). *Can J Psychiatry* 52 (8): 501-2; discussion, 503.

Brunet, A., D. S. Weiss, T. J. Metzler, S. R. Best, T. C. Neylan, C. Rogers, J. Fagan, and C. R. Marmar. 2001. The Peritraumatic Distress Inventory: A proposed measure of PTSD criterion A2. *American Journal of Psychiatry* 158 (9):1480-5.

Bryant, B., R. Mayou, L. Wiggs, A. Ehlers, and G. Stores. 2004. Psychological consequences of road traffic accidents for children and their mothers. *Psychol Med* 34 (2):335-46.

Byrne, C., B. Love, G. Browne, B. Brown, J. Roberts, and D. Streiner. 1986. The social competence of children following burn injury: A study of resilience. *J Burn Care Rehabil* 7 (3):247-52.

Cella, D. F., S. W. Perry, S. Kulchycky, and C. Goodwin. 1988. Stress and coping in relatives of burn patients: A longitudinal study. *Hosp Community Psychiatry* 39

(2):159-66.

Chapelon, J., C. Machu, B. Gatterer, S. Boyer, C. Décamme, and O. Forget et al. 2007. *Les grandes données de l'accidentologie.* Paris.

Darves-Bornoz, J. M., Alonso, J., de Girolamo, G., de Graaf, R., Haro, J. M., Kovess-Masfety, V., et al. 2008. Main traumatic events in Europe: PTSD in the European study of the epidemiology of mental disorders survey. *J Trauma Stress* 21 (5): 455-62.

Desandes, E., Clavel, J., Berger, C., Bernard, J. L., Blouin, P., de Lumley, L., et al. 2004. Cancer incidence among children in France, 1990-1999. *Pediatr Blood Cancer* 43 (7): 749-57.

De Vries, A. P., N. Kassam-Adams, A. Cnaan, E. Sherman-Slate, P. R. Gallagher, and F. K. Winston. 1999. Looking beyond the physical injury: Posttraumatic stress disorder in children and parents after pediatric traffic injury. *Pediatrics* 104 (6):1293-9.

Ehlers, A., R. A. Mayou, and B. Bryant. 1998. Psychological predictors of chronic posttraumatic stress disorder after motor vehicle accidents. *Journal of Abnormal Psychology* 107 (3):508-19.

Fuemmeler, B. F., Elkin, T. D., & Mullins, L. L. 2002. Survivors of childhood brain tumors: Behavioral, emotional, and social adjustment. *Clin Psychol Rev* 22 (4): 547-85.

Fuemmeler, B. F., L. L. Mullins, and B. P. Marx. 2001. Posttraumatic stress and general distress among parents of children surviving a brain tumor. *Children's Health Care* 30:169-82.

Fukunishi, I. 1998. Posttraumatic stress symptoms and depression in mothers of children with severe burn injuries. *Psychol Rep* 83 (1):331-5.

Green, B. L., M. Korol, M. C. Grace, M. G. Vary, A. C. Leonard, G. C. Gleser, and S. Smitson-Cohen. 1991. Children and disaster: Age, gender, and parental effects on PTSD symptoms. *J Am Acad Child Adolesc Psychiatry* 30 (6):945-51.

Greenberg, J., T. Pyszczynski, S. Solomon, L. Simon, and M. Breus. 1994. Role of consciousness and accessibility of death-related thoughts in mortality salience effects. *J Pers Soc Psychol* 67 (4):627-37.

Hall, E., G. Saxe, F. Stoddard, J. Kaplow, K. Koenen, N. Chawla, C. Lopez, L. King, and D. King. 2006. Posttraumatic stress symptoms in parents of children with acute burns. *J Pediatr Psychol* 31 (4):403-12.

High Committee of Public Health [Haut comité de la santé publique]. 1997. Santé des enfants, santé des jeunes. Paris: Ecole Nationale de Santé Publique.

Hobbie, W. L., M. Stuber, K. Meeske, K. Wissler, M. T. Rourke, K. Ruccione, A. Hinkle, and A. E. Kazak. 2000. Symptoms of posttraumatic stress in young adult survivors of childhood cancer. *J Clin Oncol* 18 (24):4060-6.

Iseri, P. K., E. Ozten, and A. T. Aker. 2006. Posttraumatic stress disorder and major depressive disorder is common in parents of children with epilepsy. *Epilepsy Behav* 8 (1):250-5.

Jehel, L., S. Paterniti, A. Brunet, C. Duchet, and J. D. Guelfi. 2003. Prediction of the occurrence and intensity of post-traumatic stress disorder in victims 32 months after bomb attack. *Eur Psychiatry* 18 (4):172-6.

Kangas, M., J. L. Henry, and R. A. Bryant. 2002. Posttraumatic stress disorder following cancer. A conceptual and empirical review. *Clin Psychol Rev* 22 (4):499-524.

Kazak, A. E. 1997. A contextual family/systems approach to pediatric psychology: Introduction to the special issue. *J Pediatr Psychol* 22 (2):141-8.

Kazak, A. E., M. Alderfer, M. T. Rourke, S. Simms, R. Streisand, and J. R. Grossman. 2004. Posttraumatic stress disorder (PTSD) and posttraumatic stress symptoms (PTSS) in families of adolescent childhood cancer survivors. *J Pediatr Psychol* 29 (3):211-9.

Kazak, A. E., L. P. Barakat, K. Meeske, D. Christakis, A. T. Meadows, R. Casey, B. Penati, and M. L. Stuber. 1997. Posttraumatic stress, family functioning, and social support in survivors of childhood leukemia and their mothers and fathers. *J Consult Clin Psychol* 65 (1):120-9.

Kelley, S. J. 1990. Parental stress response to sexual abuse and ritualistic abuse of children in day-care centers. *Nurs Res* 39 (1):25-9.

Kent, L., H. King, and R. Cochrane. 2000. Maternal and child psychological sequelae in paediatric burn injuries. *Burns* 26 (4):317-22.

Kessler, R. C., Chiu, W. T., Demler, O., Merikangas, K. R., & Walters, E. E. 2005. Prevalence, severity, and comorbidity of 12-month DSM-IV disorders in the National Comorbidity Survey Replication. *Arch Gen Psychiatry* 62 (6): 617-27.

Kornblith, A. B., J. Anderson, D. F. Cella, S. Tross, E. Zuckerman, E. Cherin, E. Henderson, R. B. Weiss, M. R. Cooper, R. T. Silver, et al. 1992. Hodgkin disease survivors at increased risk for problems in psychosocial adaptation. The Cancer and Leukemia Group B. *Cancer* 70 (8):2214-24.

Landolt, M. A., K. Ribi, J. Laimbacher, M. Vollrath, H. E. Gnehm, and F. H. Sennhauser. 2002. Posttraumatic stress disorder in parents of children with newly diagnosed type 1 diabetes. *J Pediatr Psychol* 27 (7):647-52.

Landolt, M. A., M. Vollrath, K. Ribi, H. E. Gnehm, and F. H. Sennhauser. 2003. Incidence and associations of parental and child posttraumatic stress symptoms in pediatric patients. *J Child Psychol Psychiatry* 44 (8):1199-207.

Landolt, M. A., M. Vollrath, K. Timm, H. E. Gnehm, and F. H. Sennhauser. 2005. Predicting posttraumatic stress symptoms in children after road traffic accidents. *Journal of the American Academy of Child and Adolescent Psychiatry* 44 (12):1276-83.

Laor, N., Wolmer, L., & Cohen, D. J. 2001. Mothers' functioning and children's symptoms 5 years after a SCUD missile attack. *Am J Psychiatry* 158 (7): 1020-26.

Lensvelt-Mulders, G., van der Hart, O., van Ochten, J. M., van Son, M. J., Steele, K., & Breeman, L. 2008. Relations among peritraumatic dissociation and posttraumatic stress: A meta-analysis. *Clinical Psychology Review* 28 (7): 1138-51.

Manne, S. L., K. Du Hamel, K. Gallelli, K. Sorgen, and W. H. Redd. 1998. Posttraumatic stress disorder among mothers of pediatric cancer survivors: Diagnosis, comorbidity, and utility of the PTSD checklist as a screening instrument. *J Pediatr Psychol* 23 (6):357-66.

Mason, S., and V. F. Hillier. 1993a. Young, scarred children and their mothers—a short-term investigation into the practical, psychological and social implications of thermal injury to the preschool child. Part II: Implications for the child. *Burns* 19 (6):501-6.

———. 1993b. Young, scarred children and their mothers—a short-term investigation into the practical, psychological and social implications of thermal injury to the preschool child. Part III: Factors influencing outcome responses. *Burns* 19 (6):507-10.

Mirzamani, S. M. (2005). Mothers' psychological problems following disaster affecting their children. In T. A. Corales (Ed.), *Focus on posttraumatic stress disorder re-*

search (pp. 95-121). New York: Nova Science Publishers.

Nader, K. 2008. How children and adolescents' brains are affected by trauma. In *Understanding and Assessing Trauma in Children and Adolescents: Measures, Methods, and Youth in Context*. New York: Routledge.

National Highway Traffic Safety Administration. 1999. *Traffic Safety Facts 1999- Children*. Washington, DC: US Department of Transportation.

Norris, F. H. 1992. Epidemiology of trauma: frequency and impact of different potentially traumatic events on different demographic groups. *Journal of Consulting and Clinical Psychology* 60 (3): 409-18.

Pelcovitz, D., B. Goldenberg, S. Kaplan, M. Weinblatt, F. Mandel, B. Meyers, and V. Vinciguerra. 1996. Posttraumatic stress disorder in mothers of pediatric cancer survivors. *Psychosomatics* 37 (2):116-26.

Pelcovitz, D., B. G. Libov, F. Mandel, S. Kaplan, M. Weinblatt, and A. Septimus. 1998. Posttraumatic stress disorder and family functioning in adolescent cancer. *J Trauma Stress* 11 (2):205-21.

Rizzone, L. P., F. J. Stoddard, J. M. Murphy, and L. J. Kruger. 1994. Posttraumatic stress disorder in mothers of children and adolescents with burns. *J Burn Care Rehabil* 15 (2):158-63.

Smith, M. Y., Redd, W. H., Peyser, C., & Vogl, D. (1999). Post-traumatic stress disorder in cancer: a review. *Psychooncology* 8 (6): 521-37.

Stuber, M. L., D. A. Christakis, B. Houskamp, and A. E. Kazak. 1996. Posttrauma symptoms in childhood leukemia survivors and their parents. *Psychosomatics* 37 (3):254-61.

Stuber, M.L, S. Gonzales, K. Meeske, B. Houskamp, R. S. Pynoos, and A. E. Kazak. 1994. Post-traumatic stress in childhood cancer survivors II: Family interaction. *Psychooncology* 3:313-17.

Stuber, M. L., A. E. Kazak, K. Meeske, and L. Barakat. 1998. Is posttraumatic stress a viable model for understanding responses to childhood cancer? *Child Adolesc Psychiatr Clin N Am* 7 (1):169-82.

Terr, L. C. 1991. Childhood traumas: an outline and overview. *Am J Psychiatry* 148 (1):10-20.

Williams, J., C. Steel, G. B. Sharp, E. DelosReyes, T. Phillips, S. Bates, B. Lange, and M. L. Griebel. 2003. Parental anxiety and quality of life in children with epilepsy. *Epilepsy Behav* 4 (5):483-6.

Winston, F. K., N. Kassam-Adams, F. Garcia-España, R. Ittenbach, and A. Cnaan. 2003. Screening for risk of persistent posttraumatic stress in injured children and their parents. *The Journal of the American Medical Association* 290 (5):643-9.

Winston, F. K., N. Kassam-Adams, C. Vivarelli-O'Neill, J. Ford, E. Newman, C. Baxt, P. Stafford, and A. Cnaan. 2002. Acute stress disorder symptoms in children and their parents after pediatric traffic injury. *Pediatrics* 109 (6):e90.

III

TREATMENT AND SERVICES

10

Pediatric Psychosomatic Medicine

Emotional Health in Children with Chronic Illness

Maryland Pao

Pediatric psychosomatic medicine strives, in the words of Leo Kanner (1937), "to make psychiatric understanding of sick and healthy children and their families an integral part of the pediatrician's thinking and acting." As childhood mortality from acute illness declines and medical technology makes life-prolonging advances more children are surviving into adulthood with chronic conditions. Therefore, we need to focus on fostering normal physical, motor, language, cognitive, sexual, and emotional development in children with chronic illnesses. Many factors influence adaptation to chronic illness such as the child's temperament, intelligence, and social competence, the nature and severity of the illness, the required treatment modalities, and family and community factors. Almost 20% of children with chronic conditions have behavioral and emotional symptoms. Recognition of when these symptoms are normal responses to hospitalization and illness versus when they become pathologic and impairing for children can lead to early interventions and perhaps even prevention. Pediatric psychosomatic medicine services serve to bridge the gap between psychiatric and pediatric training to improve the emotional health and quality of life of youth with chronic illness.

PEDIATRIC CONSULTATION-LIAISON

The goal is "to make psychiatric understanding of sick and healthy children and their families an integral part of the pediatricians' thinking and acting." Leo Kanner (1937).

INTRODUCTION

Our task in pediatrics is "to maximize [all] children's functional abilities and sense of well-being, their health-related quality of life, and their development into healthy and productive adults" (AAP 1993). This is a challenge in youth with chronic illness who face numerous physical, developmental, and emotional challenges along the way. In America an estimated 13%-20% of children under 18 years old have a chronic illness/special health need (Bethell et al. 2008) with at least 10% of the children having chronic conditions that impact their daily lives. In the general population an estimated 10% of children have behavioral and emotional symptoms with 20% of children with chronic conditions having such symptoms. Importantly, a child's poor adjustment to illness is not directly related to the severity of the medical condition but rather to many other factors including the child's age and developmental level, previous experience and coping skills, family response and support, and the nature of the illness and its physical consequences. Severe childhood illness may be viewed as a set of serious challenges that can either be overwhelming and lead to a sense of emotional defeat or can be overcome and lead to resilience (Turkel and Pao 2007).

A generation ago fewer children with severe chronic illness or disability survived to adulthood and issues of transition from pediatric to adult health care were rarely considered (Blum et al. 1993); but now over 90% of children with chronic conditions will survive beyond the second decade of life (Scal et al. 1999). Psychosocial outcomes for chronically ill children in adulthood include an elevated use of health care services, more days in hospital, poorer school attendance, lower academic achievement, and less permanent employment records. They are also more likely to be single and have delayed independence (Gledhill et al. 2000). The question is can these outcomes be prevented?

Consultation-liaison psychiatry, recast as psychosomatic medicine (PM) in 2003, is focused on an integrated medical model since it is clearer than ever today that biological processes affect mental states and vice versa. PM is defined as "subspecialization in the diagnosis and treatment of psychiatric disorders and symptoms in complex medically ill patients with acute or chronic medical or surgical illness in which psychiatric illness is affecting their medical care and/or quality of life (e.g., organ transplantation, cancer, renal failure, heart disease, asthma)" (Gitlin et al. 2004). In pediatric psychosomatic medicine clinicians strive to ameliorate the adversity of being chronically or seriously ill, facilitate optimum child development (which includes helping parents), and, ultimately, hope to prevent mental illness since we now understand that many mental illnesses begin in childhood. As mortality decreases with advancing technologies, chronic physical and mental illnesses in childhood are increasing, but with earlier and better recognition of mental health symptoms we can prevent and treat conditions early.

AT THE BEGINNING—PEDIATRIC PSYCHIATRY

Leo Kanner (1894-1981), the author of the first English textbook of child psychiatry in 1935, is most well known for his descriptions of children with "autistic disturbances." But in 1937 Kanner wrote an article entitled "The Development and Present Status of Psychiatry in Pediatrics" published in the *Journal of Pediatrics* on how to make psychiatry useful to pediatricians. He noted a shift in psychiatry; where the focus had been on psychopathology it gradually started to emphasize normal development and behavior which was more in the realm of the pediatrician's daily concerns. The belief that "mental hygiene" or the prevention of mental illness and delinquency could be avoided through proper education and child guidance had begun to take hold in the early 1900s. By the early 1930s pediatricians were aware that "from the ashes of malnutrition and contagious disease arise a new group of problems, the so-called behavior difficulties" (Kanner 1937).

In 1930 Dr. Kanner established the first full-time psychiatric consultation service at the Harriet Lane Home for Invalid Children in the Pediatric Department of the Johns Hopkins University Hospital in Baltimore. Specifically, he underscored the importance of proximity between the pediatric and psychiatry services. Via ongoing education such as conferences, lectures, and case presentations, he demonstrated to the busy practicing pediatrician psychiatric principles, diagnoses, and treatments; the use of multidisciplinary services; and how to work with families. Dr. Kanner observed the interplay between medical diseases and how emotions could exacerbate those diseases and understood that the need to develop evidence-based research ideas was critical (Kanner 1937).

THE FIELD OF PSYCHOSOMATIC MEDICINE

In the 21st century psychiatry is no longer isolated in asylums. Like the Kanner model, teaching psychiatry in general hospitals and medical schools is standard practice, though often limited in scope. Psychological distress in the medically ill is recognized as a universal phenomenon but how best to address it still remains unclear. Psychosomatic medicine, or the focus on connections between emotional dysregulation, stress responses, and medical illness, has existed as an area of clinical and research interest within psychiatry for nearly 100 years (Lipsett 2001). In the 1960s, PM was recognized as the clinical practice of consultation-liaison (C-L) psychiatry and had gained acceptance as an independent area of knowledge and training within psychiatry in the U.S. and abroad (Worley et al. in press). In the 1970s fellowship programs in C-L, supported by the development of NIMH training grants, began to appear within several major U.S. teaching hospitals. By the late 1990s C-L psychiatry training was required for residents in general psychiatry residency programs (Gitlin et al. 1996). In 2003 the American Board of Psychiatry and Neurology (ABPN) officially recognized psychosomatic medicine as a subspecialty of psychiatry and the first ABPN exam in psychosomatic medicine was set in June 2005.

This subspecialization of psychiatry in the diagnosis and treatment of psychiatric disorders and symptoms in complex medically ill patients encompasses treatment of patients with acute or chronic medical, neurological, obstetrical, or surgical illness in which psychiatric illness is affecting their medical care and/or quality of life. The PM consultant helps to determine if (1) patients have an underlying or premorbid psychiatric disorder; (2) patients have a psychiatric disorder that is the direct consequence of a primary medical condition or medical treatment; or (3) if they have a somatoform disorder or psychological factors affecting a general medical condition. Psychiatrists specializing in PM provide consultation-liaison services in general medical hospitals, attend medical psychiatry inpatient units, and provide collaborative care in primary care and other outpatient settings. Standards for PM fellowship training include the expectation that this expertise will encompass "persons of all ages" and "those cared for in specialized medical settings," such as pediatrics or obstetrics and gynecology (Ford et al. 1994).

Outside America, where different national health care systems and manpower and health service policies vary from that of the U.S., two types of C-L services have evolved. An evaluation of 56 C-L services from 11 countries found one type of model is a more "classical medical model" where the consultation services provided are "mono-disciplinary," while in other hospitals a "multidisciplinary" mental health model has evolved (ECLW Collaborative Study, Huyse et al. 2000). The type of model was not predicted by hospital or C-L service size. Factors such as psychiatrist and psychologist manpower, other disciplines (e.g., nurses, social workers), experienced staff, secretarial support, presence of a psychiatric emergency room and outpatient clinic, and the availability of other psychosocial services such as pastoral care, social work, and psychological medicine were considered.

CURRENT PEDIATRIC PSYCHOSOMATIC MEDICINE IN AMERICA

Pediatric consultation-liaison/psychosomatic medicine models in America include general medical hospital consultation services as well as outpatient collaborative models with pediatricians and other pediatric specialists. Reimbursement for these models remains a challenge to maintain viable clinical services (Shaw et al. 2006).

Pediatric PM differs from adult PM primarily in its focus on (1) developmental streams such as cognitive, emotional, and physical; (2) its appreciation of the essential role of the family in the child's adaptation; and (3) an approach emphasizing coping and adjustment, or anticipatory guidance, rather than psychopathology. Child psychiatrists in pediatric hospital settings can help identify parent psychopathology and help parents receive treatment. They can also help parents to understand that their lack of expectations and overindulgence can lead to the development of poor self-esteem, poor problem solving skills, and lack of achievement in children (Pao et al. 2007). In addition, helping parents develop self-reflection about their parenting styles can help parents communicate better with one another and encourage them to cooperate in the management and disciplining of their sick children and adolescents.

A consequence of advances in medical care has been that many children experience multiple, intensive, long-term hospitalizations. In 2000, approximately two million children and adolescents were hospitalized for pediatric illness (Owens et al. 2003) accounting for at least five million hospital days each year (Newacheck and Hafon 1998). Physicians and hospital staff should understand that many children with chronic conditions are "growing up in the hospital" and that these hospital experiences can profoundly affect their cognitive, emotional, social, and sexual developmental trajectories (Pao et al. 2007). Integrated multidisciplinary care in pediatrics is more important today than ever.

Training in Pediatric Psychosomatic Medicine

While there are a sizable number of child psychiatrists today who also trained in pediatrics, including those completing triple board programs (combined training in pediatrics, general and child and adolescent psychiatry), many child psychiatrists are less comfortable treating children with complex medical illnesses like HIV or those who undergo intensive medical treatments such as bone marrow transplantation. In child psychiatric training there has been a shift towards outpatient training and provision of care, fewer opportunities to work with pediatricians in inpatient hospital settings, and a significant workforce shortage in child psychiatry. Since 1999 the consultation-liaison section of the child psychiatry exam has become a less significant aspect of becoming board certified in child and adolescent psychiatry.

Currently there are several training pathways that lead to pediatric PM: (1) those with previous training in general psychiatry alone; (2) those with training in general psychiatry and pediatrics; and (3) triple board programs (Nguyen et al. 2007). A new gateway into general and child and adolescent psychiatry for those with previous training in pediatrics only, called the "Post Pediatric Portal Project (PPPP)," has been initiated at three sites since 2007 (http://www.tripleboard.org/post-pediatric-portal-pilot-project/). There are no accredited pediatric PM fellowships at this time, but the above pathways provide strong background for those interested in practicing pediatric psychosomatic medicine. Several of the 45 American PM fellowships offer specific training experiences in children and adolescents and a bibliography for pediatric PM training has been described (Pao et al. 2007). The *Clinical Manual of Pediatric Psychosomatic Medicine* was recently published by Drs. Richard Shaw and David DeMaso (2006) with a *Textbook of Pediatric Psychosomatic Medicine* currently in press.

RESEARCH IN PEDIATRIC PSYCHOSOMATIC MEDICINE

There are two general research approaches to understanding the emotional impact of medical illness in children. One approach looks at the common sequelae of early adversity including typical responses seen across a variety of medical disorders (e.g., low self-esteem, difficulty maintaining peer relationships) while the other identifies disease-specific sequelae (e.g., depression in asthma, eating disorders in diabetes, or cognitive and psychosocial problems in pediatric HIV). See Appendix 10.1 for a list of references on evidence-based pediatric C-L practice. The American Academy of Child and Adolescent Psychiatry (AACAP) Committee on the Physically Ill Child is committed to establishing a research network to facilitate research in pediatric psychosomatic medicine.

PEDIATRIC PSYCHOSOMATIC MEDICINE IN ASIA

Historically, mental disorders were mainly treated by traditional Chinese medicine (TCM) which is seen as holistic but is nonverbally based. Before 1980 there were no psychological, psychosomatic, or psychotherapeutic components in the undergraduate or postgraduate education of medical students or doctors in China, Vietnam, or Laos. Medical psychology is taught in universities separately from medical training. Pediatric PM has progressed slowly in Asia due to a lack of awareness and stigma that slows progress understanding mental health concerns particularly in children. Subspecialization in consultation-liaison psychiatry or child psychiatry came about only recently in Asia, which means there are few experts in these areas. In the East PM is sometimes seen as a "talking medicine" focusing on the personal life of patients and their relationships and less clearly as the medical-psychological field it is today.

With a population of over 1.3 billion people in China there are an estimated 30 million children and adolescents with mental health problems. The first inpatient child psychiatry unit in China was established in the late 1950s, and the specialty of pediatric psychosomatic medicine, which is referred to in China as psychological medicine, medical psychology, or consultation-liaison (C-L) psychiatry, was not developed until the late 1980s. The first medical psychology department in a general children's hospital on the Chinese mainland was set up at Tianjin Children's Hospital in 1988. Today there are approximately 30 major children's hospitals located in large or mid-sized cities that have departments of psychological medicine. Most children's hospitals have outpatient mental health clinics although some children and adolescents still receive services in adult clinics. The Children's Hospital of Fudan in Shanghai, China, provides an outpatient "Psychological Counseling Clinic" where individual therapy and group therapy are provided as well as psychiatry consultation for inpatients, which provides psychological assistance to medical inpatients and their families. In addition, psychiatric staff provide public and parent education about child and adolescent mental health issues as well as a "summer camp" for children with special medical disorders such as primary immune deficiency, diabetes, and leukemia (Gao 2008).

The professionals working in the specialty of pediatric psychosomatic medicine include child psychiatrists and pediatricians trained in child psychiatry (both referred to as psychological doctors) and developmental pediatricians. In China child psychologists and social workers generally work in major independent psychiatric hospitals rather than medical settings. There are an estimated 150 child psychiatrists working in the major psychiatric hospitals or child mental health centers in the major cities of mainland China (CCDCP 2006). Most general psychiatrists (approx 26,000) provide both adult and child mental health services. An increasing number of developmental pediatricians participate in children's mental health services in general hospitals, children's hospitals, and community health care centers throughout China. There is currently no subspecialty board certification in either child psychiatry or psychosomatic medicine (Gao, personal communication, 2009).

In one community sample in China 1695 6-11-year-old children in 12 elementary schools in the Linyi Prefecture of China were surveyed using the Child Behavior Checklist (CBCL) and Family Environment Scale (FES-CV) (validated in Chinese) (Liu et al. 1999). The prevalence of childhood psychopathology was estimated at 17.2% with risk factors including poor parenting, low birth weight, poor marital relations, and chronic physical illness (Liu et al. 1999). Psychiatrists in Chinese children's hospitals are working to describe the range of behavioral and emotional problems they see in children in order to develop targeted services (in both inpatient and outpatient settings). Risk factors for child psychopathology in China may be quite different given significant differences in Western and Chinese societies (such as TCM and family roles).

COLLABORATIVE PM TRAINING: THE ASIA-LINK PROGRAM

In adult PM, a three-year project to develop and promote psychosomatic medicine in China, Vietnam, and Laos is under way (Friezsche et al. 2008). The Asia-Link Program supported by the European Union and coordinated by Freiburg University Clinic together with Tongji University Hospital in Shanghai, begins in year 1 training 50 doctors from different fields as future teachers. In year 2 these doctors will be given a curriculum (60 hrs) emphasizing the biopsychosocial approach that includes enhancing doctor-patient communication, diagnosis, crisis intervention, basic psychopharmacology, theory, and didactic methods. In year 3 the program hopes to create a network of departments of psychiatry to provide PM training and services in general hospitals. The program outcome is pending and is sensitive to the concern that adaptations will need to be made to accommodate cultural differences.

In pediatric PM, through the development of exchange training/research programs with international partners in child psychiatry and among pediatric psychosomatic medicine specialists and pediatricians, the opportunities for multicenter clinical research and nationwide epidemiological studies in China are immense and should be realized to help China's next generation of youth.

CONCLUSIONS

There are more than 70 million children under 18 years old in America today comprising approximately 25% of the American population. An estimated 13%-20% of these children have a chronic illness and this number is only likely to increase. In pediatric psychosomatic medicine we need to promote public awareness of children's mental and physical health issues, reduce stigma, provide mental health education and training to providers in hospital and clinic settings, and promote research on children's disorders and treatments in the context of development and culture. More specifically, we can enhance parenting skills, family functioning, and social support, which has repeatedly shown to be the best predictor of good outcomes in health outcomes research. In addition to training and collaboration issues, the AACAP Committee on the Physically Ill Child is committed to establishing a research network to facilitate research in pediatric psychosomatic medicine with our partners around the globe.

APPENDIX 10.1. REFERENCE LIST
OF EVIDENCE-BASED PEDIATRIC PM

(1) Bauman LJ, Drotar D, Leventhal JM, Perrin EC, and Pless IB. A review of psychosocial interventions for children with chronic health conditions. *Pediatrics* 1997 August;100(2 Pt 1):244-51.

(2) Christie D, and Wilson C. CBT in paediatric and adolescent health settings: A review of practice-based evidence. *Pediatr Rehabil* 8(4)(2005 October): 241-47.

(3) Holden EW. Empirically supported treatments in pediatric psychology: Recurrent pediatric headache. *Journal of Pediatric Psychology* 24(2) (1999): 91-109.

(4) Janicke DM. Empirically supported treatments in pediatric psychology: Recurrent abdominal pain. *Journal of Pediatric Psychology* 24(2) (1999): 115-27.

(5) Jelalian E. Empirically supported treatments in pediatric psychology: Pediatric obesity. *Journal of Pediatric Psychology* 24(3) (1999): 223-48.

(6) Kazak AE. Evidence-based interventions for survivors of childhood cancer and their families. *Journal of Pediatric Psychology* 30(1) (2005): 29-39.

(7) Kerwin ME. Empirically supported treatments in pediatric psychology: Severe feeding problems. *Journal of Pediatric Psychology* 24(3) (1999): 193-214.

(8) Kibby MY, Tyc VL, and Mulhern RK. Effectiveness of psychological intervention for children and adolescents with chronic medical illness: A meta-analysis. *Clinical Psychology Review* 18(1) (1998): 105-17.

(9) McClellan JM, and Werry JS. Evidence-based treatments in child and adolescent psychiatry: An inventory. *J Am Acad Child Adolesc Psychiatry* 42(12) (2003 December): 1388-1400.

(10) McGrath ML. Empirically supported treatments in pediatric psychology: Constipation and encopresis. *Journal of pediatric psychology* 25(4) (2000): 225-54.

(11) McQuaid EL. Empirically supported treatments of disease-related symptoms in pediatric psychology: Asthma, diabetes, and cancer. *Journal of Pediatric Psychology* 24(4) (1999): 305-28.

(12) Plante WA, Lobato D, and Engel R. Review of group interventions for pediatric chronic conditions. *J Pediatr Psychol* 26(7) (2001 October): 435-53.

(13) Powers SW. Empirically supported treatments in pediatric psychology: Procedure-related pain. *Journal of Pediatric Psychology* 24(2) (1999): 131-45.

(14) Powers SW, Jones JS, and Jones BA. Behavioral and cognitive-behavioral interventions with pediatric populations. *Clinical Child Psychology and Psychiatry* 10(1) (2005): 65-77.

(15) Roberts MC, Lazicki-Puddy TA, Puddy RW, and Johnson RJ. The outcomes of psychotherapy with adolescents: A practitioner-friendly research review. *J Clin Psychol* 59(11) (2003 November): 1177-91.

(16) Stauffer MH. A long-term psychotherapy group for children with chronic medical illness. *Bulletin of the Menninger Clinic* 62(1) (1998): 15-32.

(17) Walco GA. Empirically supported treatments in pediatric psychology: Disease-related pain. *Journal of Pediatric Psychology* 24(2) (1999): 155-67.

(18) Gustafsson PA. "Don't blame it on the parents—Make them your allies: A family/systems approach to paediatric illness." *Clinical Child Psychology and Psychiatry* 10(1) (2005): 23-31.

REFERENCES

American Academy of Child and Adolescent Psychiatry. "Clinical parameter for the psychiatric assessment and management of physically ill children and adolescents." *J Am Acad Child Adolesc Psychiatry* 48 (2009): 213-233.

American Academy of Pediatrics, Committee on Children with Disabilities and Committee on Psychosocial Aspects of Child and Family Health. "Psychosocial risks of chronic health conditions in childhood and adolescence." *Pediatrics* 92 (1993): 876-878.

Bethell CD, Read D, Blumberg SJ, and Newacheck PW. "What is the prevalence of children with special health care needs? Toward an understanding of variations in findings and methods across three national surveys." *Matern Child Health J* 12 (2008): 1–14.

Blum RW, Garell D, Hodgman CH, et al. "Transition from child-centered to adult health care systems for adolescents with chronic conditions." *J Adolesc Health* 14 (1993): 570–576.

China Center for Disease Control and Prevention 2006. Available at http://news.sina.com.cn/c/2006-03-17/09169372113.shtml

Ford CV, Fawzy FI, Frankel BL, and Noyes R Jr. "Fellowship training in consultation-liaison psychiatry: Education goals and standards." *Psychosomatics* 35 (1994): 118-124.

Fritzsche K, Scheib P, Wirsching M, Schussler G, Wu W, Cat NH, Vongphrachanh S, and Linh NT, ASIA-Link Workgroup. "Improving the competence of medical doctors in China, Vietnam and Laos—The Asia-Link Program." *Int J Psychiatry Med* 38 (2008): 1-11.

Gao HY. "Mental Health at a General Children Hospital in Shanghai, a 9 Year Review (1999-2007)." Presented in Clinical Perspectives, Child Mental Health: East Meets West, AACAP 55th Annual Meeting 10/29/2008, Chicago IL.

Gao HY. Personal communication, 2009.

Gitlin D. et al. "Recommended Guidelines for Consultation-Liaison Psychiatric Training in Psychiatry Residency Programs: A Report from the Academy of Psychosomatic Medicine Task Force on Psychiatric Resident Training in Consultation-Liaison Psychiatry." *Psychosomatics* 37 (1996): 3-11.

Gitlin D, Levenson J, and Lyketsos C. "Psychosomatic medicine: A new psychiatric subspecialty." *Acad Psychiatry* 28 (2004): 4-11.

Gledhill J, Rangel L, and Garralda E. "Surviving chronic physical illness: Psychosocial outcome in adult life." *Arch Dis Child* 83 (2000): 104–10.

Huyse, FJ., Herzog, T., Lobo, A., Malt, UF., Opmeer, BC., Stein, B., Creed, F., Crespo, MD., Gardoso, G., Guimaraes-Lopes, R., Mayou, R., van Moffaert, M., Rigatelli, M., Sakkas, P., Tienari, P. "European Consultant-Liaison Psychiatric Services: The ECLW Collaborative Study." *Act Psychiatrica Scandinavica* 101(5) (2000): 360-366.

Kanner L. "The development and present status of psychiatry in pediatrics." *J Pediatrics* 11 (1937): 418-435.

Lipsett D. "Consultation-liaison psychiatry and psychosomatic medicine: The company they keep." *Psychosom Med* 63 (2001): 896-909.

Liu XC, Kurita Hiroshi, Sun Zhenxiao, and Wang Fuxi. "Risk factors for psychopathology among Chinese children." *Psychiatry and Clinical Neurosciences* 53 (1999): 497-503.

Newacheck PW and Hafon N. "Prevalence and impact of disabling chronic conditions in childhood." *Am J Public Health* 88(1998): 610-617.

Nguyen N, Walker A, and Pao M. "Pediatric psychosomatic medicine medicine track: Creating the pathway and the curriculum." Poster presentation at AADPRT 2007.

Owens PL, Thompson J, Elixhauser A, Ryan K. *Care of Children and Adolescents in U.S. Hospitals.* Rockville, MD: Agency for Healthcare Research and Quality, 2003.

Pao M, Ballard ED, Raza H, and Rosenstein DL. "Pediatric psychosomatic medicine: An annotated bibliography." *Psychosomatics* 48 (2007): 195-204.

Pao M, Ballard ED, and Rosenstein DL. "Commentary: Growing up in the hospital." *JAMA* 297 (2007): 2752-2755.

Scal P, Evans T, Blozis S, Okinow N, and Blum R. "Trends in transition from pediatric to adult health care services for young adults with chronic conditions." *J Adolesc Health* 24 (1999): 259–264.

Shaw RJ and DeMaso DR. *Clinical Manual of Pediatric Psychosomatic Medicine Mental Health Consultation with Physically Ill Children and Adolescents.* Washington, DC: American Psychiatric Publishing, Inc., 2006.

Shaw RJ, Wamboldt M, Bursch B, and Stuber M. "Practice patterns in pediatric consultation-liaison psychiatry: A national survey." *Psychosomatics* 47 (2006): 43-49.

Turkel S and Pao M. "Late consequences of pediatric chronic illness" *Psychiatr Clin North Am* 30 (2007): 819–835.

Worley L, Levenson J, Stern T et al. "Core competencies for fellowship training in psychosomatic medicine: A collaborative effort by the APA Council on Psychosomatic Medicine, the ABPN Psychosomatic Committee, and the Academy of Psychosomatic Medicine." *Psychosomatics* (in press).

11

Autism Spectrum Disorder and Traditional Chinese Medicine (Acupuncture)

Virginia Chun-Nei Wong and Vanessa Loi-Yan Chu

INTRODUCTION

Autism spectrum disorder (ASD), also known as pervasive developmental disorder (PDD), is a neurodevelopmental disorder characterized by three core features with deficits in communication, and in social interaction, with repetitive interests, behavior, and activities (RIBI) emerging before three years of age. In this chapter, we will at times use "autism" interchangeably with "autism spectrum disorder" (ASD).

Historical Background of ASD

"Autism" comes from the Greek word "auto-, aut-," which means "self, same, spontaneous; directed from within." The term describes conditions in which a person is removed from social interaction, hence an isolated self.

In 1911, Eugen Bleuler, a Swiss psychiatrist first applied the term "autism" to adult schizophrenia. In 1943 the term "autism" first appeared in a medical paper published by Dr. Leo Kanner (an American psychiatrist) of Johns Hopkins University based on his observation of 11 children seen between 1938 and 1943 with abnormal behavior and withdrawal from human contact. In the next year (1944) Dr. Hans Asperger (an Austrian pediatrician) in Germany used the same term to describe a group of abnormally behaving children (Tuchman and Rapin 2006).

Historically, and compared to Western medicine, there has been a dearth of scientific literature in China regarding the diagnostic features and treatment of "autism" or "autism spectrum disorder." The relative lack of publications about autism in China is likely to be linked to the fact that the disorder was not recognized by mental health professionals in China until after the second edition of the *Chinese Category of Mental Disease* (CCMD-2) published in 1995 (Clark and Zhou 2005). In China children with ASD have been medically under the care of child psychiatrists rather than child neurologists or developmental pediatricians, and educationally they have been under the care of the educational authority.

Definition and Classification of ASD and Autism

Autism is a neurodevelopmental disability that affects a person's ability to communicate, understand language, play, and interact with others. Autism is a behavioral syndrome, which means that its definition is based on the patterns of behaviors that a person exhibits. In our view autism is just an umbrella term or behavioral phenotype resulting from multiple etiologies, in the same way that cerebral palsy can be due to multiple etiologies with resultant damage to the motor regions of the brain. Autism is a neurological disability that is presumed to be present from birth and is always apparent before the age of three years. Although autism affects brain functioning there is no *one* single cause although recent evidence has shown that genetics are highly likely to explain a subtype of autism.

In the past decade "autistic spectrum disorder" (ASD) has been used increasingly as a term; it encompasses a broad definition of autism including the classical form of autistic disorder as well as closely related disabilities that share many of the core characteristics. In addition to classical autism, PDDs include the following diagnoses and classifications:

1. *Pervasive developmental disorder—not otherwise specified* (PDD-NOS), which refers to a collection of features that resemble autism but may not be as severe or extensive;
2. *Rett syndrome*, which affects girls and is a genetic disorder with hard neurological signs, including seizures, that becomes more apparent with age;
3. *Asperger syndrome*, which refers to individuals with autistic characteristics but relatively intact language abilities, and
4. *Childhood disintegrative disorder*, which refers to children whose development appears normal for the first few years but then regresses with loss of speech and other skills until the characteristics of autism are conspicuous.

Although the classical form of autism can be readily distinguished from other forms of ASD the terms "autism" and "ASD" are often used interchangeably.

Prevalence of ASD

There is evidence for an increase in the prevalence of autism, though the increasing trend might be due to the different diagnostic criteria used, different methodologies, and increasing awareness due to mass media, or even as "a ticket for reimbursed service." When the prevalence of autism was first studied in 1966 the prevalence rate was 4 per 10,000. Recently, the estimated prevalence of autism was 60 to 70 per 10,000 (Fombonne 2009) (see also chapter in this book by Steiman and colleagues).

As there is no "cure" for autism parents have been eager to seek different forms of treatments. The estimated prevalence for the use of complementary and alternative medicine (CAM) in children diagnosed with ASD ranges from 31.7% to 95% in the United States (Levy et al. 2003; Harrington et al. 2006). In 2008 a cohort study conducted by us in Hong Kong estimated that about 40% of ASD children had used CAM, with acupuncture being the most common form (see Table 11.1) (Wong 2009).

Since 1998 our group was the first research team in the world to conduct randomized control trials (RCT) of acupuncture in autism. So far we have conducted five RCT trials. As the popularity of using acupuncture for ASD among Chinese is high we reviewed the literature on the use of the acupuncture in ASD patients.

FUNDAMENTAL THEORIES OF
TRADITIONAL CHINESE MEDICINE (TCM)

Traditional Chinese medicine (TCM) is a system of health care, distinct from Western medicine, with unique diagnostic or assessment methods, treatment principles, language, and terminology. TCM consists of a wide range of philosophical concepts. Throughout 2500 years of clinical practice and modification the philosophical concepts have translated into clinical experiences with a certain degree of evidence, mainly subjective in nature.

Table 11.1:   Prevalence of the Use of Complementary and Alternative Medicine (CAM) in Children with ASD

	City/ Country	Using CAM	References
2009	Hong Kong	40.8%	(Wong 2009)
		(47.5% using acupuncture)	
2009	USA	19%	(Golnik and Ireland 2009)
2008	USA	>30%	(Levy et al. 2003)
2007	USA	74%	(Hanson et al. 2007)

The history of China dates back to at least 2000 years BC with medical culture and practices being influenced by the political authority represented by the emperor of the designated dynasty.

Yin-Yang Theory (陰陽學說)

The Yin-Yang Theory was originally a philosophical concept of ancient Chinese dealing with two opposite aspects of nature which are interrelated with each other. The Chinese believe that the universe is governed by two opposing forces. All matters in nature can be categorized by Yin and Yang. The characteristics of Yin in Chinese philosophy describes the feminine, latent, and passive principle, while the characteristics of Yang describe the masculine, active, and positive principle of the two opposing cosmic forces into which creative energy divides and whose fusion in physical matter brings the phenomenal world into being. The main components of the Yin-Yang relationship can be summarized as

1. Opposition of Yin and Yang (陰陽對立制約)
2. Interdependence/mutual rooting of Yin and Yang (陰陽互根互用)
3. Inter-consuming-supporting relationship of Yin and Yang (陰陽消長平衡)
4. Inter-transformation relationship of Yin and Yang (陰陽相互轉化)

The theory of Yin-Yang promoted the formation and development of traditional Chinese medicine (TCM) in its own theoretical system, and finally became an important component part of the basic theory of TCM. TCM believes that normal physiological functions of the human body result from the opposite but coordinated relationship between Ying and Yang. Imbalance of Yin and Yang is one of the basic pathogeneses of a disease. Yin and Yang have different clinical manifestations in symptoms and signs.

Five Phases Theory (五行學說)

Five Phases Theory (also known as Five Elements Theory) is another central philosophical theory in TCM. Based on observations, the ancient Chinese classified material things or phenomena into five categories by comparing their structures, properties, and actions. Five Phases Theory posits wood, fire, earth, metal, and water as the basic elements of the material world and these elements are in constant movement and change in relation to each other.

The ancient Chinese used the Five Phases Theory to study the connections between the physiology and pathology of the Zang Fu organs, tissues, and the natural environment.

Five Phases Theory describes not only the physiology and pathology of the human body but can also be used to interpret the relationship of the human body to the natural environment. The five elements correspond to different aspects of the natural world and the body. Furthermore, Five Phases Theory is also used to explain the physiology and pathology of the human body and to guide the clinical diagnosis and treatment.

Relationship between the Five Phases

The Mutual Engendering Cycle refers to the relationship in which each phase and its associated phenomena give rise to or promote another sequential phase.

The Mutual Restraining Cycle refers to the manner in which each phase and its associated phenomena restrict and control another phase.

Overwhelming (also known as "over-acting") refers to abnormally severe restraining of the five phases in the same sequence as normal restraining. Rebelling (also known as "insulting") refers to restraining opposite to the normal restraining sequence of the five phases.

Through engendering and restraining relationships a relative balance and normal coordination in the Five Phase Theory can be maintained.

Theory of Qi (氣), Blood (血), Fluid and Humor (津液)

The Theory of Qi, Blood, Fluid and Humor in TCM is used to understand the development, transportation, distribution, physiological function, pathological change, and mutual relations of Qi, Blood, Fluids and Humors in the human body.

In TCM, Qi is a core theory. It refers to the basic element that constitutes the cosmos and, through its movements, changes, and transformations, produces everything in the world, including the human body and life activities. In the field of medicine Qi refers to the refined nutritive substance that flows within the human body as well as to its functional activities. Blood is a kind of red liquid rich in nutrition, circulating within the blood vessels, which has the functions of nourishing and moistening the whole body. Fluid and Humor refer to all kinds of normal fluid in the body, except the Blood, also known as Body Fluids. To specify, Fluid is identified as the liquid substance that circulates with Qi and Blood while Humor refers to the thick fluid stored in body cavities such as bowels, viscera, and auricular and cranial cavities. Qi, Blood, and Body Fluids are all derived from Essence. They are the basic materials comprising the human body and maintaining life activities. Although the three have different properties, forms, and functions, they are physiologically dependent on each other and influence each other in pathology.

Visceral Manifestation Theory (臟象學說)

The internal organs and associated terminologies in TCM are very different from those in Western medicine. The organs are divided into "Zang" or "viscera" (i.e., heart, liver, spleen, lung, and kidney), where Essence and Qi are formed and stored, and "Fu" or "bowel" (i.e., gallbladder, stomach, large intestine, small intestine, urinary bladder, and triple energizers) where food is received, transported, and digested.

Meridian and Collateral (Jing (經) Luo (絡) Theory)

Meridian and collateral are a giant web system with conduits through which Qi, Blood, and Body Fluids circulate linking together different areas of our body: for example, the bowels, viscera, extremities, superficial organs, and tissues. These conduits make up a comprehensive and complex body map that supplies vital energy to every part of the body and makes the body an organic whole. Acupoints reflect the body's physical and pathological condition. These points are connected by meridians also called Jing (經) and Luo (絡). Jing means "the path"; it is the main pathway of the meridian system. The meridian connects points from the top to the bottom and internal to external. Luo means "web." The Luo meridians are a branch of the Jing meridians and are smaller but can connect all of the small parts of the body like a web. The meridian and collaterals connect the internal organs to the end of the extremities and the internal organs with the exterior of the body. With these meridians the entire human body's functions can be coordinated to keep the body in balance.

Autism Spectrum Disorder and TCM

Although in China TCM has evolved over 2,500 years we failed to find the word "autism" or "autistic" in the TCM literature. Depending on the symptoms of autism or autism spectrum disorder the clinical manifestations have been placed in different TCM syndrome categories: delay in development; speech and language problems; hearing problems; and emotion problems.

In relation to TCM, autism spectrum disorder may be considered a complex disease. Many organs or systems of the body are involved and the progress of the disease varies. The sites of the pathological changes are mainly in the "brain, heart, spleen, liver, and kidney" (in TCM the functions of the brain are dispersed across five Zang organs, including heart and liver, and are maintained by comprehensive functional interactions among the five Zang organs). Manifestations of the disease do not necessarily follow a prescribed order but depend on the pathogenic factors involved and the mechanisms affected. The possible causes can be classified according to TCM as follows:

(a) Prenatal factors:

    i. Parental psychoneurosis causes weak physique of the infantile patient and imbalance of Yin and Yang;

    ii. Viral infection or drug administrations during pregnancy affect the normal development of the fetus causing congenital insufficiency;

    iii. Birth injury and other traumas result in infantile stagnation of Qi and Blood, obstructive meridians, and perturbation due to loss of nourishment of the heart and liver.

(b) Postnatal factors:

    i. Malnutrition, or imbalanced diet, excessive ingestion of uncooked and cold food impairing the spleen and stomach leads to deficiency of Qi and Blood;

    ii. Excessive intake of fat and sweet food causes dampness, heat, and phlegm, which may block functional activities of Qi and disturb the mind;

    iii. Other primary disease or trauma give rise to imbalance of Yin and Yang;

    iv. Environmental pollution, vaccinations, harmful chemicals, etc.

Syndrome Differentiation and Treatment

Syndrome differentiation is a diagnostic process based on the comprehensive analysis of information, signs, and symptoms gathered from four bedside examination techniques (inspection, listening and smelling, inquiry, and palpation) to formulate the syndrome or pattern of the patient. There are various systems used to determine specific TCM syndromes. These all follow the principle of identifying the state of disharmony between Yin-Yang within the domain of signs and symptoms.

We found three papers published in Chinese that suggested the differentiation of syndromes for ASD (see Table 11.2) (Wu and Wu 2006; Liu and Yuan 2007; Yuan et al. 2009).

Using references from ancient TCM books or chronicles and the experiences of current Chinese medicine practitioners we have attempted to summarize the TCM method of differentiating syndromes and principles of treatment for ASD in three categories (see Table 11.3).

Table 11.2:   Summary of the Differentiation of Syndromes from Current Studies

Study	Differentiation of syndromes	Clinical Manifestation	Treatment Principle
(Yuan et al. 2009)	Liver Qi stagnation (肝郁氣滯)	Depression, eccentric and unsociable	--
	Heart-liver fire (心肝心旺)	Inability to sleep, agitation and irritability, delirium.	--
	Phlegm misting the heart orifice (痰迷心竅)	No facial expression, dementia, drooling, unclear in speech.	--
	Kidney Essence deficiency (腎精虧虛)	Paleness and emaciation, retarded growth, short stature, late closure of the fontanel, retard mentality and activity, weariness in tendons and bones.	--
(Liu and Yuan 2007)	Heart-liver fire (心肝心旺)	Inability to sleep, agitation and irritability, delirium, yellowish urine and dry stool. Red tip of the tongue with yellow coating. Rapid and string-like pulse.	Clear heart-liver fire and nourish the heart to tranquilize.
	Phlegm misting the heart orifice (痰迷心竅)	Dementia, drooling, unclear in speech. No response to voice. Enlarged tongue with white greasy coating.	Fortify the spleen to sweep phlegm, tonify the kidney, and replenish blood.
	Kidney Essence deficiency (腎精虧虛)	Paleness and emaciation, retarded growth, short stature, late closure of the fontanel, retarded mentality and activity. Pale tongue.	Enrich the kidney Essences and replenish Yin.
(Wu and Wu 2006)	Liver-kidney depletion (肝腎虧虛)	--	Enrich the kidney and nourish the liver.
	Dual deficiency of heart-spleen (心脾兩虛)	--	Nourish the heart and fortify the spleen to tranquilize.
	Yin deficiency with effulgent fire (陰虛火旺)	--	Enrich the Yin and moisten dryness.

Table 11.3. Summary of the Clinical Manifestations and Treatment Principles of Different TCM Syndromes

Syndrome Differentiation	Clinical Manifestation	Treatment Principle
Heart-liver fire syndrome (心肝火旺)	Dizziness, distending pain in the head, flushed face, congested eyes, bitter taste and dryness in the mouth, irritability, insomnia, dream-disturbed sleep.	Clear heart-liver fire and nourish the heart to tranquilize.
Syndrome of phlegm misting the heart orifice (痰迷心窍)	Mental depression, apathy, dementia, soliloquy, abnormal behavior, abrupt coma with drooling and sputum rumbling in the throat, upwardstaring of the eyes, convulsions, bleating sounds.	Fortify the spleen to sweep phlegm, tonify the kidney and replenish Blood.
Spleen Qi deficiency (脾氣虚弱)	Dizziness, fatigue, sallow face, indigestion, abdominal distension, lassitude, anorexia, and loose bowels.	Fortify the spleen and replenish Qi
Kidney Essence deficiency syndrome (腎精虧虚)	Thinness and weakness in limbs, retarded development, hypophrenia, unclosure of fontanel, slurred speech, difficulties in lifting head or sitting and standing.	Enrich the kidney Essences and replenishYin.

ACUPUNCTURE

Acupuncture is a procedure in which specific body areas, i.e., the meridian points, are pierced with fine acupuncture needles for therapeutic purposes. It has been practiced in China for more than 2500 years (Ramey and Buell 2004). During the past two decades, especially since President Nixon visited China in 1972, acupuncture has been popular worldwide with the establishment of university degrees and TCM courses in universities for Western doctors both in Europe and North America. Other folklore medicine similar to TCM had been practiced in Japan, Korea, India, and South America based on unique cultural and historical evolution. There has been growing interest in the therapeutic application of acupuncture, and increasing scientific research using an evidence-based approach to understand the pathophysiology of its mode of action.

Apart from the traditional needle acupuncture various forms of acupuncture have been developed including electro-acupuncture, laser acupuncture, and acupressure. Being a relatively simple, inexpensive, and safe treatment acupuncture has been well accepted by Chinese patients as well as Caucasians in Europe and North America. Acupuncture has been widely used for various chronic neurological disorders such as stroke, pain, Parkinson disease, and Alzheimer disease as an alternative treatment approach. Over the past decade acupuncture has also been increasingly practiced in many Western countries.

Acupuncture involves the complex theories of regulation of Yin-Yang balance, visceral, Qi, Blood, and Body Fluids. By stimulating various meridian points disharmony and dysregulation of organ systems are corrected to relieve symptoms and restore natural internal homeostasis. Many studies in animals and humans have demonstrated that acupuncture can cause multiple biological responses, both locally close to the site of application, or distally (mediated mainly by sensory neurons) to many structures within the central nervous system. This can lead to activation of pathways affecting various physiological systems in the brain as well as in the periphery.

From our literature search we have summarized the types of acupoints reportedly used in the treatment of ASD. There has been a lack of consensus regarding the number or combination of acupoints, duration of treatment, or use of outcome measures in the literature surveyed. Altogether 50 acupoints have been used, with 17 on the head scalp, 14 on the upper limbs, and 19 on lower limbs (see Figures 11.1, 11.2, and 11.3).

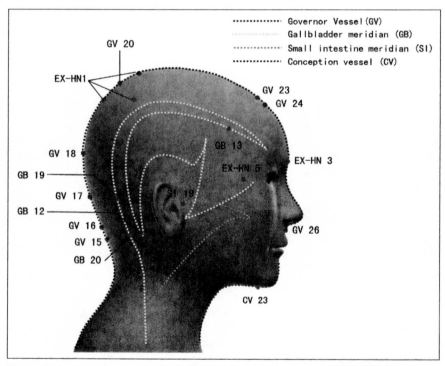

Figure 11.1. Acupoints on the Scalp Reportedly Used in the Treatment of ASD

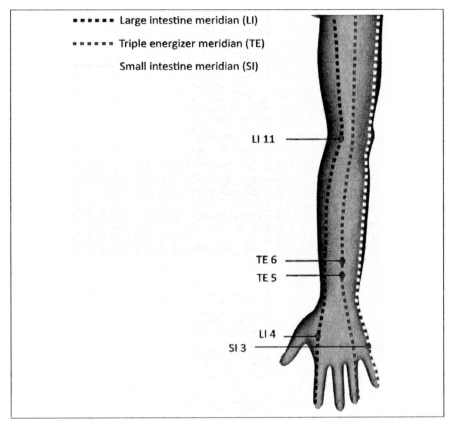

- ■ ■ ■ ■ ■ **Large intestine meridian (LI)**
- ■ ■ ■ ■ ■ **Triple energizer meridian (TE)**
- **Small intestine meridian (SI)**

LI 11

TE 6
TE 5

LI 4
SI 3

Figure 11.2.   Acupoints on the Upper Limbs Reportedly Used in the Treatment of ASD

Scalp Acupuncture

Scalp acupuncture is an acupuncture technique which was fully developed in the last century based on the theory of TCM, acupuncture techniques, clinical experience, holographic theory, and a modern knowledge of the representative areas of the cerebral cortex. The main principle behind it is that the specific functional parts of the brain can be affected by stimulating identified areas on the surface of the scalp. It is believed that there is a close relationship between the functions of the cerebral cortex and the scalp's therapeutic zones. By stimulating the scalp we are able to adjust the functions at the corresponding areas of the cerebral cortex to treat disease. This technique is used widely in China for neurological and psychological disorders.

For ASD there are ten studies that have used scalp acupuncture for children with ASD. The points which they used are summarized in Table 11.4.

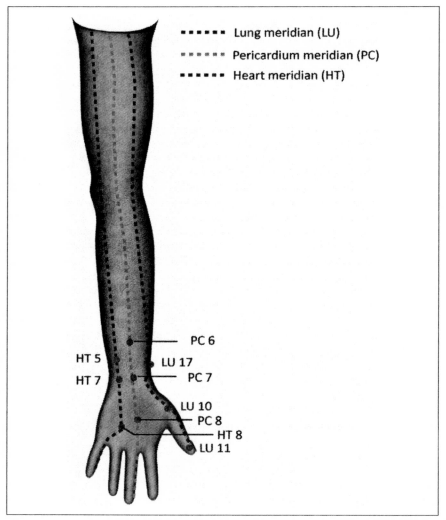

Figure 11.3.   Acupoints on the Upper Limbs Reportedly Used in the Treatment of ASD

Tongue Acupuncture (TAC)

In 1998 and based on the results of pilot studies of individual cases of ASD, our research team was the first in the world to use tongue acupuncture for ASD (Wong 2003; Wong et al. 2001; Wong et al. 1999; Wong, Sun, and Wong 2000, 2001). TAC is a technique that stimulates points on the tongue in order to cure disease. It is based on one of the most ancient

Table 11.4. Location of the Common Stimulation Areas of Acupuncture Area

Area		Location	References
語言二區	Speech 2	A vertical line 2.0 cm posterior and inferior to the parietal tubercle 3.0 cm in length.	(Fang, Wang, and Wang 2008) (Yan et al. 2007) (Wang et al. 2007) (Wang, Shang, and Wei 2006)
語言三區	Speech 3	A horizontal line starting at the midpoint of the vertigo and hearing area and running posteriorly 4.0 cm each in length.	(Fang, Wang, and Wang 2008) (Yan et al. 2007) (Wang et al. 2007) (Wang, Shang, and Wei 2006)
感覺區	Sensory area	The line parallel to and 1.5 cm posterior to the motor area.	(Yan et al. 2007)
視區	Vision area	Two lines 1.0 cm lateral to the midpoint of the external occipital protuberance, parallel to the anterior-posterior midline, and 4.0 cm in length extending superiorly.	(Yan et al. 2007)
暈聽區	Vertigo and hearing area	A horizontal line 1.5 cm above the apex of the ear and 2.0 cm anterior and 2.0 cm posterior with a total of 4.0 cm in length.	(Yan et al. 2007)

medical books in China—*Yellow Emperor*. As the tongue is connected to the Zang Fu through the 14 meridians and collaterals, by observing its color, thickness, dryness, superficial growth, and smell, the tongue can reflect the Zang Fu's physiology and pathology as well as Qi and Blood functions related to internal conditions. Furthermore, in the Zang Fu theory the tongue reflects conditions of the heart, which is the "master organ" controlling all the other internal organs. Hence, a close relationship is believed to form between the tongue, Zang Fu organ systems, and the meridians and it is thought that indirectly the tongue is linked by meridians to all the organs and parts of the body. By stimulating points on the tongue there can be a direct effect on organs throughout the whole body. There are almost 30 acupoints on the tongue (15 points on the surface of the tongue and 13 points underneath the tongue) corresponding to various organs and parts of the body. More importantly, some of these points have been found to connect to different regions of the brain (especially the cerebellum) through rich neural-vascular pathways inside the tongue.

Jin's three-needle technique was developed in 1979 by Professor Jin who is a TCM practitioner in China (Yuan and Luo 2004). The main characteristic of this acupuncture is the use of three points to treat one specific disease. According to Professor Jin one should not overneedle. Hence, he took the prototypical treatment methods for each common illness and, based upon empirical usage on the basis of TCM, determined the historically preferred three acupoints. This information was then statistically analyzed and used in clinical research thereby determining the treatment efficacy of the acupoints in question. According to the results of our search Jin's three-needle technique was widely used with ASD patients. There are seven studies, and the commonly used points and their locations are addressed in Figures 11.4a and 11.4b.

Applying Acupuncture to ASD

Acupuncture has been widely recognized as a valuable health care treatment. Clinical studies and related research on acupuncture have been un-

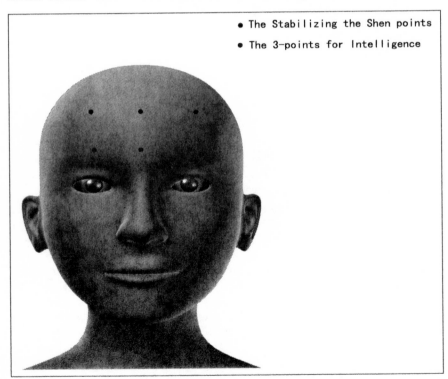

Figure 11.4a. Commonly Used Acupoints for the Treatment of ASD with Jin's Three-Needle Technique

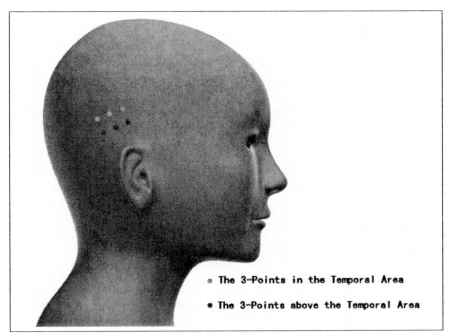

● The 3-Points in the Temporal Area

● The 3-Points above the Temporal Area

Figure 11.4b.   Commonly Used Acupoints for the Treatment of ASD with Jin's Three-Needle Technique

dertaken by independent groups, but the quality of research still varies considerably. We searched and reviewed articles reporting the use of TCM for ASD published in Chinese and other languages over the past 20 years. Most Chinese articles suggested a beneficial effect of acupuncture on ASD. There are 23 studies researching the use of acupuncture on patients with ASD. The types of interventions are body acupuncture (with a diverse use of acupoints), scalp acupuncture, auricular acupuncture, electro-acupuncture, and tongue acupuncture.

Among all these studies, seven papers were published in English (Chen, Wu-Li, and Wong 2008; Allam, ElDine, and Helmy 2008; Wong 2009; Chen and Wong 2009; Wong and Sun 2009a, 2009b; Wong and Sun 2002) and the remaining in Chinese. Nine are RCTs (Allam, ElDine, and Helmy 2008; Wong 2009; Wang et al. 2007; Wong and Sun 2009a, 2009b; Wang, Shang, and Wei 2006; Chen, Wu-Li, and Wong 2008; Zhang et al. 2005; Chen and Wong 2009), eight are case series (Chen, Wu-Li, and Wong 2008; Jia, Sun, and Fan 2008; Jiang and Wang 2005; Ju, Shi, and Shi 2008; Liu et al. 2008; Luo, Lu, and Liu 2006; Xi, Liu, and Ai 2007; Zhang 1997), and five are controlled studies (Ma, Yuan, and Rui 2006; Yuan et al. 2007). Two randomized controlled trials (Wang, Shang, and Wei 2006; Wang et al. 2007) may be describing the same study because the design, number of participants, duration of study, and site are exactly the same.

The scientific quality of some of these studies has been problematic. The general methodological problems have included lack of sample size calculation to ensure a sufficient power for statistical comparison, unclear inclusion criteria, ill-defined possible etiological factors, and age unreported. Nor have the duration of treatment and other adjunctive treatments been specified. The endpoint assessment and follow-up periods have been too short or even not reported in some studies. Moreover, the acupuncture and related treatments or interventions were too heterogeneous to analyze (varying form of acupuncture, point selection, and use of TCM herbal medicine), making it difficult for us to make direct comparisons (see Table 11.5).

Our RCT Trials for Autism

From July to September 1999, the author (V. Wong) performed a pilot study with 30 children with autism using tongue acupuncture and demonstrated improvement in core (i.e., language, social communication, cognition) and secondary features (i.e., hyperactivity, attention, aggression, temper tantrum, sleep, functional independence) (Wong and Sun 2002). Results have shown that among these 30 respondents the majority showed functional improvement of various degrees depending on the age and severity of their disabilities. Some improvement was noticeable within the tongue acupuncture sessions, especially for drooling, spasticity, ataxia, and poor balance in walking. Functional improvement was noted after one to two courses of tongue acupuncture. Most children tolerated the treatments well, with only occasional pain and minor bleeding in some patients.

After this study, Wong performed three more trials of acupuncture for ASD (Chen and Wong 2009; Wong and Sun 2009a, 2009b). There follows the abstracts for our two TAC studies on autism.

Randomized Control Trial of Acupuncture versus Sham Acupuncture in Autism Spectrum Disorder (Wong and Sun 2009)

Objective: We aim to study the efficacy of acupuncture versus sham acupuncture in children with autism spectrum disorder (ASD). *Methods:* A single-blind randomized control trial was conducted on 50 children. These children were randomly assigned to a treatment group with tongue acupuncture (40 sessions over 8 weeks) or a control group (sham tongue acupuncture to non-outpoints in the tongue). *Results:* There was improvement in both treatment and control groups on all assessed measures but more so in the treatment than control group: (1) eye-hand coordination, perfor-

Table 11.5. Studies on Acupuncture on ASD Patients (1997–2009 June)

Study	Study type	Age	ASD Diagnosis	Acupuncture	Tui Na	Chinese Herbal Medicine	Other intervention	Outcome measure	Results
(Wong 2009)*	RCT (T: 18; C: 18)	3–12 yrs	DSM-IV ADI-R ADOS	Body and auricular acupuncture for 24 sessions over 8 weeks	--	--	--	ADOS ABC ATEC RERLRS WeeFIM SPT CGIS Parental report	Improvement in ABC and RFRLRS and significant improvement in CGIS
(Wong and Sun 2002)*	RCT (T: 15; C: 15)	3–15 yrs	DSM-IV ADI-R	Tongue acupuncture for 40 sessions over 8 weeks	--	--	--	WeeFIM PSI RFRLS CGIS	Significant improvement in RFRLS, CGIS, PSI, and WeeFIM
(Wong and Sun 2009)*	RCT (T: 25; C: 25)	3–11 yrs	DSM-IV ADI-R CARS	Tongue acupuncture for 40 sessions over 8 weeks	--	--	--	GMDS RFRLRS RLDS SPT WeeFIM	Improvement in various developmental and behavioral aspects
(Wong and Sun 2009)	RCT (T: 21, C: 9)	3–16 yrs	DSM-IV ADI-R CARS	Tongue acupuncture for 40 sessions over 8 weeks	--	--	--	ATEC RLDS SPT WeeFIM CGIS PET scan	T had significant improvement in behavior, language, functional status, CGIS (p=0.0003), and cortical cerebral metabolism using ^{18}F-fluorodeoxyglucose PET

Table 11.5. Studies on Acupuncture on ASD Patients (1997–2009 June) (contd.)

Study	Study type	Age	ASD Diagnosis	Acupuncture	Tui Na	Chinese Herbal Medicine	Other intervention	Outcome measure	Results
(Chen and Wong 2009) *	RCT (T: 30; C: 25)	3-18 yrs	DSM-IV ADI-R ADOS	Electro-acupuncture for 12 sessions over 4 weeks	--	--	--	WeeFIM PEDI Leiter-R CGIS ABC RFRLRS RLDS Standardized parental report	Significant improvement in WeeFIM, PEDI, CGIS
(Yuan et al. 2009)	Controlled study (T: 35; C: 34)	2-8 yrs	DSM-VI CARS > 42	Body and scalp acupuncture 30-60 min, daily for 120 treatments, total 2 treatment courses, 2 weeks rest between each treatment course	--	--	--	CARS	Total effective rate after 1st treatment course: 85.7% Total effective rate after 2nd treatment course: 100%
(Jia, Sun, and Fan 2008)	Cases series (n=34)	2-9 yrs	ABC CCMD-3	Electro-acupuncture	--	--	--	SPECT image	Efficacy: 78.95%

Table 11.5. Studies on Acupuncture on ASD Patients (1997–2009 June) (contd.)

Study	Type / Cases	Age	Criteria	Acupuncture	Duration	Chinese Herbal Medicine	Speech therapy	Significant relations	Total effectiveness
(Ju, Shi, and Shi 2008)	Cases series (n=13)	3–8 yrs	Version 10 ICD - 120	Body and scalp acupuncture	30 min, twice per day for 3 months	Chinese Herbal Medicine three times per day for 3 months	Speech therapy 30-60 mins for 3 months	Sign-significant relations	Total effectiveness rate: 85%
(Fang, Wang, and Wang 2008)	Controlled Studies (T: 16; C:13)	--	CCMD-3 ABC score >67	Scalp acupuncture Body acupuncture	v	--	T: ABA Sensory Integrated therapy Speech therapy Game therapy C: conventional intervention	ABC	Treatment group had significant difference after treatment
(Liu et al. 2008)	Case Series (n=38)	3–11 yrs	ASD criteria CARS score≥16	Electro - scalp acupuncture 30 treatments for 3 months	--	--	--	CARS By symptoms (cannot be identified)	Effective: 78.9%
(Chen, Wu-Li, and Wong 2008)	Case study (n=2)	11 yrs	DSM-IV ADI-R ADOS	Electro-acupuncture for 24 treatments	--	--	--	ABC RFRLRS WeeFIM CGI-I Scale Parental report Monitoring for safety	Improvement in some core features

Table 11.5. Studies on Acupuncture on ASD Patients (1997–2009 June) (contd.)

Study	Study type	Age	ASD Diagnosis	Acupuncture	Tui Na	Chinese Herbal Medicine	Other intervention	Outcome measure	Results
(Allam, ElDine, and Helmy 2008)	RCT (T: 10; C: 10)	4-7 yrs	DSM IV CARS ≥ 30	Scalp acupuncture twice weekly	--	--	--	Language test	Highly significant improvements in attention and receptive, significant improvement in expressive semantics.
(Xi, Liu, and Ai 2007)	Case series (n=32)	1.5-10 yrs	Autism	Electro-acupuncture for 9 months	--	--	--	ATEC	Significant improvement in ATEC score
(Yan et al. 2007)	Controlled study (T: 20; C: 20)	2.5-8 yrs	Autism ABC CARS PPVT	T: Body and scalp acupuncture, 60-90 Min treatments	--	--	T and C: ABA Sensory integrated training	C-PEP	Total effective rate same as control group
(Wang et al. 2007; Wang, Shang, and Wei 2006)	RCT (T: 30; C: 30)	3-9 yrs	ICD-10 CCMD-3	Electro-acupuncture for 4 months	--	--	Behavior therapy	ABC PPVT	Total effective rate: 86.7%
(Yuan et al. 2007)	Controlled study (T: 40; C: 40)	2-14 yrs	DSM-IV	Body and scalp acupuncture for 120 Min treatments	--	--	--	C-PEP	Significant effective in cognitive, fine motor, gross motor, and oral speech function

Table 11.5. Studies on Acupuncture on ASD Patients (1997–2009 June) (contd.)

(Luo, Lu, and Liu 2006)	Case series (n=35)	<10 yrs	DSM-IV	Body and scalp acupuncture for 120 Min treatments	--	--	ABC	Total effective rate: 82.9%
(Ma, Yuan, and Rui 2006)	Controlled study (A: 15; B: 29; C:10)	<12 yrs	Autism ICD-10	Group A & B: Body and scalp acupuncture	Group B: graphic training	--	ABC ADC	Group B: Significant improvement in body movement, social communication, and language factor
(Jiang and Wang 2005)	Case series (n=11)	--	Not specific	Body acupuncture for 3 months	Acupoint injection with vitamin B6	--	Not specified	Total effective rate: 81.81%
(Zhang et al. 2005)	RCT (T: 20; C: 10)	<12 yrs	DSM-IV	Body and scalp acupuncture for 16 weeks	--	--	Sign-significant relations	Total effective rate: 65%
(Zhang 1997)	Case series (n-12)		Not specified	Acupuncture (50-200 Min treatment)	--	--	--	4 clinical effective; 4 effective; 4 no effect

* RCT trials performed by our research team.

Key: ABA: Applied Behavioral Analysis; ABC: Aberrant Behavioral Checklist; ADC: Autism Development Checklist; ADI-R: Autism Diagnostic Interview, Revised; ADOS: Autism Diagnostic Observation Schedule; ADS: Autism Development Checklist; ATEC: Autism Treatment Evaluation Checklist; CARS: Childhood Autism Rating Scale; CCMD-3: Chinese Classification of Mental Disorders and Diagnostic Criteria, Second Edition; CGI scale: Clinical Global Impression-improvement Scale ; C-PEP: Chinese Version of the Psychoeducational Profile; DSM-IV: Diagnostic and Statistical Manual of Mental Disorders, 4th Edition; GMDS: Griffiths Mental Developmental Scale; ICD-10: The International Statistical Classification of Diseases and Related Health Problems 10th Revision; PEDI: Pediatric Evaluation of Disability Inventory; PET scan: Positron Emission Tomography Scan; PPVT: Peabody Picture Vocabulary Test; PSI: Parental Stress Index; ERLRS: Ritvo-Freeman Real Life Scale; RLDS: Reynell Language Developmental Scale; SPECT image: Single Photon Emission Computed Tomography image; SPT: Symbolic Play Test; WeeFIM: Functional Independence Measure for Children.

mance and practical reasoning on the Griffiths Mental Developmental Scale; (2) sensory-motor, social, effectual, language, and total score of the Ritvo-Freeman Real Life Scale; (3) Comprehension language age on the Reynell Language Developmental Scale; and (4) total score and language age on the Symbolic Play Test. The only statistically significant improvement in the treatment as compared to the control group was seen in the self-care and cognition domains of the Functional Independence Measure for children. *Conclusion:* We have demonstrated that a short course of acupuncture had efficacy in improving various developmental and behavioral aspects of children with autism. The long-term efficacy in functional gain needs to be further explored.

Randomized Control Trial of Using Tongue Acupuncture in Autism Spectrum Disorder Using PET Scan for Clinical Correlation (Wong and Sun 2009)

Background: The therapeutic approach of traditional Chinese medicine to autism spectrum disorder is a functional one. *Objective:* We aimed to use tongue acupuncture (TAC) to assess for any change in brain function. *Method:* A randomized control trial was performed on 21 autistic boys—treatment (T: n=12; receiving daily TAC for 8 weeks) or control (C: N=9; no acupuncture). They were matched for severity and cognitive/functional levels. *Results:* The treatment group had significant improvement on behavior (p=0.0211); language (p=0.0211); functional status (p=0.0011); Clinical Global Impression Scale (p=0.0003); and cortical cerebral metabolism using ^{18}F-fluorodeoxyglucose Positron Emission Tomography (p=0.0451). *Conclusion:* A short course of TAC can improve functional aspects of autism spectrum disorder.

Acupuncture for Children with Autism Spectrum Disorder: Randomized Control Trial (Chen and Wong 2009)

This was a randomized, double-blind, sham-controlled, clinical trial to study the efficacy, safety, and compliance of short-term electro-acupuncture for children with ASD.

Children with ASD were randomly assigned to the electro-acupuncture (EA) group (n=30) or the sham electro-acupuncture (SEA) group (n=25) matched by age and severity of autism. The EA group received EA for selected acupoints while the SEA group received sham EA to sham acupoints. A total of 12 acupuncture sessions over 4 weeks were given. Primary outcome measures included the WeeFIM®, Pediatric Evaluation of Disability Inventory (PEDI), Leiter International Performance Scale-Revised (Leiter-R), and Clinical Global Impression-Improvement (CGI-I) scale. Secondary outcome measures consisted of the Aberrant Behavior Checklist (ABC), Ritvo-Freeman Real Life Scale (RFRLS), Reynell Developmental Language Scale

(RDLS), and standardized parental report. Data was analyzed by Mann-Whitney test. There were significant improvements in the language comprehension domain of the WeeFIM® (p=0.02), the self-care caregiver assistant domain of PEDI (p=0.028), and the CGI-I (p=0.003) for the EA group compared with the SEA group. As for the parental report, the EA group also showed significantly better social initiation (p=0.01), receptive language (p=0.006), motor skill (p=0.034), coordination (p=0.07), and attention span (p=0.003). More than 70% children with ASD adapted to acupuncture easily, while 8% had poor acupuncture compliance. Mild side effects with minor superficial bleeding or irritability during acupuncture were found. A short 4 week (12 sessions) course of electro-acupuncture is therefore useful to improve specific functions in children with ASD, especially language comprehension and self-care ability.

In 2007 the author (V. Wong) began a systematic review for the Cochrane Library to determine the effectiveness and safety of acupuncture with a published protocol for autism (Cheuk, Wong, and Chen 2009). We searched for randomized controlled trials either comparing acupuncture (including acupressure, laser acupuncture, or electro-acupuncture) with placebo, sham, or no treatment, or comparing acupuncture plus other treatments with the same other treatments.

In 2008 an assessor-blinded, randomized controlled trial with crossover design was performed in Hong Kong to study the sustainability of the acupuncture effect (Wong 2009). Thirty-six patients diagnosed with ASD were randomly allocated to the treatment (n=18) and control groups (n=18). A total four acupoints (GV 20, EX-HN3, HT 7, SP 6) and one auricular acupoint (brain point) were chosen for 24 sessions of acupuncture over 8 weeks. The results showed that acupuncture can be helpful to improve core features such as communication skills, social skills, stereotype behavior, and irritability in children with ASD.

CONCLUSION

The effectiveness of acupuncture has stood the test of time as it has survived through thousands of years. TCM acupuncture treatments for autism have been conducted over the past ten years with some beneficial effects on core symptoms of ASD, though there is no suggestion from any research that complete cure is possible. Some trials have shown patients to improve to such a degree that a fairly normal life was possible.

The current practice of acupuncture in China is still evolving and new techniques are adopted as research and clinical practice push the frontiers of knowledge further. There is still a lack of consensus about acupuncture techniques for autism and more research is needed to establish the existence of functional acupuncture areas and to validate their inclusion in an integrated TCM and Western medicine model treatment program for autism.

In 2008 a pilot project for the integration of TCM (acupuncture) and Western medicine for traumatic brain injury (TBI) or acquired brain injury (ABI) was officially approved and launched in our Children Habilitation Institute in the Duchess of Kent Children's Hospital. We have been using our concept of "integration of TCM and Western medicine" for children with various neurodevelopmental disabilities over the past decade, of which autism is the pioneer project. There is still a long way to go but we are sure that an "integrated program of TCM and Western medicine" for early intervention of children with autism is the way to go.

Acknowledgments

We would like to thank the Tung Wah Group of Hospitals for their funding and support for some of the acupuncture projects (2004-2008). We also thank Mr. Spencer Ng for drawing the figures of acupuncture points and meridians.

REFERENCES

Allam, H., N. G. ElDine, and G. Helmy. 2008. Scalp acupuncture effect on language development in children with autism: A pilot study. *J Altern Complement Med* 14 (2):109-14.

Chen, W. X., L. Wu-Li, and V. C. Wong. 2008. Electroacupuncture for children with autism spectrum disorder: Pilot study of 2 cases. *J Altern Complement Med* 14 (8):1057-65.

Chen, W. X. L., and V.C.N. Wong. 2009. Acupuncture for children with autism spectrum disorder: Randomized control trial. *The Journal of Child Psychology and Psychiatry* (in press).

Cheuk, D. K. L., V. Wong, and W. X. Chen. 2009. Acupuncture for autistic spectrum disorder *Cochrane Database of Systematic Reviews* (2).

Clark, E., and Z. Zhou. 2005. Autism in China: From acupuncture to applied behavior analysis. *Psychology in the Schools* 42 (3):285-95.

Fang, F., Q. L. Wang, and C. Q. Wang. 2008. 16 cases of autistic children with integrated traditional Chinese medicine and western medicine treatment. *Chinese Journal of Practical Nervous Disease* 11 (10): 115-16.

Fombonne, E. 2009. Epidemiology of pervasive developmental disorders. *Pediatr Res* 65 (6):591-98.

Golnick, A. E., and Ireland, M. 2009. Complementary alternative medicine for children with autism: a physician survey. *Journal of Autism and Developmental Disorders* 39 (7): 996-1005.

Hanson, E., Kalish, LA., Bunce, E., Curtis, C., McDaniel, S., Ware, J., and Petry, J. 2007. Use of complementary and alternative medicine among children diagnosed with autistic spectrum disorder. *Journal of Autism and Developmental Disorders* 37 (4): 628-36.

Harrington, J. W., L. Rosen, A. Garnecho, and P. A. Patrick. 2006. Parental perceptions and use of complementary and alternative medicine practices for children with autistic spectrum disorders in private practice. *J Dev Behav Pediatr* 27 (2 Suppl):S156-61.

Jia, S. W., T. T. Sun, and R. Fan. 2008. [Visualized study on acupuncture treatment of children autism using single photon emission computed tomography]. *Zhongguo Zhong Xi Yi Jie He Za Zhi* 28 (10):886-9.

Jiang, W. H., and Y. H. Wang. 2005. [Acupoints selected by Danjie methog for treatment of autistic children with stereotyped behaviors]. *Medicine Industry Information* 2 (14):93.

Ju, W., X. M. Shi, and X. S. Shi. 2008. [Acupuncture, massage-based treatment for 13 autistic children with language disorder]. In *Proceedings of 3rd National Children's Rehabiliataion Academic Conference and 10th National Symposium of Cerebral Palsy*. China.

Levy, S. E., D. S. Mandell, S. Merhar, R. F. Ittenbach, and J. A. Pinto-Martin. 2003. Use of complementary and alternative medicine among children recently diagnosed with autistic spectrum disorder. *J Dev Behav Pediatr* 24 (6):418-23.

Liu, G. , and L. X. Yuan. 2007. [The etiology and syndrome differentiation of child autism in Traditional Chinese Medicine]. *Liaoning Journal of Traditional Chinese Medicine* (34):9.

Liu, Z. H., H. Y. Zhang, C. T. Zhang, and D. Jing. 2008. [Clinical research of head acupuncture for autistic children]. In *Abstracts of WHO Congress on Traditional Medicine, Satellite Symposium on Acupuncture and Human Health*. China.

Luo, G. F., Z. R. Lu, and G. Liu. 2006. [Thirty-five children with autistic disorder treated by Jin's three needles]. *Chinese Acupuncture and Moxibustion* 26 (4):632.

Ma, R. L., Q. Yuan, and J. Rui. 2006. [Effect of acupuncture combined behavior intervention on children with autism]. *Zhongguo Zhong Xi Yi Jie He Za Zhi* 26 (5):419-22.

Ramey, D, and P.D Buell. 2004. A true history of acupuncture. *Focus on Alternative and Complementary Therapies* 9:269-273.

Tuchman, Roberto, and Isabelle Rapin. 2006. *Autism: A Neurological Disorder of Early Brain Development*. London: Mac Keith Press/ICNA.

Wang, C. N., Y. Liu, X. H. Wei, and L. X. Li. 2007. [Effects of electroacupuncture combined with behavior therapy on intelligence and behavior of children of autism]. *Zhongguo Zhen Jiu* 27 (9):660-2.

Wang, C. N., S. Y. Shang, and X. H. Wei. 2006. [The influence of electroacupuncture plus behavior therapy on social adaptive behavior ability in autism children]. *Shanghai Journal of Acupuncture and Moxibustion* 25 (12):91-2.

Wong, C. L. 2009. Acupuncture and autism spectrum disorders assessor-blind randomized controlled trial. Paediatrics and Adolescent Medicine, The University of Hong Kong, Hong Kong.

Wong, V. 2003. Trial of Traditional Chinese Medicine (Tongue Acupuncture or TAC) in Visual Disorders: A Pilot Study. In *5th Congress of European Paediatric Neurology Society (EPNS)*. Taormina Area, Italy, 22-25 October, 2003: European Journal of Paediatric Neurology.

Wong, V., and J. G. Sun. 2002. Research on Tongue Acupuncture in Children with Autism. In *Joint Congress of ICNA and AOCNA 2002—The 9th International Child*

Neurology Congress & the 7th Asian & Oceanean Congress of Child Neurology, Satellite Symposium on Autism / Neuromuscular Disorders Hong Kong. 18-19 September, 2002: Brain & Development.

Wong, V., J.G. Sun, Q.Y. Ma, and E. Yang. 2001. Double Blind Randomized Placebo-Controlled Trial Using Tongue Acupuncture in Children with Autistic Spectrum Disorder. In *4th European Paediatric Neurology Symposium.* Baden-Baden, Germany, 12-16 September 2001: European Journal of Neurology.

Wong, V., J.G. Sun, Q.Y. Ma, E. Yang, C. Y. Yeung, and R. Li. 1999. Use of Traditional Chinese Medicine (TCM) (Tongue Acupuncture) in Children with Neurological Disorders—Pilot Study of 100 Cases. In *3rd EPNS Congress – European Paediatric Neurology Society.* Nice, France, 7-10 November, 1999: European Journal of Paediatric Neurology.

Wong, V., J. G. Sun, and W. Wong. 13-15 November, 2000. Pilot Study of Efficacy of Tongue Acupuncture in Neurologically Disabled Children with Severe Drooling Problem. Paper read at 5th World Conference on Acupuncture (WFAS), at Seoul, Korea.

———. 2001. Randomized control trial of using tongue acupuncture in children with autistic spectrum disorder. In *17th World Congress of Neurology.* London, United Kingdom, 17-22 June, 2001: Journal of the Neurological Sciences.

Wong, V. C. 2009. Use of complementary and alternative medicine (CAM) in autism spectrum disorder (ASD): Comparison of Chinese and Western Culture (Part A). *J Autism Dev Disord* 39 (3):454-63.

Wong, V. C. N., and J. G. Sun. 2009. Randomized control trial of acupuncture versus sham acupuncture in autism spectrum disorder. (in press). *J Altern Complement Med.*

———. 2009. Randomized Control Trial of using Tongue Acupuncture in Autism Spectrum Disorder using PET scan for clinical correlation (In Press). *J Altern Complement Med.*

Wu, H., and Z. Y. Wu. 2006. [Trinity of Chinese Medicine treatment of autism]. *Journal of Chinese Medicine* 3 (11):116-7.

Xi, Y. F., Y. Y. Liu, and Z. Ai. 2007. Efficacy of intelligence-increasing acupuncture method for improving linguistic function in autism children. *Shanghai Journal of Acupuncture and Moxibustion* 26 (5):7-8.

Yan, Y. F., Y. Y. Wei, Y. H. Chen, and M. M. Chen. 2007. Effect of acupuncture on rehabilitation training of child's autism. *Zhongguo Zhen Jiu* 27 (7): 503-5.

Yuan, Q., and G. M. Luo. 2004. *Chinese-English explanation of Jin' 3-needle technique* Shanghai: Shanghai ke xue ji shu wen xian chu ban she.

Yuan, Q., T. Q. Chai, J. Y. Lang, R. C. Wang, and Z. F. Wu. 2007. [Effect of acupuncture for autism in children: An observation of 40 cases]. *Journal of Guangzhou Univeristy of Traditional Chinese Medicine* 24 (3):208-11.

Yuan, Q., R. C. Wang, Z. F. Wu, Y. Zhao, X. J. Bao, and R. Jin. 2009. [Observation on clinical therapeutic effect of Jin's 3-needling therapy on severe autism]. *Zhongguo Zhen Jiu* 29 (3):177-80.

Zhang, Q. M., R. Y. Yu, J. Pang, Y. F. Zhou, Y. Zhou, and R. Jin. 2005. Effect of acupuncture in improving intelligence and language disorder of autistic children. *Chinese Journal of Clinical Rehabilitation* 9 (28):112-3.

Zhang, S. K. 1997. [Clinical observational study of 12 children with autistic disorder treated by acupuncture]. *Zhejiang Journal of Traditional Chinese Medicine* (6):207.

12

Development of Child Mental Health Services in Central and Eastern Europe

Dainius Puras and Robertas Povilaitis

INTRODUCTION

This chapter will provide an overview, with special focus on contextual factors, of the situation in the field of child and adolescent mental health services (CAMHS) in the region of Central and Eastern Europe (CEE). Through numerous projects, programs, and international NGOs, as well as informal networks the authors have been exploring CAMHS in this unique part of the world and will present their insights based on a qualitative analysis of CAMHS in the region. It was decided to use a narrative style to describe the situation and to rely more on the experience and participation in the process of change, as well as an analysis of the contextual factors and tendencies in the development of the field of child and adolescent psychiatry (CAP) and CAMHS, rather than to present the statistical analysis of quantitative data. This decision was based on the assumption that given the unique background of this region, a qualitative rather than quantitative analysis was relevant. Furthermore, we wanted to describe the opportunities, challenges, and obstacles at all possible levels (e.g., the level of clinical interaction between clients and professionals, the community level, the national and international level). Yet another argument for the design and style of presentation chosen by the authors is that, as will be presented later, many countries in the region have faced and still continue to face serious limitations in relation to the evaluation of services and policies. This is why it is hardly possible to present hard scientific data on the status of existing services and policies in CAMHS/CAP fields. We firmly believe that during the paradigm shift that has been going on during the past two decades in

CEE a qualitative approach to and analysis of the context surrounding CAMHS facilitate an open discourse about the systemic challenges.

The main goal of this chapter is to reveal the unique situation of the field of CAMHS in the region. There is no doubt that the region is experiencing a prolonged and dramatic paradigmatic transition in the fields of human service such as the field of CAP and CAMH. On the one hand, convincing evidence exists that well-known indicators of child mental health such as rates of suicidal behavior or violence against children and bullying are very high in most countries in the region. On the other hand, the performance level of the child mental health care systems in many CEE countries remains very low. The problem is not simply related to lack of resources or lack of political will to invest more resources in child mental health; the prevailing attitudes of decision makers and the general population seem to be an even bigger challenge. Serious concern needs to be raised over the poor mental health of children and youth in the countries of Eastern and Central Europe and the lack of adequate and effective responses from their respective governments in relation to mental health. In many CEE countries huge resources are still invested in the system of ineffective services such as large residential institutions for children of all ages and with different problems and disorders. Many innovative services, based on a modern public health approach, have relied mainly on international donors and, therefore, encounter sustainability problems because international foundations are in the process of leaving the region; meanwhile the region's governments are often reluctant to secure funding for innovative services.

It is of utmost importance to reveal the basic obstacles to the development and implementation of effective child mental health policies in the CEE countries. If the political will for basic change in child mental health and related systems continues to be lacking and both financial and human resources are ineffectively invested by national governments the situation may reinforce a "vicious circle" based on the institutionalization of children, social exclusion, a culture of dependence and learned helplessness among parents, and children and youth who have problems in their social and emotional development. The threat of such a scenario is high in many countries of the region—especially in the current financial crises.

The rich experience of innovative projects, programs, and services has been accumulated in CEE countries demonstrating the expansion of human and social capital in citizens and organizations able and willing to develop effective child mental health approaches. However, the analysis of both indicators of child mental health and indicators of performance for the child mental health care systems reveals a picture which raises serious concerns. Lack of funding for effective preventive child and family mental health interventions appears to be just a secondary negative outcome of the prevailing attitudes. This conclusion challenges the traditional view which emphasizes lack of financial resources in CEE countries as the basic obstacle for developing a modern mental health service. Concrete examples of successes and failures related to the implementation of modern preventive approaches in the field of child mental health in the CEE countries will be presented.

HISTORICAL BACKGROUND

The situation in the field of child and adolescent mental health in Central and Eastern Europe deserves special attention. This is a huge region covering 30 new democracies with a population of around 400 million. The region is extremely diverse culturally and socioeconomically. It is obvious, for example, that Slovenia and Turkmenistan are very different countries and this is why making any generalizations about the situations in 30 countries is a risky exercise. One group of countries—the 15 comprising the former Soviet Union—were influenced by totalitarian ideology (although the extent of influence varied), while the so-called satellite countries of Central Europe and the Balkan countries of the former Yugoslavia experienced the influence to a lesser degree. In the Central European countries of Poland, the Czech Republic, Hungary, the Slovak Republic, and the former Yugoslavia there were more possibilities to introduce modern methods. What makes the context of change in all these countries similar is that after having been under communism for 50-70 years they are all facing a unique process of transition from a totalitarian system to democracy. The period from 1990 onwards, when sociopolitical changes started, has been marked by an impressive combination of successes, challenges, and failures in many fields, including CAMHS. A brief historical background of Soviet political ideology and its influence on psychiatry provides insight into the historical development of child psychiatry and its impact on the reforms to CAMHS today.

The countries in Central and Eastern Europe have historically possessed child and adolescent mental health services that focus on a biomedical model of mental health problems with little consideration for the social and environmental factors affecting the mental health of children and adolescents. Soviet political ideology exerted a strong influence on the development of services, the training of professionals, and the provision of care for children and adolescents. Under communism the CEE countries developed a unique system of mental health care for both children and adults. Different from the so-called developing or third world countries this system benefitted from a relative advantage of Soviet ideology in the fields of health policy and social security; a rather impressive amount of financial and human resources was invested in the health and social services. However,

different from the developed countries of the Western world, relevant resources were predominantly invested in numerous residential institutions
for clients with different kinds of mild and severe problems. State policy
was based on the model of social exclusion of vulnerable groups. In cases
of either families being in crisis or a child developing any problem the
usual solution was to institutionalize the child. The official indicator of
good performance in this system was the high percentage of "organized
children" (which meant institutionalized children) with any kind, including mild cases, of developmental or psychosocial disabilities. Community-
based services were prevented from developing by the very fact that Soviet
ideology declared psychosocial problems to have been successfully solved
by the political system. This is why the development of psychosocial components of care was blocked and the CAMH field was dominated by the
concepts of defectology and child psychoneurology.

Child psychiatry in CEE countries comes from various medical backgrounds (general medicine, general psychiatry, pediatrics). Traditionally,
professionals have had insufficient training to identify mental disorders
and problems at an early stage or to develop treatment programs that take
into account the child or adolescent's social and environmental condition.

CAP initially was part of child psychoneurology and was developing on
the basis of a narrow biomedical model which was represented by clinical
neurology from the middle of the twentieth century. In the middle of the
1970s throughout the Soviet Union child and adolescent psychiatry was
recognized as a specialty, independent of child neurology. Since then, and
until now, this specialty has been struggling for independence from adult
psychiatry with different success in different countries. While adult psychiatry in the Soviet Union was famous for an extreme broadening of the criteria for schizophrenia (which resulted in the political abuse of psychiatry),
child and adolescent psychiatry was looking for other ways of interpreting
the possible causes of emotional and behavioral disorders in children. Most
frequently different types of diagnosis were used, reflecting a former link
with child neurology, such as organic brain syndrome or organic-type consequences of hypothetical mild brain damage during pregnancy, birth, or
early infancy. Again, it is important to remind ourselves that these trends
were a direct result of the ideological statements made by a totalitarian state
according to which the psychosocial causes of these disorders had already
been eliminated.

Both inpatient and outpatient CAP services were predominantly based
on pharmacological treatment. Professional groups of clinical psychologists
started to emerge and slowly grow from the 1980s onwards. Social work as
a specialty and separate field did not exist until 1990 when sociopolitical
change began in the region. Among the weaknesses in the former system
one could mention a low level of development of the teamwork approach

particularly as the development of non-medical specialities (e.g., psychology, social work, etc.) was poor in many countries.

The services for children with developmental disabilities developed under the influence of defectology, which was the Soviet equivalent of special education. The level of "defect" was identified in each disabled child in order to decide if it was cost-effective to invest in his education as future cheap labor force. This is why mildly retarded children were usually referred to special schools while cases of moderate and severe mental retardation were diagnosed by defectologists as "uneducable." Parents were given strong advice by professionals to abandon these children and place them in state institutions for the rest of their lives.

Interestingly, by labeling them as mildly mentally retarded a large group of children suffering from social and emotional deprivation were also placed in special boarding schools. In this way the Soviet system was hiding social problems and instead presenting them as problems emerging from in the child's brain.

Psychiatric services for children and adolescents developed along the same lines as basic health services, as a highly centralized, bureaucratic, vertical system with an absence of planning based on public health needs. The system relied heavily on large institutions such as psychiatric institutions, institutions for children with disabilities, institutions for orphans and "social orphans" and correctional institutions for managing the problems of juvenile justice. There was little emphasis on keeping the child within the family or community and there was a heavy reliance on inpatient care.

One major difference between the development of child psychiatry and general psychiatry services was the multi-agency aspect of child services. A number of services were provided in schools, e.g., schools for the deaf and blind, boarding schools for mentally disabled children, homes for children with severe physical disabilities—all of them under the responsibility of the Ministry of Education. Services in polyclinics, dispensaries, hospitals, and infant homes for disabled children were administered under the auspices of the Ministry of Health. The Ministry of Labour was responsible for family benefits and institutions for children with severe mental disabilities, and the Ministry of the Interior was delegated responsibility for delinquents and young offenders.

The basis of the Soviet system of health care was local polyclinics established in every community. The polyclinics functioned as mass screening centers for identifying diseases, prevention, and immunization, as well as being a referral point for specialized care. When a child was born the local physician assessed the child and a record of growth and development was kept throughout his/her life. Special attention was paid to early signs of developmental disorders, hearing or sight impairment, and the detection of disabilities. A polyclinic also had a number of specialists including, among others, a speech therapist and sometimes a child psychiatrist.

Many human resources were used in this kind of system. Without deeper analysis the impression may be that this could have been an effective system. However, several systemic obstacles of an ideological nature prevented the Soviet system of child mental health care from being effective. Even if problems were identified at an early age, this often resulted in social exclusion and institutionalization of children. Thus, children with developmental or physical disabilities, abused children, or children with parents with substance abuse problems could be sent to special institutions and schools for children with specific problems. In some cases this would be day schools, but often children with learning or physical disability would be provided long-term residential care in large institutions. In Soviet times parents were advised to send their children to an institution and choices were often limited for financial reasons. Children were diagnosed at a very young age and often the diagnoses would remain for the rest of their lives. Education and care were provided in special institutions separate from communities, families, and mainstream educational services.

Services were developed based upon the disorders or disabilities identified among children. The emphasis was on developing a comprehensive set of services for each "disorder." There was little emphasis on including a socio-environmental explanation for a particular problem. Problems were diagnosed and treatment was administered, either in hospitals, dispensaries, schools, or institutions, but the case management process did not include a wider analysis of the child's family or community environment. Thus, if the "family environment" was viewed as problematic the child was taken out of the environment and put into a "sanatoria" for respite from the family or, in numerous cases, into an orphanage.

The system was functioning and, in many ways, it provided the needed services. Every child's physical needs were assessed, treated, or referred accordingly. In this respect, every child was looked after by the state despite a very narrow definition of "mental health" which neglected social-environmental factors. Mental health promotion and prevention for children and adolescents did not exist within this structure. Mental health services were controlled by the political ideology. If mental health problems were supposed to only have a biological base then there was nothing to promote or prevent.

Paradoxically, Soviet ideology strongly emphasized the need to prevent as a priority in the general health system. This resulted in rather good indicators of children's physical health (e.g., rather low newborn mortality rates, good coverage in vaccination, and good control of infectious diseases, etc.). However, the concept of hygiene (public health) in the Soviet system did not include mental health. Only biological risk factors were considered as the possible cause of mental health problems (the psychosocial risk factors were supposed to be "eliminated" by ideology); therefore, the mental health field was reduced to the biological treatment of mental disorders. Important components such as mental health promotion and prevention of mental health problems did not exist in the Soviet public health system.

From its beginning, the existing regime had expected mental illness to vanish under socialism because it was considered that psychosocial risk factors were a product of the unjust social structure of capitalism. After that assumption failed and mental illness remained a problem in the Soviet Union most psychiatric illnesses were attributed to narrow biological etiology and explained as disturbed biological brain functioning. This biological model best suited the totalitarian way of thinking. Puras (1994) describes how the field of child psychiatry in Lithuania was controlled by ideology and, therefore, the psychological problems of children and families were claimed by official state ideology to not exist with only biological interpretations permitted in clinical practice, training, and research.

The Soviet "state" ideology and its influence on the development of mental health care services, treatment, and the theoretical orientation of psychiatrists resulted in a heavy reliance on hospitalization and medically based approaches to CAMHS. This ideology has in many ways posed a barrier to the development of new theoretical approaches; for example, the concept of attachment is unknown in many countries and is not used in practice but the ideology's effects remain heavily present in the health care reforms of the last two decades.

OVERVIEW OF THE CHANGES IN THE CEE REGION DURING 20 YEARS OF TRANSITION

In 1990, after dramatic changes throughout the whole region of Central and Eastern Europe huge opportunities for the development of modern approaches in the field of CAMH and CAP emerged.

The Field of Legislation

New laws were adopted by national parliaments in the field of the rights of the child and childhood policies. The UN Convention on the Rights of the Child was ratified by all countries in the region. The changes in legislation facilitated the development of new services. Also, with the new spirit of "glasnost" many questions were raised about the situation of children and the violation of their rights in closed institutions.

As it appeared later, 20 years of change were not sufficient to implement the basic principles of the rights of the child in everyday life in most of the

CEE countries. During recent years the UN Committee on the Rights of the Child has expressed serious concerns about the situation of mentally disabled children and children who are in conflict with the law in many CEE countries. In response to the countries who presented reports on the implementation of the convention during 2007-2009 (i.e., Serbia, Romania, Bulgaria, and other countries) the UN Committee on the Rights of the Child (2009) recommended the development and implementation of comprehensive policies in the field of child mental health and children with mental disabilities.

Development of Services

The biggest gap that needed to be filled was to introduce community-based services for child protection and family support. In most countries of the region the social welfare system had no tradition of solving social problems at the community level. During the last decade of the twentieth century a network of child protection agencies was established. For the first time a new professional group of social workers appeared on the scene. First attempts to work therapeutically with families at risk were introduced after many years of a culture of blaming, moralizing, and punishing parents for lack of competence and parenting skills.

However, this process turned out to be complicated. At times the skills possessed by the new professionals were found to be insufficient to maintain therapeutic relations with parents. The quality of training for the new generation of professionals became problematic because of the lack of experienced trainers who could introduce the modern concepts of working with families based on a supportive therapeutic approach. For example, in some CEE countries the concept of supervision is still ignored by those who make decisions and manage services.

Due to the above mentioned obstacles the management of cases of child abuse still often resulted in the solution inherited from the former system— that is, to protect the rights of the child by separating him/her from the parents and placeing him/her into long-term institutional care. Services for the psychosocial rehabilitation of parents who were known to abuse their child still remain very weak or non-existent in many CEE countries.

In the field of CAP services progress was achieved at both inpatient and outpatient level. Inpatient units have been decreasing in size and improving the quality of care by introducing multidisciplinary teamwork and psychosocial therapies in addition to traditional biological treatments. Outpatient services became more decentralized and were equipped with different psychosocial therapies. In some countries teamwork was introduced as the basic method of outpatient care. Despite the positive trends many challenges still remain in the provision of CAP services. In some countries child psychiatry does not exist anymore as a medical speciality and general psychiatrists (usually without adequate training in the field of CAP) take over the management of children with mental health problems.

In all CEE countries, with different degrees of success, innovative demonstration services were established as first alternatives to the tradition of institutional care. These innovations have been a joint effort between national/municipal authorities and the newly founded non-governmental organizations, including the societies for parents who have mentally disabled children. New services included day care centers for moderately and severely retarded children, early intervention services for infants with disabilities, workshops, and independent living centers for youngsters and young adults with mental disabilities. During the first decade of transition (1990-2000) considerable financial support was received from international foundations such as UNICEF, the Open Society Foundation and its national branches, Global Initiative on Psychiatry, and other organizations to support the newly established community-based services.

Despite all this progress many children with disabilities in the CEE region still remained in residential institutions (Browne et al. 2006). Family support services at the community level and methods for integrating disabled children into the system of education have been developed, but in most countries they still are not effective enough to stop the process of institutionalizing children with existing and perceived disabilities.

Promotion/Prevention

There has been an increasing awareness about the importance of activities aimed at the promotion of child mental health and prevention of mental health problems. In all countries many new initiatives were started to prevent problems like alcohol and drug use, suicides, violence, etc. Particularly active in this field was the emerging NGO sector. However, many of the programs that were developed and implemented were of unknown effectiveness. The sustainability of these preventive programs is threatened by lack of political will and an absence of CAMHS policies.

The most serious challenge for the region is the lack of evidence in relation to CAMHS policies. They either do not exist or if approved, there is no tradition of independent monitoring and sustainable implementation. The WHO (2005) recommends developing and implementing CAMHS policies so that the allocated resources are used in an evidence-based and rational way. The mix of services should include all obligatory components: self-care, informal community care, mental health services, thorough primary health care, community mental health services, psychiatric services in general hospitals, and long-stay facilities for severe cases which need highly qualified specialist care. The existence of such an organization of services would ensure, as an obligatory condition, that specialized services are not used for mild cases and resources are used rationally.

The systemic problem for the CEE region is not the quantity of resources but the fact that financial and human resources are used ineffectively because of the absence of "filters" (tiers). For example, the lack of involvement by GPs in the provision of child mental health care creates the problem that specialized mental health care services are overloaded with referrals for mild cases. In this situation no resources are left to effectively manage more serious cases.

Another obstacle to the effective management of resources is the inherited lack of a culture that emphasizes monitoring and evaluation of policies and services. The tradition in the former system was that for many decades statistics and data collection systems reflected processes but not outcomes. For example, the number of beds, doctors, admissions to inpatient care, and outpatient visits was presented as evidence of an effective system. Outcomes such as improvement in mental health and the quality of the CAMHS system performance were not measured.

For example, in Lithuania the only existing tier of provision for outpatient mental health services is the system of municipal mental health centers which are part of primary health care funded by the capitation system. This is why a referral from the GP is not needed and both adults and children with mental health problems have a right to direct access to specialized mental health care. The establishment of these centers in 1997 was based on an intention to increase accessibility and ensure that all cases of mental health problems and disorders were managed effectively by multidisciplinary teams. After 12 years it appears that these centers do not have the capacity to manage complex cases which need a longer therapeutic process and bigger teams. Also, a negative result of this system was the fact that general practitioners were not involved in child mental health care.

The process of transition in CEE countries was marked by an unprecedented crisis of mortality and morbidity in the general population. The mortality rates are significantly higher in CEE countries compared to other European countries. Analyzing this public health crisis reveals a close relationship between this phenomenon and unexpected and prolonged psychosocial stress (Cornia and Paniccia 2001). The changes in the social, economic, and political environment required coping skills which were not developed during the totalitarian system. This dramatic change resulted in feelings of hopelessness and helplessness with a large proportion of the population perceiving themselves as victims of change. According to the Eurobarometer *European Social Reality Report* (European Commission 2007) the populations of former EU15 countries (old EU member states) were happier then populations in the new member states. For example, almost half of respondents in Denmark (49%), Ireland (46%), and the Netherlands (43%) reported being very happy. Conversely, in the new EU countries representing the CEE region only a small minority of population reported being very happy: Lithuania (13%), Estonia (12%), Latvia (12%), Slovakia (10%), Romania (9%), and Bulgaria (8%).

Training of Child Mental Health Professionals

For many years "biomedical interventions" have been the main mode of treatment for children with emotional and developmental disorders in the former Soviet countries. New educational programs for child psychiatrists have been developed in a number of CEE countries which include the psychosocial aspects of mental health and the development of alternative therapies to "medical" interventions.

New EU member states have fulfilled EU requirements and moved to residency programs in all medical specialties. For example, in Lithuania there is a possibility for medical school graduates to choose four-year residencies in general (adult) psychiatry or four-year residencies in child and adolescent psychiatry. However, in some CEE countries there are still serious problems with the autonomy of child and adolescent psychiatry as an independent medical specialty. In some CEE countries this specialty does not exist anymore while in other countries the idea is to hand over the management of child mental health disorders to general (adult) psychiatrists. In some countries of Eastern Europe, although the specialty of child and adolescent psychiatry exists, the training programs are very short and do not meet international requirements.

To date, there has been a lack of emphasis on the valuable role general practitioners can play in early identification of mental health problems and disorders among children and adolescents. Family doctors have not been trained in early detection of mental health problems because the health care structure was based on a number of specialized services and the majority of cases were referred directly to child psychiatric services. There are thousands of children whose mental disorders or problems go unidentified for a variety of reasons, one of which is professionals lacking the appropriate training to identify problems at an early stage. Training general practitioners would not only improve early identification of problems and disorders but might also reduce the number of referrals to specialized services for children whose mental health problems can be managed at the primary care level. If properly trained, child psychiatrists could play an active role providing consultation to general practitioners so that they could more effectively manage cases of child mental health problems. Unfortunately, in most CEE countries this change has not yet occurred.

Using the skills of newly developed professionals and integrating professionals such as nurses, social workers, and psychologists into the active care of CAMH are regarded as important steps in developing a broad range of services.

Nurses in the CEE region have been under-represented in the care of children and adolescents with mental health problems or disorders. Traditionally, nurses have been subordinate to psychiatrists and have not played an important role in the process of care and treatment. Now they are slowly being recognized as a valuable resource and new educational curricula have been set up in a number of countries. Training is required to upgrade skills and broaden nurses' knowledge about the psychological and social dimensions of child mental health problems, the involvement of parents in the management of children's problems, and the development of community services.

Social work schools have been set up in all CEE countries. The first generation of social workers are now working in different settings with at risk children and families. The main problems are linked to the quality of training and the ratio between the number of social workers and doctors in the teams. In many CEE countries there are still more child psychiatrists than social workers in outpatient services. This staff ratio factor reduces the possibility of developing effective psychosocial interventions for children and families at risk.

LITHUANIA AS AN EXAMPLE OF A COUNTRY IN TRANSITION

The case of Lithuania as a classic country in transition is presented because of its unique combination of achievements and challenges during the process of reforming CAMHS in this country. On the one hand numerous innovations have been implemented in service development, professional training, and policy formulation in Lithuania. On the other hand after 20 years since the launch of reforms serious gaps still remain in policy development and service provision.

Mental Health Policy

There have been several attempts to introduce modern methods of evaluation to the mental health system. As part of an international mental health policy, programs, and services project the "country profile" instrument was used to evaluate mental health policy and services in the Republic of Lithuania. An independent group of Lithuanian researchers carried out the quantitative and qualitative analysis of the mental health system. This analysis included evaluation of the context, resources, processes, and outcomes. As a result of the research the country's profile was produced, clearly identifying the existing gaps (Puras et al. 2004). The analysis of the contextual factors revealed high levels of social pathology (including violence, suicide, and other self-destructive behavior) with stigmatizing attitudes from the general population towards mentally disturbed persons, disabled children, dysfunctional families, and other vulnerable groups. The analysis of existing data about resources invested in the mental health care system raised questions for policy makers about the effectiveness of the traditional way of investment. The largest proportion of physical and human capital appeared to be concentrated in psychiatric institutions, with large numbers of beds, psychiatrists, and ever-increasing funding for medications, while other components of care, such as community-based child mental health services, were not being developed. There was a strong tradition of neglecting psychosocial interventions in health service funding schemes. Statistical accounts keep the tradition of treating processes as outcomes, while a modern assessment of service, programs, and policy outcomes is lacking. The number of children placed in different state institutions, number of outpatient visits and inpatient cases, and other quantitative data remain, because of tradition, the indicators of effective system performance. This is how self-feeding service systems emerge and protect themselves finding supportive arguments for their further development instead of critically analyzing their effectiveness. These gaps, in the absence of evidence-based policy making, were leading to ineffective investment reinforcing the system of residential institutions and excessive medicalization. The results of the analyses were especially important for the CAMHS. The findings from this country profile were suggested by the research team as an argument for policy makers for mental health care reform.

It took several years for the analysis to be used in policy formulation. After the WHO Ministerial Conference on Mental Health in 2005 the minister of health created a task force for the development of a national mental health policy. After two years of debates the policy was finally approved by the Parliament in 2007. This policy document is based on modern principles such as the need for a flexible spectrum of community-based services, an evidence-based balance in the biopsychosocial paradigm, the evaluation and monitoring of policies and services, the protection of human rights, and promotion of mental health and prevention of mental health problems. The national mental health policy also emphasizes the need to invest in evidence-based approaches.

In the two years since the national mental health policy was approved there has been not much success at the level of implementation. The near future will show if Lithuania is ready to implement modern approaches in the field of child and adolescent mental health and move to a new level in the culture of evaluating and monitoring policy and services. One of the particularly important tasks over the next years is to restore balance in the biopsychosocial paradigm. Ironically, after 50 years of the ideologically

driven dominance of the biomedical component and neglect of psychosocial interventions Lithuania, and the whole CEE region, experienced one
more wave of reductionistic biomedical approaches in managing complex
societal problems such as the prevention of destructive and self-destructive
behavior. Governments were reluctant to move to a modern public health
approach and to invest in modern psychosocial technologies but new biomedical technologies (the new generation of medications) have been reimbursed as a first priority. This resulted in a further increase in the dispropor-
tions of the biopsychosocial paradigm; in 2007 investments in biomedical
technologies (i.e., medications) in the field of mental health care from
obligatory health insurance funds exceeded investments in psychosocial
interventions (i.e., psychotherapies) by more than 200 times. This tendency
has been particularly threatening for the modern development of child and
adolescent mental health services which need an especially strong component of psychosocial interventions.

Development of CAMH Services

Lithuania, like other post-communist countries, has inherited from the
previous system a highly centralized, medicalized, and dehumanizing system of services for all groups of troubled children and adolescents, i.e.,
mentally disabled, socially and emotionally deprived, psychiatrically, emotionally, or psychosocially disturbed ones. There were no alternative services
available other than the large institutions such as infant homes (orphan-
ages), children's homes, special boarding schools for mild mental retardation and socially deprived children, psychoneurological institutions for
moderately and severely mentally retarded, closed correctional institutions
for juvenile delinquents, and large understaffed inpatient psychiatric units
for children within general psychiatric hospitals. Starting in 1990 the political, economic, and social changes introduced in Lithuania provided the
possibility to develop, for the first time in the nation's history, an effective
and modern system of child mental health services.

At the beginning of the 1990s it was commonly understood among politicians, professionals, and the general public that new approaches needed
to be introduced in the field of child mental health care to gradually replace
the existing system of institutionalizing children and medicalizing social
problems.

In 1991 the Child Development Center was established in Vilnius as a
demonstration clinic affiliated with Vilnius University for the implementation of modern CAMHS policy and practice. In the first years a lot of progress was made restoring the balance within the biopsychosocial paradigm.

The first years of change in the field of CAMH, since 1990, have been very
promising. During first five years, pilot models for new systems of services

have been developed. In 1998, the program Development of Community-Based Services for Children with Developmental Disorders in Lithuania developed by the Vilnius Child Development Center received a Health for All award from the World Health Organization for the best national program among community-based women and children's health projects. All these activities have been accomplished with the active participation of the academic department, Center of Child Psychiatry and Social Pediatrics at Vilnius University.

From the very beginning the philosophy of the center was based on the general concept that alternative approaches must be developed in order to gradually replace the existing medicalized and stigmatizing system of institutions. To achieve this goal emphasis has been placed on several tasks:

- To develop demonstration models within the center's clinic with an emphasis on multidisciplinary teamwork and active involvement of parents;
- To replicate positive experiences accumulated in the center through the outreach programs in the city of Vilnius and throughout the country;
- To initiate new training programs for professionals working with troubled children and their families;
- To facilitate interagency and interdisciplinary cooperation at different levels (e.g., governmental and municipal agencies, NGOs, and professional groups);
- To lobby, using the results of the center's activities and those of other organizations, to change the priorities in mental health and social policy of the government and municipalities;
- To initiate research projects in the field; and
- To analyze international experience in the field and creatively use the best practices from developed countries, as well as avoiding practices which have no evidence base.

The center is a combination of a demonstration clinic and research and training center, which, in cooperation with governmental, professional, non-governmental organizations, and international partners is lobbying for the development of a model of effective and economic services for children and adolescents with different cognitive, emotional, and psychosocial disorders. Having analyzed the experience of different schools in the field of child and adolescent psychiatry, i.e., developmental, social, and behavioral pediatrics, pediatric rehabilitation, special education, clinical child psychology, and social work, the center is facilitating the development of best practice in the field of child mental health throughout Lithuania.

One of the priorities is the reasonable de-medicalization of services (keeping in mind the historical legacy of the Soviet system to hide social problems under the labels of medical conditions) and add psychosocial and educational components to the system of care, without losing the strengths of a medical model while also challenging the tradition of medicalizing social problems.

Another priority is a creative search for the optimal balance between specialized services and more non-specific interventions that might be developed within primary health care, emerging community social welfare services, and schools. The experience of developed European countries has proved that it is of utmost importance to develop several tiers within the CAMH system so that effective prevention programs and the strong involvement of primary care services (e.g., GPs, schools, network of support services for children and families at risk) allow only the more complicated cases to reach specialized CAMH services; otherwise resources will be used ineffectively.

Pursuant to the philosophy of the center, special emphasis has been made of empowering the family, which for many years had been stigmatized, blamed, and demoralized for having exceptional children or for the lack of good parenting skills. At a minimum, they had been excluded from the therapeutic process. The staff of the center have had very positive working experiences with parents of disabled children and parents who have difficulties coping with childrearing. Promoting and strengthening the competence of parents and mobilizing protective factors and resilience within each child, family, and community are one of the cornerstones of the philosophy of the center.

The urgent need to develop a new social policy, with emphasis on new long-term prevention programs for at risk young children and their families, was again presented to the government. While public opinion about parents who fail to properly take care of their children is as "bad parents" and often results in demands for repressive measures the philosophy of the model emphasizes the need to share responsibility for failures in parenting between parents, the community, the general public, and local and national authorities.

In the very difficult socioeconomic transition towards democracy and a market economy, when many families face enormous economic, psychological, and social difficulties, both the general public and the authorities are more prone to resort to finding scapegoats for social tragedies (e.g., suicides, street children, criminality, violence, child abuse, etc.). In this situation there is a danger of allocating limited funds to strengthen the repressive and segregated institutions for disadvantaged groups as opposed to investing in community-based preventive services for children and families. During these political debates the center and its allies (non-governmental organizations and, recently, municipalities interested in budget decentralization) have been actively lobbying for the development of an infrastructure of preventive community-based services for children and families at risk.

The first training programs, with support from foreign professionals, were organized in 1990s and several attempts to initiate national projects were made. The basic structure of the clinic as a demonstration center was developed based on a multidisciplinary team of professionals, active involvement of parents, and the introduction of psychosocial, psychotherapeutic, and psychoeducational interventions. This minimized the use of excessive pharmacological treatment which in the former system was the only treatment option for a variety of disorders, including emotional and behavior problems, but also mental retardation, autism, and other developmental disabilities.

It is important to mention that the combination of different fields (e.g., care for children with developmental disabilities and children with emotional and psychosocial disorders, as well as children at risk in general) was based on the belief that certain important "common denominators" existed among the fields that traditionally have been separated in developed countries. Both children's disabilities and psychosocial (e.g., mental, emotional, and behavioral disorders) have been similarly ignored by the previous system. Both fields—child and adolescent psychiatry and developmental pediatrics—need a new infrastructure based on the involvement of the educational and social welfare systems and incorporating a new approach towards families, who have previously been stigmatized and demoralized, as well as new training programs based on teamwork and community involvement.

In general, reforms in services for disabled children have been significantly more effective when compared to changes in the field of child psychiatry and the management of psychosocial problems, such as prevention of child abuse, juvenile delinquency, or the problem of street children. In the field of developmental disabilities, after the concerted efforts of a joint coalition of parents' organization, reform-minded professionals, and national as well as municipal authorities, a positive "self-fulfilling prophecy" effectively worked demonstrating that it is possible to implement a community-based system of services as an alternative to the traditional system of segregated institutions. However, in the field of social problems of childhood and adolescence (e.g., prevention of juvenile delinquency, child abuse, suicidal behavior, etc.) the signs of learned helplessness still prevail among stakeholders and the principal investments are usually made only of the level of tertiary prevention. Thus, a vicious circle still tends to prevail, as resources are mainly used to reinforce ineffective approaches of stigma, social exclusion, and institutionalization.

From 1997 onwards the Lithuanian health system moved to a new system of health insurance that was a serious challenge to the implementation of modern ideas in the field of CAMHS. Health insurance was supposed to cover health care services in the traditional understanding of the medical model, i.e., short-term inpatient treatment and pharmacotherapy, which meant that only a small part of the model of services developed within the center would be paid for by the national health insurance fund. The activities of the center and its ambitions to replicate the model throughout the country have been further threatened because of its emphasis on multidisciplinary and preventive approaches which health insurance authorities are reluctant to recognize as health care services. Despite some unavoidable losses, both the structure and philosophy of the center survived. Even more, there has been moderate success in replicating services throughout the country during subsequent years. Thus, more than 30 outpatient early intervention teams for infants and preschool children with developmental disabilities have been established throughout the country.

In 2000, an international training program for professionals in the field of child mental health and developmental disabilities was developed and an application was submitted together with the Global Initiative on Psychiatry to Dutch foundations. Usually it included two- to eight-week internships for professionals from the former Soviet Union in the center and other demonstration sites of the model. Professionals from Russia, Ukraine, Moldova, Georgia, Azerbaijan, Belarus, and countries of the former Soviet Central Asian countries had a unique opportunity to learn from the achievements and challenges of the Vilnius model. During recent years this training program was experiencing difficulties related to its funding because major donor organizations have left the CEE region.

In 2008 the IACAPAP leadership decided to have its traditional regional study group for early career child psychiatrists from Eastern and Central Europe in Vilnius. This was recognition of the achievements of the Vilnius model. The study group led by the president of IACAPAP Professor Per-Anders Rydelius was extremely successful. While discussing the cases presented by young professionals from ten countries participants shared challenges that exist at the clinical and systemic (societal) levels. It was brought to everyone's attention that CAMH services in many CEE countries are under threat of being underdeveloped in the face of the economic crisis and a new wave of medicalizing health services. Some participants, even if representing the new generation, have been following the traditional model of viewing a patient as a purely medical case. As it became obvious during the discussions that this style of management of everyday practice, even if not effective in the vast majority of cases, was a method of self-defense for professionals because the broader view is confronted by an absence of intersectorial approach and lack of client-tailored services in the community.

In cooperation with the Lithuanian Welfare Society for Persons with Learning Disabilities ("Viltis"), the Child Development Center has successfully participated, since 1991, in the national program of integration of disabled persons. As a result of this cooperation the process of integrating mentally disabled children into the educational system began throughout the country. The center served as a resource and training center for starting and implementing the integration process.

There was a growing awareness among families of children with developmental or psychiatric disorders, the general public, and politicians that the traditional medical model and the search for a miraculous medical or mystical cure can be replaced by realistically developed individual treatment or rehabilitation programs which must be run by local teams of professionals in partnership with the family.

More than 50 methods of assessment, therapy, and rehabilitation, including those well known in developed countries but never before used in Lithuania and the CEE region, were first implemented in the center and are now used throughout the country. These include methods for assessing the child and the family, different modalities of psychotherapeutic interventions, and methods of psychosocial support and rehabilitation for families and children. The general trend was to accept all evidence-based approaches and not become too dependent on any one particular school of thought or clinical practice.

The first problem was the situation of children with developmental disabilities including mental retardation and autism. A strong coalition of professionals, parents' organizations, and reform-minded politicians was successful in convincing the national authorities to develop a network of community-based services for these children as an alternative to the traditional system of large residential institutions. The Child Development Center was driving this process with the provision of professional knowledge and skills, with special focus on early intervention services for infants and preschool children with developmental problems and disabilities. This field has developed now as developmental (social) pediatrics, with a network of community-based teams throughout the country. Thus, a good foundation was prepared for integrating disabled children into the education system and society in general.

In the field of CAMH the specialty of child and adolescent psychiatry was well established with a four-year postgraduate (residency) program. Currently there are 80 specialists in CAP working in outpatient and inpatient services. The Lithuanian Society of Child and Adolescent Psychiatrists is actively involved in numerous national and international activities which promote international standards in the field of CAP and CAMH. After long debates with the health insurance authorities relatively good agreements have been achieved so that the cost of inpatient and day care units includes teams of professionals working with children in need. A pilot service for intensive one-week crisis intervention programs was opened and it is also covered by health insurance despite the fact that referred cases usually do not have a medical diagnosis. This was an important victory in convincing national authorities that health insurance funds should be used for effective and flexible management of urgent psychosocially challenging cases. Outpatient services are represented by child psychiatrists, psychologists, and social workers who are employed by municipal mental health centers and funded by health insurance on the basis of capitation principle.

In terms of the quality of CAMH services and policies a considerable shift has been made:

- From superficial biomedical treatment to evaluation and treatment plans based on a biopsychosocial paradigm.
- From large understaffed inpatient units with a high risk of violating the basic rights of children to small inpatient units with therapeutic environments and a better balance between psychosocial and biomedical interventions.
- From the former approach to assist vulnerable children and families through exclusion and institutionalization to the introduction of pilot models based on the philosophy of social inclusion, respect for the human rights of the child, and support for vulnerable families through therapeutic interventions.

However, after 20 years of attempts to change the system of services there is an increasing understanding that the effects of the former ineffective system are still huge and modern interventions still often lose the battle for funding to traditional services which rely on the concept of social exclusion, stigma, and institutionalization.

Prevention of Bullying in Schools

During the last five years there has been a significant increase in society's awareness about school violence especially bullying. The peak of the increasing awareness was the international conference "Modern Approaches in Prevention of Violence and Bullying in Schools" that took place in Vilnius in 2007. The problem of bullying was addressed in a special international meeting in the Parliament of Lithuania (January 2007) and the Office of the President (April 2007). The prime minister of Lithuania formed a task force to prepare an action plan for the prevention of school violence (May 2007). The representatives of foreign institutions including the Nordic Council of Ministers and the United Kingdom and Netherlands embassies and several socially responsible corporates supported the bullying prevention initiatives.

According to data from the International Study of Health Behaviour in School-Aged Children (HBSC Study) the rates of bullying victimization and the scope of bullying among schoolchildren in Lithuania were one of the highest since the study started in 1994 (Zaborskis and Vareikienė 2008). Data from the HBSC Study conducted in 2006 showed that the rate of bullying victimization for girls was the highest in Lithuania (26.5%) and for boys Lithuania had one of the highest rates (27.97%). Similarly, the percentage of boys bullying others was the highest in Lithuania (30.3%); girls bullying others was also one of the highest (16.6%). The high prevalence of bullying made us look into the reasons behind it more comprehensively.

The study used the Olweus Bully/Victim Questionnaire and compared the results from schools in Vilnius and Bergen. The prevalence of experiencing bullying and bullying others was much higher in the Vilnius schools compared to the results from the Bergen study (Povilaitis 2008). The study in the Vilnius schools, among pupils aged 9-16 years, showed that 32% of pupils experienced bullying and 13.8% bullied others.

Due to effective awareness raising and lobbying from NGOs there was increasing understanding among policy makers that bullying is a problem of strategic importance. The National Programme for Helping Children and Preventing Child Abuse 2008-2010 included evidence-based methods for preventing bullying in schools, i.e., Olweus Bullying Prevention Program. The program in Lithuania started to be implemented in 2008. At the first stage of implementation 30 instructors in Lithuania were trained and they implemented this program in 30 schools from three regions. At the second stage of implementation 30 new instructors will be trained in other municipalities. Between 2008 and 2010 the program will reach 90 Lithuanian schools in various regions.

The Olweus Bullying Prevention Program lasts for 18 months in every school, and all school staff are familiarized with the key principles of the program and provided with needed materials. The staff are also properly trained and instructor consultations are available to them. All school staff, students, and their parents are involved in different activities of the program. During implementation the core components of the program are implemented at the school, class, and individual level.

This case of implementing evidence-based preventive methods nationally is a good example of success where all stakeholders (NGOs, professionals, researchers, municipal, and national authorities) agree to follow modern public health principles such as prioritizing, allocating needed resources, and applying evidence-based approaches.

EXPERIENCE FROM THE CAMHEE PROJECT

In 2004, ten new countries became members of the European Union. Eight of these countries belong to the region discussed in this chapter—the Czech

Republic, Slovakia, Hungary, Poland, Slovenia, Estonia, Latvia, and Lithuania. Later, two more countries from the region, Bulgaria and Romania, also joined the EU. This fact created a fascinating opportunity for those ten countries to change the context of the developing CAMH field and to use all advantages—financial and contextual—available to them as full members of the EU. One of the examples how EU accession can be used for positive change in the CAMH field is the idea of the CAMHEE project. This is how the idea of the CAMHEE project was born.

Since 1994, when eight countries from the CEE region—Poland, Hungary, the Czech Republic, Slovenia, the Slovak Republic, Estonia, Latvia, and Lithuania—joined the European Union, this process of an enlarged European Union presented a new window of opportunity to the CEE region for further developing modern approaches in the field of CAMH and related issues. The idea behind this is that if managed effectively, the process of EU enlargement can facilitate progressive change not only in the new EU member states but also, through the European Neighbourhood Policy, to contribute to positive changes in the broader region of Eastern Europe.

One of the first attempts to use this opportunity was the CAMHEE project which was carried out by 35 partners in 16 EU countries during the years 2007-2009. When this chapter for the IACAPAP monograph was in the process of being finalized the CAMHEE project was not yet completed. However, it is important to present in this chapter not the results, but rather the process of initiation and launch of the project and cooperation between partners in identifying critical points for development in the CAMH field in Europe and globally.

The project funded by the EU Public Health program "Child and Adolescent Mental Health in Enlarged EU: Development of Effective Policies and Practices" (CAMHEE) started in January 2007 and will last until the end of 2009. This project aims to provide a set of recommendations and guidelines for effective child and adolescent mental health (CAMH) policies and practices in the European Union with special emphasis on the new EU countries and in light of the Declaration and Action Plan endorsed by the WHO European Ministerial Conference on Mental Health. To achieve this, it was decided that the project will develop four main objectives:

1. To create a network of partners within the European Union for the adopting and implemention of modern effective public health approaches in the new and applicant EU countries.
2. To develop guidelines and recommendations for national and municipal (regional) policies in participating countries in the field of CAMH based on the evidence obtained through independent analysis of each country's situation, including the analysis of context, resources, processes, and outcomes.

3. To initiate and support activities in the new and applicant member states in the field of CAMH, with special focus on the implementation of effective and evidence-based policies and practices based on involvement and participation of children, families, and communities.

4. By networking to share the experiences and knowledge accumulated by the joint activities of all the project partners in order to advise the European Union and member states on mental health promotion and mental disorder prevention among children and adolescents, with a special focus on managing the changes needed in new member states to move from inherited patterns of institutionalization and medicalization to modern public health approaches based on the involvement of children, youth, parents, and communities.

The idea to apply his project proposal to the EU Public Health program was a very good example of the positive effects of EU enlargement and the European mental health agenda. Immediately after the WHO European Ministerial Conference on Mental Health "Facing the Challenges, Building Solutions" a decision was made by all the main stakeholders and interest groups in the field of CAMH in Lithuania that with the support of the Lithuanian Ministry of Health, a group of interested partners representing governmental agencies, universities, NGOs, and professional groups would use this unique momentum and invite other EU and applicant countries to join their efforts in attempting to contribute to the better mental health of children and adolescents in Europe with special emphasis on the process of enlargement and CAMHS in the new EU countries. Many partners in the EU and applicant countries reacted with enthusiasm and agreed to join this initiative. It is important to mention that the self-confidence of the Lithuanian network of partners considerably increased after the commitment of the Ministry of Health of Lithuania to contribute to co-financing the project. Later this commitment was shared by the Vilnius municipality. It was a sign of the emerging understanding of national and municipal authorities of their responsibility to recognize the new public health priorities, such as child mental health, and facilitate modern public health approaches in this field.

Lithuania is a new EU member state which has made remarkable improvements in economic development and establishing democracy and rule of law during the last 15 years of change. However, in the field of CAMH many indicators (like prevalence of suicides, bullying, or rates of children living in state institutions) are among the highest in Europe. There is increasing awareness of the fact that child mental health has become a public health priority and that EU accession has to be used for effective decisions and changes in this field. The CAMHEE project aimed to develop and implement new approaches in policy and practice to give a chance to new (like Lithuania) and applicant EU countries to implement in a systematic and evidence-based way modern public health approaches in the field of CAMH, based on the principles of health promotion, social inclusion, tolerance for vulnerable groups, deinstitutionalization, support for protective factors, resilience, autonomy, and civic participation. Only with the financial support for joint European activities and exchanges of experience and knowledge between the "new" and "old" member states will basic changes take place in child mental health systems leading to its liberation from political and professional isolation and integration in general public health, social, and education policies and practices.

One of the ideas from the CAMHEE project was that with the help of modern systems analysis methods developed in the EU would obstacles and opportunities for implementation of the modern policies and practices in the field of CAMH be identified. After having made a scientifically based "diagnosis" of the CAMH systems in participating countries the recommendations for effective policy and practice for the CAMH systems will be developed. Work by the partnership networks will facilitate a better quality of CAMH policies and practices in the whole EU. Apart from the main theme of the project, analysis of child mental health policies in EU countries, three specific topics were selected for more in-depth analysis:

1. The prevention of destructive and self-destructive patterns of behavior in school settings;
2. The development of modern approaches to parent training, with special emphasis on parents who have mental disorders or represent other risk groups; and
3. The development of effective community-based activities in the field of CAMH as alternatives to the tradition of institutionalization and social exclusion, and the provision of tools for economically evaluating this process.

As was expected partners from both "old" and "new" EU countries formed effective networks and are in the process of developing recommendations which, hopefully, will be used effectively by politicians, professionals, parents, and children in the European Union.

The CAMHEE project involved 35 associate partners from Austria, Belgium, Bulgaria, Estonia, Finland, Germany, Greece, Hungary, Latvia, Lithuania, Norway, Poland, Romania, Slovenia, Spain, and the United Kingdom. As was outlined in the project design the partners represented very different groups of stakeholders—universities, state agencies and institutions, and non-governmental organizations. The idea behind this design and partnership composition was the idea that the field of CAMH needs a broad intersectorial approach and involvement on an equal basis from all important stakeholders. The participation of NGOs was especially welcomed because CEE countries need to strengthen the civil society and the principle of citizen participation including children and youth at risk of mental health problems and their families.

Preliminary results from the CAMHEE project revealed existing systemic gaps in crucial aspects of the CAP/CAMHS field, i.e., parent training, prevention of destructive and self-destructive behavior, and management of services. Only through a self-critical analysis of these systemic challenges will good opportunities for developing modern services, based on evidence and protection of children's rights, emerge and be effectively used.

CHALLENGES AND OBSTACLES FOR FURTHER DEVELOPMENT

Despite numerous achievements, 20 years of dynamic change did not manage to eliminate the huge effects of the Soviet legacy in the field of health and social policy, including CAMH. Development of the CAMH field is a perfect reflection of the level of democracy and civil society in each country. While aspects of the physical health of children such as prevention of infant mortality and morbidity, vaccination, and prevention of infectious disorders have already been adequately addressed during the Soviet period (and were further developed as priorities during the transition period) many problems in the field of CAMH still lack the political will to be managed in a comprehensive way.

One of the systemic gaps identified in Lithuania, and in many other CEE countries, is an inherited lack of culture concerning evaluation and monitoring of policy and service. The Soviet tradition was to focus on statistics which reflected process rather than results. Until now this gap has not been filled because research and evaluation activities in the field of CAMH were not funded. This gap leads to further gaps such as lack of evidence-based policies, weak components of mental health promotion and prevention of disorders, a low level of involvement from GPs in the field of CAMH, and an absence of tiers in the system of services. In such a situation there is always a threat that even limited resources may be used irrationally, i.e., if mild cases are not managed by preventive programs and primary care then many of them will reach the specialized services, thus challenging the capacity of services to effectively manage the severe cases.

Another challenge which is worth mentioning is the lack of political will to invest more in modern approaches, while the traditional system of services based on the culture of stigma, helplessness, and social exclusion is still often protected by state funding. The process of transition in all CEE countries appeared to be very painful and resulted in high rates of destructive and self-destructive behavior among all ages of population (including children and youth) and a lack of tolerance within the population to vulnerable groups, i.e., families at risk of social problems or troubled youth. In this situation the threat of reinforcing the vicious circle of ineffective investments still remains, i.e,., where a considerable part of the population de-mandings "simple solutions" and pushes politicians to rely on the system of repressive institutions and exclusion. This is a very important challenge for all new democracies in Europe. The advocates for the field of CAMH need to be active in promoting modern approaches and in protecting human rights and especially the rights of children. With other partners of broad coalition (e.g., NGO sector, other professional groups, reform-minded politicians, mass media) the problems of the mental health of children and adolescent will be addressed in a more effective way.

CONCLUSION

The field of CAMH in the CEE region is struggling to further implement the principles of scientific evidence, a modern culture of evaluation, a good balance in the biopsychosocial paradigm, and modern ways of protecting children's rights. In the current situation when CAP, as a medical specialty, is competing with many other and more influential medical specialties it is of utmost importance to strengthen the preventive aspects of CAMH as a new public health priority for the twenty-first century. Much has been achieved, but to achieve a broader public health and participatory approach has to be added to the traditional development of child and adolescent psychiatry as a medical specialty.

REFERENCES

Browne K., Hamilton-Giachritsis C., Johnson R., & Ostergren M. Overuse of institutional care for children in Europe. *British Medical Journal* no. 332 (2006): 485-87.

Cornia G.A. and Paniccia R. *The Mortality Crisis of Transitional Economies.* London: Oxford University Press, 2001.

Currie C. et al. *Inequalities in Young People's Health: HBSC International Report from the 2005/2006 Survey.* Copenhagen: WHO Regional Office for Europe, 2008.

European Commission. *European Social Reality Report.* Special Eurobarometer 273, 2007.

Jenkins R., Tomov T., Puras D., Naneishvili G., Kornetov N., Sheradze M., et al. Mental health reform in Eastern Europe. *Eurohealth* 7 no. 3 (2001): 15-21.

Povilaitis R. Prevalence of bullying in two Vilnius schools (in Lithuanian). *Visuomenės Sveikata* 41 no. 2 (2008): 33-38.

Puras D. Child and adolescent psychiatry in Lithuania. In H Remschmidt & H. Van Engeland (Eds.), *Child and Adolescent Psychiatry in Europe.* London: Springer-Verlag Telos, 1999: 205-12.

Puras D. Treatment approaches in Lithuanian child psychiatry: Changing the attitudes. *Nordic Journal of Psychiatry* 48 no. 6 (1994): 397-400.

Puras D. Development of child mental health services in Lithuania: Achievements and obstacles. *Medicina* 38 no. 4 (2002): 363-69.

Puras D., Germanavicius A., Povilaitis R., Veniute M., & Jasilionis D. Lithuania country profile. *International Review of Psychiatry* 16 no. 1-2 (2004): 117-25.

Shatkin J.P. & Belfer M.L. The global absence of child and adolescent mental health policy. *Child and Adolescent Mental Health* 9 no. 3 (2004): 104-8.

Thornicroft G. & Tansella M. *The Mental Health Matrix. A Manual to Improve Services.* London: Cambridge University Press, 1999.

UN Committee on the Rights of the Child, 2009 at http://www2.ohchr.org/english/bodies/crc/ (accessed June 26, 2009).

World Health Organization. *Atlas of Health in Europe*, 2008 at http://www.euro.who.int/document/e91713.pdf (accessed June 26, 2009).

Zaborskis A. & Vareikienė I. *Bullying in Lithuanian Schools by HBSC Study: Trends in 1994-2006 and Cross-National Comparisons.* (Paper presented at the International Conference—Modern Approaches in Prevention of Violence and Bullying in Schools (Vilnius, December 2007)).

World Health Organization. *The World Health Report 2001—Menal Health: New Understanding, New Hope.* WHO, 2002.

World Health Organization. *Child and Adolescent Mental Health Policies and Plans.* WHO, 2005.

13

An Historical Approach to the Discovery and Promotion of Child Mental Health

Jean-Yves Hayez

DEFINITION

For a child good mental health[1] is a state of his psyche and his behavior which expresses the existence of three aspects that are "good enough"[2] (Cloutier 1966; Chiland and Young1993):

a) The absence of any psychopathological problem or psychiatric illness as is usually diagnosed;

b) The coexistence of a reasonable ability to adjust and an ability to rebel against anything which, in the child's soul and consciousness, makes no sense or is unfair. By suggesting that describing these two potentialities in specific terms might be an indicator of good mental health we can work around two opposing stumbling blocks.[3] The first would be that we refer to "normality" as the central indicator of mental health according to which the "good" child would be one who conforms to the rules and expectations of his parents and society. In this case, the work done to improve mental health would be of the "hygienist" type.[4] Another aspect is about confusing mental health and anarchy. There are a number of (natural?) universal laws upon which human social interaction is based and to which we are all subject. A (large?) part of the group's rules is of value because it allows its members to coexist without insecurity;

c) The existence of a "positive self-image." The self, as a unique and precious individual, is incongruence with its own aspirations and is authentic. This is combined with a pleasure in experiencing existence and finding meaning in it, and a feeling of happiness that is "good enough": *"I am what I am, and I am happier being that than the opposite!"*

For each of the listed dimensions there is a gradient between acquisition and non-acquisition, and thus a grey area between good and poor mental health that is defined by the subjectivity of those children or adults who have to evaluate it. We are used to this uncertainty; the mass of so-called objective criteria to which we regularly refer does not really suppress it in reality. There are differences between the perceptions and expectations of children and those of adults. Adults use their power to impose their own representations of mental health. They project, whether consciously or un-consciously, their dreams and needs in these representations; "The child who works hard and succeeds at school is a child who is in good mental health!" We need to bear this clearly in mind; no category of human is free of projections that stem from personal history or culture with respect to what is good for another person. This applies to professionals just as much as to other people (Laplantine 1993). We are also too reluctant to listen to our children when they suggest, at least intuitively, how they "think" about their mental health. We could, therefore, pay more attention to them while still not leaving all the power in their hands. The lazy child could tell us "I am fine as I am; there is no point in working." He could be delightfully egoistical and reject the idea of exerting the least effort to develop his own resources and participate in building the human race. Of course, this is just not possible. Education with its conversations, invitations, and demands still has an essential role to play. It remains a sign of good adult mental health that the parents' dreams for their children define the path for them, up to a certain point. We should, therefore, try to remain humble, skeptical, open-minded, and prepared to listen to what parents, children, or col-leagues from cultures other than our own are saying to us about child men-tal health. In this way we will be willing to constantly question in ourselves what we consider to be realistic knowledge about the child.

This interrogation and investigation should involve regular and in-depth discussions in the form of "consensus conferences" that bring together the viewpoints of everyone concerned—children, educators, society, and professionals—in a non-hierarchical situation. Such discussions should put together the fragile and constantly changing edifice that holds the most valuable representations of child mental health in a given context.

THE FOUNDATIONS OF A CHILD'S MENTAL HEALTH

The progressive elaboration of this health partly depends on the quality of the child's "equipment." It is thus a constitutional aspect of his being result-ing from the embodiments of his individual genetic inheritance.[5] With reference to a much more mysterious form of transmission that transcends the material it is also not impossible for there to be basic psychic equipment: a non-material gift that makes it possible for everyone to have specific "spiritual traits." These constitutional, genetic, and perhaps spiritual aspects make up most of our cognitive characteristics, temperament,[6] and potential mental equipment in terms of aggressivity, sexuality, anxiety or recklessness, etc. With reference to this mental equipment, we have to assume that all children are "predisposed to" depression, agitation, very average intellectual productivity, heightened sexual interest, poor sleep patterns, etc. Mental health programs, therefore, have to aim at identifying and accepting these predispositions that influence subsequent choices and differentiation. Without resignation and stagnation and with the positive help of friends and family anyone can make sure up to a certain point that their own differences do not weigh too heavily on others. On the other hand it is of value not to take a utopian approach; the idea of integrating everyone into the same educational environment is very probably a destructive utopian idea. By respectfully providing special locations or moments in life for those who are most different and who cannot keep up with the pace or demands of other people we are not ipso facto stigmatizing them.

A child's mental health is also influenced by his environment. Specifically, this means the positive or adverse stimuli arising from a rapidly changing material, family, or social environment, and the relationships that he may cement with other humans and with which he becomes imbued in order to construct his personality.

First a few words about the influence of the family but limiting ourselves to the historical perspective of the article. All mental health professionals emphasize just how important the quality of the family is for the child's development, but they haven't always been gentle or even objective towards it. In particular, for a long time they only highlighted the risk factors and psychopathological aspects issuing from the family and, what is more, they have had excessive faith in linear causal links viewing the child merely as a passive victim.[7]

We had to wait nearly until the introduction of systemic thought in the 1980s before we were reminded that the family could also be a place of resources and that the child played an interactive part in determining what happened to him. Particularly since 1990, the nuclear family has increasingly "fallen apart" and many alternative types of family have appeared. A number of professionals then found their critical spirit blunted and they found themselves unconditionally praising one or other of these new structures systematically positioned as beneficial for the child's welfare. As the pendulum returned we started to condemn the institutional placements that were once used without thinking and to preach the need to keep the child in his family at almost any cost. Those who dare to say that this new approach can sometimes be toxic (such as Berger in France) are soon regarded as merely quixotic.

The nature of relationships between the child and school, other living environments, and society as a whole represents another category of influencing factors to which we can apply the same reasoning as for the family.[8] We can never emphasize enough that the high level of instruction that has been well integrated by the child is a powerful factor for human advancement. Therefore, mental health programs must aim at providing positive schooling that is adaptable, creative and demanding, and open to everyone without distinction of sex, race, or class.

Finally, here are a few words about the influence of change on the child's mental health (Anthony and Chiland 1983).[9] Some people feel that the biological and psychological changes in the world and society have been too fast, to say the least, and are becoming too much to bear for humans, particularly young ones. This leads to pathological structures and conduct that express the human's stress and disorganization including various anxiety, depressive, or narcissistic disorders and conduct disorders in adolescents. Conversely, others believe that children have adapted very quickly and are enjoying these rapid transformations and the flow that carries them along: e.g., children from the most flexible new families, children of the Internet generation, children who believe, *"You like it? Just do it!"*

Finally, others have adopted a cautious position of uncertainty; the children could adjust and be happy in the new environments but it is happening too quickly and not everything is to their advantage. For example, when so many adults claim that they have the right to do exactly what they want, whatever the price, it leads to a crisis of values in young people.

Let us now consider these ultimate individual factors, namely reflective consciousness, freedom of thought and choice, and the partial power to create one's own ideas and own projects (Harter 1983). Although influenced by his constitutional equipment and his relations with others, the child goes further to differentiate himself. The child is constantly building an internal world of thought, aspirations, and plans: how can he represent himself and his life; what does he really expect from himself and from others; which relations to develop with his parents and his friends; what should be his own values; and how to manage sociability and ego-centricity, work and pleasure, and so on.

Rutter (1983) describes this as a "comprehensive psychological consistency, a sort of internal model of cognitions about ourselves, our relationships, our past or our future, that forms the basis for our responses to our perceptions." For example, if this internal world is high in self-esteem, the child will find it easier to appear resilient and will be less likely to be destabilized by assaults from the outside world.

P. Jeammet concluded the 11th International Congress of Child and Adolescent Psychiatry and Associated Disciplines in 1986 by stating: "If we think that it would be possible to objectivise how the brain works, the life of relationships, etc, then we are forgetting exactly what distinguishes the human being, namely his capacity for self-reflection and thus his belonging to the world of value . . . It would be illusory and dangerous to underestimate the fundamental importance for every child of giving meaning to his life and being able to integrate in relation to essential references, such as his parents, his family or his culture."[10]

THE REFERENCE MODELS

Two reference models quickly gained acceptance to exactly define and discuss what is meant by mental health. These two models came into conflict during certain periods (Joshi 1975), but have been regarded as complementary in others. One is the "medical" model; the other is the "psychoeducational (or psychosocial)" model.

The medical model is derived from the idea that a cause, which is more often external than endogenous and is often known but sometimes remains mysterious, disturbs the working of a "good" human, physical or psychic "nature." It therefore causes a problem that leads at the very least to maladjustment.

In some periods this model was promoted very heavily (*"Specific learning difficulties can only be explained by brain dysfunctions"*), while in others it leaned more towards the social world ("socioscientific" moments) (Amiel–Lebigre 1993 and Gagnalons-Nicolet). In these more integrationist times the model referred more to stress as a diffuse social "cause" of disturbance and to the available social supports such as remediation factors. Greater place was also given to the child's energy, his combativeness and predisposition towards "coping with" (Blanchet et al. 1993).

Looking after mental health using this model is "to do prevention": both primary prevention (fighting directly against the cause or doors of penetration, e.g., via education or health), secondary prevention (e.g., fighting against the first signs of stress), and even tertiary prevention. The subject's responsibility for his own future is assessed in very different ways, and is sometimes limited to accepting or refusing to take medication.

Over recent years this medical model has increased in popularity once more and has been radicalized by the ever-present debate on genetics and its deployment. When they are in the ascendant genetic psychiatrists can be the most radical and, through their claims and ultra-complicated diagrams and tables, choose to objectivize the person as being defined by his genes. So why is this medical model still so successful? Because, in good faith and with reference to their culture, doctors have been hard at work lobbying to ensure that it is applied and because the pharmaceutical industry supports them with its disinterested motives. Another reason is that it doesn't upset

the social order and because it is simple in comparison to the other un-
ashamedly complex models (Laplantine 1992). It also has the appearance
of being scientific; the data appear to be objective and legitimate and contain easily checkable facts (Frankard and Renders 2004).

The psychoeducational (or psychosocial) models represent human life as
a much more complex reality. Apart from a few mental illnesses that are
unarguably linked to the brain they regard psychic life as a jungle in which
it is almost impossible to decide with any certainty which would be the
natural healthy components. Rather it is a swarm of forces in a constant
state of flux in relation to the social aspect and the body. In this case, the
phenotypical application of genetics merely constitutes one element among
many others. As for adjustment and maladjustment to the environment,
both are regarded as learned attitudes. Promotion of mental health inspired
by these models takes this into account as it also relies on the person's
strength, energy, combativeness, and ability to bounce back. Back in 1966
G. Canguilhem emphasized the existence of a "personal normativity" to
which the person devotes all his or her strength.

Does an integrative biopsychosocial model remain a utopian dream?
Although many professionals support the idea of our biopsychosocial
nature[11]—"*The human being is his body; he is his psyche; he is society*"—
they are reluctant to accept any reference model that might naturally
follow from it. This is a complex model shot through with uncertainty.
It rejects the principle of hierarchies, ever-apposite laws and equipropor-
tionality between "causes." Each person is a DIY project or patchwork,
and we have to rebuild the identity of each individual subject. If we apply this model, research into and the promotion of mental health would
largely be subsumed into the same programs for general health (Chiland
and Young 1993). This practice is starting to gain ground in Europe in
certain medical centers or "homes" for young people. In the emerging
countries, many primary health centers are attempting to implement it
to better effect.

APPLICATIONS IN THE FIELD

Let us now review the main resources used to promote child mental health,
listing them by their target audience and objectives. Many applications are
directed at children and aim to

1. Make use of their potential, e.g., early years stimulation programs;
   workshops that promote creativity, self-expression, artistic or sporting
   abilities, communication, etc.
2. Help them to acquire a well-integrated knowledge. Educating children

is the basic mission of any school but governments often assign additional tasks to them (e.g., civics or sex education). There are also broader or multifocal information or consciousness-raising campaigns (e.g., prevention of physical or sexual abuse, promotion of the rights of children). Adolescents as a target group have received considerable investment: campaigns against racism, homophobia, all types of addiction; small-group meetings to discuss non-violence or girl/boy relationships, sexuality, and responsible parenting. Unfortunately, whatever method promoters use to get their message across, these encounters with their public all too often appear to be a hierarchical transmission of knowledge, just like at school.

3. Listen to them talk about their mental health and take on board what they are saying (e.g., "advice" from young people in certain schools, residential institutions, and even in towns and villages). As we have already mentioned it is relatively rare for adults to really listen and take account of what they hear even when they do not exclude the possibility of sharing ideas and continuing to educate. And if by chance the children have been heard they often notice that their point of view is not taken on board because their expectations will upset the existing social order too much or will require money that is earmarked for other priorities.

4. Use the children themselves; turn them into mental health practitioners. This is also unusual. The child-to-child programs that do exist, particularly in emerging countries, relate more to the promotion of physical health. Nevertheless, certain practices in Latin America do concern mental health. These confer on mature and intelligent adolescents the status of *lideres* (leaders) for the less informed members of their community.

Many other applications are aimed at the adults in charge of day-to-day education, starting with the parents. The objectives that we have reviewed with respect to the child also apply to these adults, with a few minor differences:

1. For example, listening aimed at adults is much more common and diversified than listening aimed at children. On the Internet, in particular, there are a vast number of forums that offer a listening and supportive ear, and allow affected adults to come together and develop their own ideas about mental health, sometimes with the help of professionals. These professionals often feel it is important to encourage parents to express exactly what they mean by a "successful" child and to discuss their mutual representations (Frankard and Renders 2004).

2. With respect to the transmission of knowledge, it is important to remember that in the 1970s in France a number of high level professionals, such as Françoise Dolto, decided to pass information to and communicate with parents using the mass media (Dolto 1985).
3. Finally, and more specifically, many programs encourage concerned adults to improve the affective and educative contribution that they make to children by increasing the protection factors and reducing the risk factors (see also below).

Finally, some programs are directed at the social community as a whole. Their objectives are similar to those described in the paragraphs above, again with a few minor differences:

1. As far as improving living conditions is concerned, we sometimes concentrate on marginalization and poverty in a rather too reductionist manner. We should ask ourselves more about the impact on the child of numerous contemporary social aspirations, at least in industrialized countries. These include performance at school and in general and the need to achieve the desired results at all costs; the right—almost the duty—that everyone has to do what they want and the weakening of parental authority; the equivalence of all new forms of family; a sort of negation of the condition of child (e.g., over-consuming children, sick children asked to personally make key decisions, young adolescents allowed the freedom to manage their current ideas of transsexuality, recriminalization of justice for minors, etc.).
2. As far as improving information is concerned, there are many campaigns aimed at raising the awareness of the community as a whole in the field of child mental health.

On the other hand, it is much more unusual for childhood professionals to come together and take the initiative to inform or question the decision makers, particularly the political decision makers, about the needs of children. Nevertheless, the decision makers' main motivation is rarely child welfare; they are more preoccupied with making savings or upholding their image in society by emphasizing the security aspects.

This security ideology sometimes percolates through without the scientists' awareness and sometimes with their active collaboration (Foucault 1992).[12] It can be seen, for example, in plans for early screening for delinquent "tendencies" or in the broad-brush recriminalization of adolescents. It also exists in some programs to rehabilitate young people in difficult urban environments in which collaboration between the police, local authorities, and social workers sometimes resembles tight social control.[13]

A FEW WORDS ABOUT THE TOPIC OF
MENTAL HEALTH IN EMERGING COUNTRIES

Basically, everything described above concerns these countries as well (Graham 1980). We have already said that in the primary health centers the idea of global health could be at work, sometimes more than in the industrialized countries, and this is a very good thing. The same applies to the aim of community health being managed by the community that is directly affected. A great deal will still have to be energetically invested in the long term: literacy, early years stimulation, schooling, fight against poverty and child labor when it takes place without dignity or involves exploitation, the search for true equality between boys and girls, and the promotion of responsible parenting.

There is also the need to battle the scourge of physical diseases and inadequate hygiene since these can impair mental functioning. These initial investments can be followed by large-scale campaigns like those run by UNICEF and other well-known NGOs, including the promotion of children's rights, fight against abuse, domestic violence, addiction, etc.

A FEW HISTORICAL MILESTONES

To describe these milestones we shall first identify the three main lines that sometimes cross or superimpose along their length[14]:

1. Child mental health as an integral part of public health and society's aspirations;
2. The child's "moral" suffering, whether psychopathological or sociopathological, as the object of concern for carers;
3. Child and adolescent psychiatry as a specific medical discipline.

Before and Around the Second World War

No Specific Concept of Child Mental Health

1908: C. W. Beers, a former psychiatric hospital patient, established the first mental hygiene society in Connecticut (USA) to raise public awareness of the unenviable lot of the mentally ill (cited in Cloutier 1966). His initiative spread across the world.

1948: The International Committee for Mental Hygiene changed its name and become the World Federation for Mental Health.

The WHO put forward its famous definition of health, no longer as the absence of disease, but as an overall state of physical, mental, and social well-being.

In the 1950s, respected researchers such as M. Jahoda in the United States and F. Cloutier in France developed the concept of "positive mental health" which attempts to recognize and develop the person's resources rather than prevent the raising of pathology. They also emphasize the limits and risks associated with the concept of normality. Finally, according to them, and many others, it is an internal state of well-being or perceived happiness that defines mental health. They also attempt to find objective and identifiable criteria to "break down" what this state of overall satisfaction means (Cloutier 1966; Jahoda 1950, 1958).

Birth of Child and Adolescent Psychiatry

In France, the individual initiative of Itard[15] is often mentioned. He attempted to re-educate Victor the wild (autistic?) child from Aveyron and therefore believed it would be possible to mobilize the child's failing and deviant psyche.

In the early twentieth century the French psychiatrists who were writing about the child did so in an adultomorphic way, with strong organic/constitutionalist beliefs[16] (Lebovici 1995).

Georges Heuyer breaks away from this background to bring child and adolescent psychiatry to the baptismal font. From 1925 onwards he managed an "annex clinic of neuropsychiatry" intended for children at the Salpetrière Hospital in Paris.

Despite his conventional training, this enlightened spirit surrounded himself with people whose thinking was very different from his own and he soon invited the psychoanalyst Eugénie Sokolonicka to come and work beside him. As it received a difficult welcome from the medical world, the experiment did not last long. But he started again more positively after the war with Sophie Morgenstern; this was the prelude to the Parisian School of Child Psychoanalysis. In 1937 Heuyer organized the first international conference of child psychiatry (as part of a mental hygiene conference) with the Swiss Tramer and North American Leo Kanner[17]. In 1948 he took the first university chair of child psychiatry at the same time as E. J. Anthony in Saint Louis (USA).

The Initial Influence of Psychoanalytical Psychotherapies Applied to the Child

Nevertheless, as a side issue and even before this medical discipline had been established, the mental suffering of children had already been identified, invested in, and cared for by a new category of psychotherapist—the psychoanalysts. Very quickly, Freud established a link between the influences of childhood and the current suffering of adults. The founding father had even analyzed little Hans[18]. This encouraged his pupils to take an interest in children using an approach that is anything but medicalized; straight away they started to listen to each child as a unique subject capable of identifying his inner world, and considered whether appropriate media could be used to communicate with him. It was also very quickly understood that an active interest needed to be taken in the family and social situation.

As a matter of interest, in 1927 Anna Freud published her "Introduction to the Technique of Child Analysis," and in 1938, after immigrating to London, she established the Hampstead Clinic dedicated to child therapy. These were therapies in which she was convinced of the need to introduce educational aspects and aim to achieve psychosocial adjustment.

Around 1920, Melanie Klein published her "Notes on the Development of a Small Child," while in 1927 she theorized on her use of play techniques in her sessions, from which she interpreted the symbolic aspects.

These major founding fathers and mothers quickly gained a following and we cannot cite all the early accepters who acted towards the child with great respect and enthusiasm on both sides of the ocean, even as far away as Argentina.

From 1950 to 2000

Child Mental Health Is Given a Name and Studied

In 1948, and around the time of the definition of health by the WHO, child mental health came on the scene as the result of a serious social problem; the United Nations Economic and Social Council, having become aware of the suffering experienced by war orphans, asked John Bowlby, an expert at the WHO, to research into the needs of "homeless" children. Up to 1950 Bowlby worked very actively and his results, which were published in 1951 in English and 1954 in French, remain incredibly significant (Bowlby 1951, 1954). He described the attachment drive, the great importance of material care, the existence of early sensitive periods needed to benefit from this care, and the syndromes associated with maternal shortcomings. He probably appeared too harsh in his criticism of what the residential institutions could provide as parental substitutes.

Whatever it was, his work not only gave rise to a large number of other, sometimes polemic, studies around theories of attachment; it also inspired, and still inspires, massive programs of prevention (he called it "prevention of family failure") associated with the quality of mothering and care for babies and infants.

The late 1950s onwards saw the rapid growth of mental health centers, initially in industrialized countries. When they started many put a lot of work both into the care they provided (which we shall discuss below) and into mental health promotion,[19] often on behalf of groups that were geographically close together (conferences, groups of parents, homework clubs, etc.). Over the course of time many mental health centers placed emphasis on their care mission and reduced, if not totally dropped, the prevention aspect.

Thus the promotion of mental health largely passed into the hands of more specific teams made up of professionals other than psychotherapists. Unfortunately, these services became diversified, if not fragmented, by location, reference culture, objectives, and social mandate. Many splits and rivalries developed. Even though general and agreeable coordination is most likely an idealistic illusion, it is important to remember that the opposite is not always very far from the truth; the road to hell is paved with idiosyncratic intentions.

Nor ignore the idea that, in the choice of major themes considered to be important, there are non-logical phenomena of mode and repetition by one side about what the others say. Some topics have become rather unpopular for no particular reason, while others are on the rise: maternal care, addiction prevention, stress, abuse in general (which was quickly reduced to sexual abuse), and today the new "social warning lights" of behavioral disorders and security.

In France, from the 1970s onwards Colette Chiland was a champion for the promotion of child mental health. She led this promotional work alongside her work as a therapist for suffering children often in association with other clinicians such as C. Koupernik in France or E. J. Anthony in the United States. Together they drew up a number of basic concepts.

First, C. Chiland drew attention to the risk of establishing an ideal picture of the child in good mental health, since this ideal can be infiltrated by religion or moral thinking. Rather, she suggested referring to detailed descriptions of children who feel that they are healthy, who are developing well and appear happy. She thus comes down firmly on the side of positive mental health.

As a corollary, Chiland and the other members of her team explored the subject of the child's vulnerability and strength, with its opposite extremes—great fragility and invulnerability (Chiland 1970; Anthony, Chiland, and Koupernik 1980, 1982). The authors emphasize the strong constitutional aspect of these "states of mind" (2nd op. cit., 1980, p. 538) and, in this respect, they describe a very close relationship with temperament[20]. However, they also emphasize the influence of external factors that quickly become known as risk or protection factors[21]; one key protection factor is still the quality of mothering and the climate of confidence in which it takes place.

Many later studies concentrated on describing the risk and protective factors in particular situations. They were followed by prevention programs, although these were sadly fewer in number than the research studies.

In addition, the concept of resilience to a large extent replaced the concept of strength or invulnerability, although it did lose some of its initial more restrictive meaning as a way to describe the way of bounding back after major unhappiness.

Many other psychiatrists and therapists developed important projects centered on promoting child mental health, e.g., early stimulation, raising awareness in the community of the needs of children, against maltreatment, etc. Others concentrated on defending the rights of children as they felt that recognizing their rights would make a powerful contribution to improving their mental health.

There are too many to mention them all! On behalf of all, I will mention three names: Françoise Dolto and her communication with the general public; the original and creative Briton Donald Winnicott, a free-thinking and optimistic man who believed in the natural tendency towards health present in all of us, and in man's capacity to find a solution—his own solution; and finally, in Boston, Raquel Cohen and her considerable work about mental health and disasters.

Child and Adolescent Psychiatry Becomes Accessible and Moves Away from the Medical Model

Let us return to the outpatient centers for mental health and the other similar institutions referred to by other terms that have been established and grown up since the 1950s. These have always been intensely dedicated to their care mission and, therefore, assumed responsibility for recognized psychiatric illnesses or serious psychopathological problems. But they have also been asked to help maladjusted children, to smooth off annoying relational rough edges, and return the power to the expectations of adults (parents, school, etc.). They are all too often expected to do this at little cost and with no questioning of their behavior by the adults who run these centers. Many teams had a policy of welcoming all such requests but of subtly working to give back to the child his status as subject and to bring into play the attitudes of adults.

Very quickly, these centers understood the need for multidisciplinary teams[22] and to work in networks with the other professional partners in the geographical environment. In many countries they have even been wholly or partly integrated, either flexibly or by coercion, into public health policies in which the state divides up the available care by geographical sector[23](Duché 1995).

These centers and the private consultations had to be supplemented in order to look after cases too serious for outpatient treatment. This period also saw the appearance of the first hospitals specifically offering child psychiatric services or very similar therapeutic residential centers. They were often located on a dedicated site and looked more like large, welcoming buildings than austere hospitals. At the start they were inspired by the ideas of psychoanalysis overlapping somewhat with those of institutional therapy: for example, Bruno Bettelheim's orthogenic school in Chicago. Sometimes they were original, wild, and bordering on Marxist, e.g., the communes of Fernand Deligny in Corrèze. Sometimes they were not far from being an unpleasant totalitarian ideology e.g., Maud Mannoni and Bonneuil.

All of them at least had the merit of taking very disturbed children into a highly dynamic and enthusiastic environment and greatly increasing the effort and resources devoted to improving their condition. And the child psychiatrists continued to work their way into all the networks intended to help children with psychological problems: institutions for re-educating handicapped people, those for social cases, and general hospitals on pediatric and maternity wards, or even the world of justice for minors.

Has child and adolescent psychiatry moved away from the original medical model? Yes, in a large number of countries up to the early 1990s it was primarily a psychotherapeutic and social world, and it did not truly center on identifying specific morbid entities.[24] The medical discipline was almost annexed by the psychotherapy schools and methods. We illustrate this using the metaphor of the ocean with its succession of waves and underwater currents:

(a) Up to the 1980s, the predominant waves were still those of psychoanalysis.

Psychoanalysis by the grand masters: Anthony, Solnit, Cohen, Graham, Cramer, the founding fathers of the Paris school (Lebovici, Diatkine, Soulé, Kreisler, Chiland, Misès), Gautier and Lemay in Quebec, and all those I could not mention by name. For them, the relationship between the child and his family was always a cause for concern, as were the introjections of parental images and genesis of his intrapsychic conflicts but as we have already said the family was most often regarded as the seat of psychopathology rather than a place of positive resources. Psychoanalysis, as they conceived it, could be very open to the school and society but sometimes barricaded itself into a psychotherapeutic ivory tower that could be equally purist and recondite.

Unfortunately, the psychoanalysis of discord also arose; this occurred mostly in France with the Lacan school. Françoise Dolto was part of this while having taken liberties in relation to the sometimes extreme ideas of the master and, more particularly, those of his sons and daughters.

This psychoanalysis[25] regularly appeared all-powerful, contemptuous towards other approaches, and inflationist in its desire to explain everything about people on the basis of its models and concepts. One of its most dramatic errors related to the way it modeled autism and associated pathologies. Other more recurrent and common errors related to its underestimating the part that the body "in itself" plays in the child's moral suffering; this is all too often reduced to conflicts between instances or dysfunctional introjections of parental images.

(b) Above and below this impressive but sometimes too well-ordered ocean of ideas there are threaded modest underwater currents.

The models and methods of "institutional therapy" which had been applied to certain residential centers for disturbed children. We have already mentioned them briefly.

The discovery in 1952 of the first specific psychotropic drug of the modern age, e.g., chlorpromazine, and developments in the field of psychopharmacology that followed. For a long time, many child psychiatrists have remained quite reticent about the use of psychotropic drugs for children with a very few exceptions; the strongest neuroleptics for the clearly psychotic, weaker neuroleptics for certain aggressive/impulsive disturbed children, and medication for Tourette syndrome. Things have changed radically since 1990.

In the 1970s it was the British (e.g., Laing) who were behind a sort of revolution that shook the institutions but it did not last very long. Their movement was known as "anti-psychiatry." It claimed that it was the dysfunction of the family and society, even the care institutions, that were primarily responsible for the problems experienced by the mentally ill. The movement did not, however, have a great direct influence on child and adolescent psychiatry which was already frequently open to society. One exception to this rule is Italy where it had probably been the cause of de-institutionalization and a desire for radical integration of the handicapped and mentally ill of all ages into ordinary society.

At this time of the great rise of psychoanalytical orthodoxy we have to salute the independent spirits who had the courage to affirm their truly "somatopsychic" convictions as they were well and truly integrated into their writing and practices. Prime examples of this are Julian de Ajuriaguerra and his Geneva school, and Yvon Gautier and Michel Lemay and their school in Quebec.

Between 1970 and 1980 we saw the appearance and blossoming of systemic theories. As a term borrowed from cybernetics the system essentially refers to the circular and retrospective effects associated with phenomena that occur in the whole.

The systemists promoted family therapy as the main means of helping children with problems. They used very diverse techniques, but they all ultimately attempted to improve family relationships as a whole, e.g., via communication, and they refused to center on the so-called ill person who, in their eyes, is never anything more than a "designated patient" for the convenience of the system.

Systemic professionals rapidly split into quite a few "tribes" which never really attempted either to unify their thoughts or to enter into conflict with one another. Typical examples are the work of S. Minuchin, M. Bowen, and V. Satir in the USA; the Palo-Alto school (Watzlawick et al.); Bosromeny-noch in Hungary; M. Selvini and M. Andolfi in Italy; and so on. Occasion-ally, even they could get carried away and became exaggerated in their models, e.g., schizophrenia and the double parental message, excessively rigid concept of the symptomatic patient, etc.

The systemists were slower to gain acceptance in the French-speaking world than in North America or Italy but, little by little, they created "an-other" recognized place "beside" the psychoanalysis movement without entering directly into conflict with it.[26]

Child and Adolescent Psychiatry Becomes Medicalized Again

In the early 1990s psychoanalysis, with the other psychodynamics-inspired therapies snapping closely at its heels, started to be attacked with increasing vigor. This battle was centered in the USA and the countries in its sphere of influence. Why was this? There were probably several concurrent factors: the conflict of generations between scientists,[27] the new discoveries about the brain and genes, the subtle lobbying from the pharmaceutical industries, the arrogant intransigence of some psychoanalysts, and their refusal to have their work assessed, etc. The child psychiatrists thus started to adhere more and more strictly to a medical model, the main tenets of which are listed below:

1. Many child problems can be explained primarily by the special features of the way the brains work and, even more basically, from the random factors arising from genetics.
2. It is important to make "objective" nosological classifications. The di-agnostic and therapeutic procedure must be based on robust statistical proof, i.e., evidence-based medicine.
3. The only valuable research is the experimental family. Clinical research based on simply describing cases and interactions is not scientific.
4. What needs to be improved is the disturbing symptom which will have rapidly perceptible results rather than the structure of the personality.
5. The treatment is thus based on medication, often brief periods of cog-nitive or cognitive-behavioral therapy, and, if necessary, education for the parents.

The cognitivist ideas and the therapeutic methods that they inspire are thus very well integrated into this new way of looking at problems. There were already some famous forerunners back in the 1990s, e.g., M. Rutter in Brit-ain, but they did not really form a school. Today, on the other hand, when many psychological phenomena have been rechristened, "neuropsychologi-cal" cognitivism is royally positioned.[28] It works not simply to describe this neuropsychology but also as the therapeutic means of choice to identify and change ideas and emotions which, according to them, are only effective or at least workable in the conscious field. It is therefore applied to children, either individually or in small groups, sometimes rather simplistically. And discussing education with the parents with a view to improving effectiveness in the short term may also be referred to as applied cognitivism.

As for behaviorism, this is another therapeutic complement to the neuropsychological and cerebral perspectives on mental illness but it will probably never become used as an isolated corpus of specific techniques. It will remain as a complementary therapy to the cognitivist method.

In the French-speaking world the psychotherapeutic and medical paths continue to be equally popular. It is impossible to predict whether the complementary aspects will be researched, whether a sort of polite split will persist, or whether one will consume the other. Some of the statements made by the neo-organicists are probably well founded. Psychiatrists/psychotherapists have for too long underestimated the part played by the brain and genes, and the usefulness of medicines. Many are now returning to this aspect. We can nevertheless fear for the status of the child as subject; he is often encountered in an individual therapeutic relationship and is always full of surprises. The medical model is too keen to objectivize him through the medium of its questionnaires and standard evaluation matrices and its research into behavioral indicators. Although it might be interesting to attempt to resolve the symptoms, looking to rally the personality might also be a passionate, enriching, and even essential adventure.

CONCLUSION

Did the year 2000 bring with it any significant changes? In its 2001 report on health around the world the WHO states that everywhere mental health policies are a sort of poor relation and are even non-existent in 40% of countries. The situation is even worse when we just consider the mental health of children and adolescents.

The WHO recommends having a global vision of health and integrating responsibility for "mental health" problems right from the start into primary health care. In industrialized countries this will involve improved training for general practitioners, pediatricians, and other frontline providers.

The WHO also recommends relying more on community mental health, specifically returning the health of the community back to the responsibility of that community. It is likely that emerging countries will be able to go much further in this direction than other countries quite simply because, in many places, communities remain active in a consistent manner. Everywhere in the world schools may take a positive part. More could be done in the field of citizenship and mental health provided that the time is really freed up to allow them to do this.

This important WHO report still contains a double message with respect to the human being. It reads, "The single important thing needed to understand the human being is biology and, essentially, genetics which accounts for what becomes of the brain. And it is only the brain that counts." And a few pages later: "The body and the mind are as important as one another. The human being is fundamentally psychosomatic (we have even suggested 'bio-psychosocial')." Every day we see the effects of this dual message in the field. It works at the very heart of our concept of care and our programs of prevention. In our actions, we vacillate from one concept to the other; the latter is more "theoretical" than specifically operational. A few very top-flight professionals (almost philosophers) are looking for convergence and complementarity between the language and realities of the neurosciences and psychoanalysis. But we are still a long way from being able to provide clear results and, even less, applications for the field. However, those who believe that psychogenesis is the dominant factor are not dead even if this is not mentioned by the WHO. So when will there be greater integration?

NOTES

My grateful thanks to Professor Anne-Christine Frankard, PhD (Université catholique de Louvain-Belgium).

1. Good enough? This is a new application of D. W. Winnicott's famous expression when he affirmed that the really good mother is nothing more than one who assumes she is good enough (Winnicott 1971).

Likewise E. Erickson suggested that, "as always in the health field, we can only hope to get close to something that appears to be optimum in the way of things. Such an optimum is never achieved in poor health" (p. 26 in Anthony and Chiland 1983).

2. Unless otherwise specified in this article, the term "child" is used to describe all minors, babies, children, and adolescents.

3. Back in 1976, A. J. Solnit wrote that "mental health is) a relative concept . . . a balance that constantly has to be reinvented between experience and individual expression and adjustment to the demands of family and community and to changes in the environment, which varies over time and across cultures."

4. A. J. Solnit also said (in 1976): "We misuse and abuse knowledge when we attach unjustified importance to norms and standardised objectives and when we regard achieving such objectives as a proof of mental health and not achieving them as a proof of illness."

5. With respect to what is "truly" constitutional, we can add the earliest marks derived from our initial relationships with our first caregivers: given their repetitive nature they can fix in us, in a largely irreversible manner, the initial outlines of images and representations that will have the same effect as the genetic components of the temperament.

6. Temperament? Back in 1993, J. C. Young noted that "clinicians struggle to objectivise the psychobiological equipment that derives from the prenatal genetic matrix, using concepts such as temperament that can never be entirely satisfactory" (p. 98 in Chiland and Young, 1993).

7. In 1980, P. Graham emphasized that "(our) interventions are intended to reinforce the feeling of power parents and children have towards their lot in life, and not to suppress this power. Too many therapies are applied . . . in such a way that reduces their ability, rather than increasing it."

8. A. J. Sameroff stated in 1975 that "the (interhuman) experience can be explored, not only as something that moderates biological organisation, but also as something that contributes fundamentally to the adjustment of the individual; if it is well-organised and synchronised with the biological functions, the end result will be (overall) health."

9. In this work, Neuhauer lists the main macrosocietal changes: overpopulation, migration, industrialization, mass education, the sexual revolution, and the transformation of family structures. He also mentions the changes in our biology (earlier puberty). He is not yet aware of the impact that environmental damage will have on life on the planet.

10. We must be careful not to use this reality of the *self-system* for perverse purposes. Indeed, in the world, the most conservative political forces grumble at the idea of intervening in the family and society, and strenuously insist on the concept of individual responsibility. They nearly go as far as to claim that, even if there is a mental suffering, it is because the individual is unable or finds it difficult to motivate himself, without consideration for the social responsibility (Sameroff et al. 1982).

11. In this respect, P. Jeammet said: "The respective domains of the innate and the acquired must be conceived as potential and more or less open futures, which are determined only as a result of more or less random encounters with the environment. The weight of any structure, whatever the level on which it is organised, can only be evaluated as a function of the response from the people around" (p. 593 in Chiland and Young 1993).

12. Bear in mind the strong and still-relevant assertion that A. J. Solnit made in 1976: "The current state of our knowledge is not yet enough to justify the use of diagnostic or prognostic criteria for mental health or mental illnesses as the basis for coercive State intervention into the intimate family situation."

13. Our concern does not mean that we support the complete opposite: indeed, mental health programs cannot ignore the topic of social adjustment. To a certain extent, we have made it one of the criteria for good mental health.

14. We are aware of the limits of our erudition in describing this vast field, particularly with respect to the work carried out in distant countries of the globe. We therefore ask that the reader forgive us for being a university practitioner and not an historian. We would love to hear from our readers if they are able to fill in any gaps or correct inaccuracies in this part of the paper.

15. Itard published his work in 1801 and 1806.

16. Sancte de Sanctis, for example, talks of *dementia praecocissima* to describe infant/juvenile schizophrenia, by analogy with the concept of *dementia praecox* put forward by Kraepelin.

17. A few years later (1943) he would identify autism. His primary study of cases remains an incredibly up-to-date document.

18. He did this indirectly via reports from his father. This doesn't really matter as he regarded the child as a subject speaking for himself.

19. As already mentioned, "mental health promotion" refers to a positive concept of mental health and to the psychoeducational model. "Prevention" refers more to the medical model. For the sake of simplicity, the two terms are used interchangeably in the rest of the text.

20. Temperament will later be defined better (Pichot 1995), and other authors will continue to study these relationships (e.g., invulnerability—easy-going temperament (Maziade 1986; Thomas and Chess, 1977)).

21. For example, read M. Rutter (1987): "People's reactions to stress and adversity are modified by prior experiences which either increase their vulnerability or protect them from deleterious effects."

22. With "the" fundamental trinity, child psychiatrist–psychologist–social worker, occasionally joined by other re-education and therapy of the body specialists.

23. In France, for example, with Serge Lebovici and Roger Misès in the 1970s.

24. Apart from the field of psychosis, perhaps, in which for a long time each practitioner has worked more or less on the basis of his personal classification.

25. This is almost inevitable for a discipline that is in the ascendant. What happened with psychoanalysis was not its sorry privilege. It was merely surpassed by the new single reference medical models that were occupied with moving along the same lines.

26. There are, moreover, some psychoanalysts who want to work with the entire family group, but without recourse to systemic models. Nathan Ackerman was a pioneer of this in the United States, and there are still small schools of "psychoanalytical family therapy."

27. The importance of this irrational factor appears obvious to us, but is not always easily admitted by the fighters.

28. Neuropsychologists? Of course, they have always existed! The human being does not think and does not experience his emotions independently of activation by his brain, and it is not always possible to detect which is the chicken and which the egg in what we produce as ideas, feelings, behaviors, and brains' activation.

REFERENCES

Amiel-Lebigre F. & Gagnalons-Nicolet M. *Entre santé et maladie.* Paris: PUF, 1993.

Anthony E. J., Chiland C., & Koupernik C. *L'enfant à haut risque psychiatrique,* Volume 3. Paris: PUF, 1980.

Anthony E. J. & Chiland C. *Parents et enfants dans un monde en changement,* Paris: PUF, 1983.

Anthony E. J., Chiland C., & Koupernik C. *L'enfant vulnérable,* Volume 4. Paris: PUF, 1982.

Blanchet L., Laurendeau M.-C., Paul D., & Saucier J.-F. *La prévention et la promotion en santé mentale. Préparer l'avenir.* Quebec: Gaëtan Morin, 1993.

Bowlby J. *Maternal care and mental health.* Geneva: World Health Organization, Monographic Series, 1951.

Canguilhem G. *Le normal et le pathologique*, 3rd Edition. Paris: PUF, 1966.

Chiland C. *L'enfant de six ans et son avenir*, coll. Le fil rouge, Paris: PUF, 1970.

Chiland C. & Young J. G. *Nouvelles approches de la santé mentale. De la naissance à l'adolescence pour l'enfant et sa famille*. Paris: PUF, 1993.

Cloutier F. *La santé mentale*. Paris: PUF, 1966.

Dolto F. *La cause des familles*. Paris: Laffont, 1985.

Duché D. J. Histoire de la psychiatrie de l 'enfant. In S. Lebovici, R. Diatkine, & M. Soulé (Eds.), *Nouveau traité de psychiatrie de l 'enfant et de l 'adolescent*. Paris: PUF, 1995.

Foucault M. *Histoire de la folie à l'âge classique*, Paris: Gallimard, 1961 (2nd edition, 1992).

Frankard A.-C. & Renders X. *La santé mentale de l'enfant: Quelles théories pour penser nos pratiques?* Brussels: De Boeck, 2004.

Garnezy N. Vulnerability research and the issue of primary prevention, *Amer. J. Orthopsychiat.* 41(1) (1971):118-132.

Graham P. Epidemiological approach to child mental health in developing countries. In E. P. Purcell (ed), *Psychopathology of children and youth: A cross cultural perspective*. New York: Josiah Marcy, 1980, 293-298.

Harter S. Developmental perspective on the self-system. In E. M. Hetherington & P. H. Mussen (Eds.), *Handbook of child psychology. Vol. 4: Socialization, personality and social development*. New York: Wiley, 1983.

Jahoda M. Toward a social psychology of mental health. In M. J. E. Senn (Ed.), *Symposium on the Health Personality*. Josiah Marcy Jr. Foundation, 1950.

Jahoda M. Current concepts of positive mental health. New York: Basic Books, 1958.

Joshi P. Fondements théoriques de la nouvelle perspective en santé mentale. *Annales Médico-Psychologiques* 129(4) (1975): 497-536.

Laplantine F. Anthropologie des systèmes de représentation de la maladie. In D. Jodelet (Ed.), *Les Représentations Sociales*. Paris: PUF, 1989 (3rd edition, 1993).

Laplantine F. *Anthropologie de la maladie*. Paris: Payot, 1992.

Lebovici S. Psychiatrie générale et psychiatrie de l 'enfant et de l 'adolescent. In S. Lebovici, R. Diatkine, & M. Soulé (Eds.), *Nouveau traité de psychiatrie de l'enfance et de l'adolescence*. Paris: PUF, 1995.

Maziade M. Etudes sur le tempérament. Contribution to the study of psychosocial risk factors in children. *Neuropsychiatrie de l'Enfant* 34 (8-9) (1986): 371-382.

Osborn A. F. Resilient children. *Early Child Development and Care* 62 (1990): 23-47.

Pichot P. Retour au tempérament: Clinical and theoretical lecture. Histoire du concept de temperament. *Revue Internationale de Psychopathologie* 17 (1995): 10.

Rutter M. Psychopathology and development II: Childhood experience and personality development. *Australian and New Zealand Journal of Psychiatry* 24 (1983):513-531.

Rutter M. Continuities and discontinuities from infancy. In J. Osofsky (Ed.), *Handbook of Infant Development*. New York: Wiley, 1987 (2nd edition).

Sameroff A. J. *Primary prevention and psychosocial disorders: A contradiction in terms*. An original paper presented at the council meeting of the American Psychological Association, Los Angeles, 1975.

Sameroff A. J., Safer R., & Elias P. K. Socio-cultural variability in infant temperament ratings. *Child Development* 53 (1982): 164-173.

Solnit A. J. Changing psychological perspective about children and their families. *Children Today* 5 (3) (1976):124-141.

Thomas A. & Chess S. *Temperament and development.* New-York: Brunner/Mazel, 1977.

WHO. Report on mental health in the world in 2001. Summarized reference text. May be downloaded from http://www.who.int/whr/2001/fr/index.html.

Winnicott D. *De la pédiatrie à la psychanalyse.* Paris: Payot, 1971.

Index

About the Contributors

Ms. **Charlotte Allenou**, MA. Laboratoire du Stress Traumatique (JE 2511) Services Universitaires de Psychiatrie, Hôpital Purpan-Casselardit, Toulouse, France.

Mr. **Charles Baily**, MA.

Professor Emeritus **Cornelio G. Banaag, Jr.**, MD. University of the Philippines, Manila, Philippines.

Professor **Philippe Birmes**, MD, PhD. Laboratoire du Stress Traumatique (JE 2511) Services Universitaires de Psychiatrie, Hôpital Purpan-Casselardit, Toulouse, France.

Ms. **Rossana Bisceglia**. University of Toronto, Department of Human Development and Applied Psychology, Toronto, Ontario, Canada.

Dr. **Rodrigo Chazan**. Child and Adolescent Psychiatric Division, Hospital de Clinicas de Porto Alegre, Federal University of Rio Grande do Sul, Porto Alegre, RS, Brazil.

Dr. **C. Cheung**, PhD. University of Toronto, Department of Human Development and Applied Psychology, Toronto, Ontario, Canada.

Dr. **Vanessa Loi-Yan Chu**. The University of Hong Kong, Queen Mary Hospital, Hong Kong, China.

Professor **Eric Fombonne**, MD, FRCPsych. Department of Psychology, Montreal Children's Hospital, Montreal, QC, Canada.

Dr. **Tamsin Ford**, MRCPsych, PhD. MRC Clinician Scientist Child Health Group, Institute of Health Services Research, Peninsula College of Medicine and Dentistry, St. Lukes Campus, Exeter, United Kingdom.

Professor **M. Elena Garralda**, MD MPhil, FRCPsych. Academic Unit of Child and Adolescent Psychiatry, Imperial College London, London, United Kingdom.

Professor Emeritus **Jean-Yves Hayez**, MD, PhD. Catholic University of Louvain, Wavre, Belgium.

Dr. **Schuyler W. Henderson**, MD, MPH. Columbia University, New York, NY, United States.

Dr. **Franck Hazane**, MD, PhD. Service Universitaire de Psychiatrie de l'Enfant et de l'Adolescent, Toulouse, France.

Professor **Jennifer Jenkins**, PhD, C.Psych. University of Toronto, Department of Human Development and Applied Psychology, Toronto, Ontario, Canada.

Dr. **Kazu Kobayashi**, MD. Seiryo Research Institute of Developmental Disorders/Seiryo Clinic Kobayashi, Kobe, Japan.

Dr. **Bertrand Olliac**, MD. Department of Child and Adolescent Psychiatry, Centre Hospitalier Esquirol, Limoges, France.

Dr. **Maryland Pao**, MD. National Institute of Health, Bethesda, Maryland, United States.

Dr. **Guilherme Polanczyk**, MD, PhD. Department of Psychology and Neuroscience, Duke University, Durham, North Carolina, United States.

Dr. **Robertas Povilaitis**. ChildLine, Vilnius, Lithuania.

Dr. **Dainius Puras**, MD. Centre of Child Psychiatry and Social Peadiatrics, Vilnius University, Vilnius, Lithuania.

Professor **Jean-Philippe Raynaud**, MD, PhD. Professor of Child and Adolescent Psychiatry, Service Universitaire de Psychiatrie de l'Enfant et de l'Adolescent, CHU de Toulouse, Toulouse, France.

Dr. **Lisa Reisinger**, PhD. Department of Psychology, Montreal Children's Hospital, Montreal, Canada.

Professor **Luis Augusto Rohde**. Child and Adolescent Psychiatric Division, Hospital de Clinicas de Porto Alegre, Federal University of Rio Grande do Sul, Porto Alegre, RS, Brazil.

Professor **Per-Anders Rydelius**, MD, PhD. Karolinska Institute, Astrid Lundgren Children's Hospital, Stockholm, Sweden.

Dr. **Kapil Sayal**, MRCPsych, PhD. Section of Developmental Psychiatry, University of Nottingham, Queen's Medical Centre, Nottingham, United Kingdom.

Dr. **Sadaaki Shirataki**, MD, PhD. Seiryo Research Institute of Developmental Disorders/Seiryo Clinic Kobayashi, Kobe, Japan.

Dr. **Rebecca Simon**, PhD. Department of Psychology, Montreal Children's Hospital, Montreal, QC, Canada.

Dr. **Mandy Steiman**, PhD. Department of Psychology, Montreal Children's Hospital, Montreal, QC, Canada.

Ms. **Emily Swinkin**, BSc(Hons). University of Toronto, Department of Human Development and Applied Psychology, Toronto, Ontario, Canada.

Professor **Virginia Chun-Nei Wong**, MBBS, MRCP, FRCP, FRCPCH, DCH, FHKAM, FHKCPaed. Department of Pediatrics and Adolescent Medicine, The University of Hong Kong, Queen Mary Hospital, Hong Kong, China.

Professor **Stevan Weine**, MD. University of Illinois at Chicago College of Medicine, Chicago, Illinois, United States.

Dr. **Yi Zheng**, MD. Deputy President, Beijing Anding Hospital, Capital Medical University, Beijing, China.